...S SYMPTOMS

THE GUIDE TO YOUR CHILD'S SYMPTOMS

The complete home reference, from birth to adolescence

US EDITORS

Donald Schiff, M.D., F.A.A.P.
Professor of Pediatrics
University of Colorado School of Medicine
Attending Physician
The Children's Hospital, Denver

Steven P. Shelov, M.D., M.S., F.A.A.P.
Chairman of Pediatrics
Maimonides Medical Center
Professor of Pediatrics
State University of New York in Brooklyn

UK EDITOR

David Haslam, F. R.C.G.P.

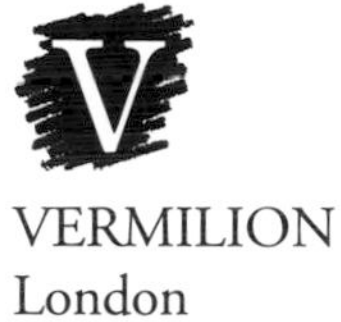

VERMILION
London

1 3 5 7 9 10 8 6 4 2

First published in the United States in 1997 by Villard Books,
a division of Random House, Inc., New York
First published in the United Kingdom in 1999 by Vermilion
an imprint of Ebury Press
Random House, 20 Vauxhall Bridge Road, London SW1V 2SA

Random House Australia (Pty) Limited
20 Alfred Street, Milsons Point, Sydney, New South Wales 2061, Australia

Random House New Zealand Limited
18 Poland Road, Glenfield, Auckland 10, New Zealand

Random House South Africa (Pty) Limited
Endulini, 5A Jubilee Road, Parktown 2193, South Africa

Random House Group Limited Reg. No. 954009

A CIP catalogue record for this book is available from the British Library.

ISBN 0 09 181603 3

Printed and bound in the United Kingdom at the University Press, Cambridge

Co-Editors
Donald Schiff, M.D.
Steven P. Shelov, M.D., M.S.

AAP Board of Directors Reviewer
Stanford A. Singer, M.D.

American Academy of Pediatrics

Executive Director
Joe M. Sanders, Jr., M.D.

Associate Executive Director
Roger F. Suchyta, M.D.

Director, Department of Communications
Linda L. Martin

Director, Division of Public Education
Lisa R. Reisberg

Project Manager, Division of Public Education
Mark T. Grimes

Project Coordinator, Division of Public Education Hope Hurley

Technical Advisers
William Lord Coleman, M.D.
Edward M. Gotlieb, M.D.
Terry F. Hatch, M.D.
Harold Koller, M.D.
Moise Levy, M.D.
Douglas Moodie, M.D.
Edwin C. Myer, M.D.
Peter Pizzutillo, M.D.
Jack T. Swanson, M.D.

Contributors
Diane L. Barsky, M.D.
Robert B. Cady, M.D.
William J. Cochran, M.D.
George J. Cohen, M.D.
Michael K. Farrell, M.D.
F. Lane France, M.D.
Howard L. Freedman, M.D.
Derek Fyfe, M.D.
Donald S. Gromisch, M.D.
Jerome A. Hirschfeld, M.D.
Hector C. James, M.D.
Michael Jellinek, M.D.
Robert Kay, M.D.
Allan S. Lieberthal, M.D.
Jeffrey M. Maisels, M.D.
William Oh, M.D.
J. Routt Reigart, M.D.
Anthony J. Richtsmeier, M.D.
Martin Sachs, D.O.
I. Ronald Shenker, M.D.
Katherine C. Teets Grimm, M.D.
Hyman C. Tolmas, M.D.
Patricia A. Treadwell, M.D.
Susan B. Tully, M.D.
David E. Tunkel, M.D.
Michael Welch, M.D.
Robert A Wiebe, M.D.
Eugene S. Wiener, M.D.

Acknowledgments
Editorial production by
DSH Editorial, Inc., a division of
G. S. Sharpe Communications, Inc.

Editorial Director
Genell J. Subak-Sharpe, M.S.

Managing Editor
Rosemary Perkins

Writers
Rosemary Perkins
Nicole Freeland

Copy Editor
Susan Hansen

Designers
Tanya Krawciw
Andrew Skalsky
Danusia Wasylkiwskyj

Illustrations
Briar Lee Mitchell
Michael Peterson
Judy Speicher

Secretarial Support
Debbie Carney
Barbara Stucky

Technical Support
Dushan G. Lukic
Debra Rabinowitz

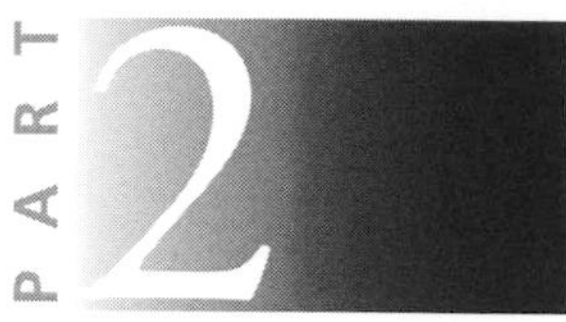

Illustrated First Aid Manual and Safety Guide

It's often said that rearing a happy, healthy, well adjusted child is one of the most demanding and challenging of all human endeavours. Fortunately, it's also the most rewarding. What is more miraculous and exhilarating than the birth of a baby? Still, caring for a newborn is a demanding round-the-clock undertaking that's a learning process for both the parents and the newcomer. Before long, however, parents learn to interpret a baby's cries, grins, frowns, and many other cues, gaining confidence in their judgement and parenting skills. Amazingly, from the moment of birth, babies are learning at an even faster pace than their parents – not only how to interpret cues from their care-givers, but also so much about the big new world they've entered.

Modern science is constantly confirming what parents have always known – babies thrive on love and attention, and the groundwork laid in the first few years of life determines in large part adult values and success. But as every parent will tell you, now and then you'll come up against a situation in which you need help. In this era in which grandparents and other traditional substitute care-givers may not be available, it's important to realize you're not alone. For starters, your GP is someone you can turn to for advice on everything from soothing a colicky infant to handling the inevitable colds, earaches, sore throats, and other common childhood ailments. Forming a solid working partnership with your GP, and also the whole primary health care team including health visitors and nurses, can help reinforce your judgement as you build confidence in your own parenting skills.

From time to time, every parent must evaluate a child's symptoms and decide what action to take. For the first few months, it's a good idea to contact your GP if you fear that something is amiss. Before long, you'll be able to judge whether the problem is one you can easily deal with yourself or whether you should seek your GP's care. This book is designed to help you distinguish minor everyday problems from more serious conditions, and to suggest a reasonable course of action. It's important to stress, however, that no book can replace your own good judgement and your GP's expertise – both critical elements in ensuring what's best for your child.

HOW TO USE THIS BOOK

The Guide to Your Child's Symptoms is divided into two major sections: an A to Z directory of the 100 or so most common childhood symptoms and an illustrated first aid manual and safety guide. There's also an extensive index.

PART 1 DIRECTORY OF COMMON CHILDHOOD SYMPTOMS

Making up the bulk of the book, this section presents easy-to-follow charts for the most common childhood symptoms. The directory itself is divided into three sections according to age: early infancy (the first 3 months), later infancy and childhood, and adolescence. In each section, the symptoms are listed alphabetically according to their common names and each chart follows a similar form.

CHART TITLE The line at the top of each chart gives the common everyday name of the symptom; for example, cough, stomachache, or runny nose, with the medical terms (if they are different) listed below.

IN GENERAL This introductory paragraph presents a brief overview of the symptom, summarizing at the outset the important facts that parents should bear in mind.

☎ CALL YOUR DOCTOR IF... This highlighted box lists the circumstances that warrant a prompt call to your GP. Read through it before going on to the rest of the chart.

WARNING This section, also included in the introduction to each chart, provides important information about what you should or should not do when treating a particular symptom.

QUESTIONS TO CONSIDER Each chart is built on a series of questions designed to help parents distinguish the most prominent features of an illness. The questions begin with the most frequent characteristics and progress along the lines that your GP might use.

IF THE ANSWER IS... If the questions posed in the first box seem to describe what's happening with your child, assume the answer is yes, and move horizontally across to the next box. If not, assume the answer is no and move down to the next set of questions. Go vertically down the page until you find questions that most nearly describe your child's situation, then move horizontally across the page.

POSSIBLE CAUSE IS... This box gives the most likely cause of the symptoms.

ACTION TO TAKE If the problem is one that you can probably deal with at home, this box briefly outlines the action you can take. Frequently, however, the advice is to call your doctor, along with a brief summary of what he or she might do to arrive at a diagnosis.

ILLUSTRATED BOXES In some of the charts, you'll find an illustrated box that provides additional information about a particular illness.

PART 2 ILLUSTRATED FIRST AID MANUAL AND SAFETY GUIDE

This part of the book is designed to help parents deal with the unexpected – everything from minor cuts and scrapes to life-threatening emergencies. The first section – The Basics of First Aid – is divided into two parts: ADMINISTERING FIRST AID: LIFESAVING TECHNIQUES, which deals with such medical emergencies as choking and CPR, and

Frequently Used First Aid Measures, which covers less dire situations – bites and stings, cuts and scrapes, bruises and sprains.

Make it a point to review this section before the need arises; when faced with a medical emergency, there's no time to consult this or any other book. From time to time, review this section to refresh your memory on the steps you should take if confronted with an emergency. Make sure that baby-sitters and other care-givers are also well versed in how to administer first aid, and don't forget to have an up-to-date list of all emergency numbers prominently displayed beside every phone in your household.

Next comes the Guide to Safety and Prevention. Included in this section are important measures to prevent injuries as well as a room-by-room guide to 'child-proofing' your home. There are also safety checklists for your car, garden, playgrounds, holiday spots, and other areas you're likely to visit with a young child.

The Guide to Food Safety addresses a growing problem – making sure that the foods you provide for your family are not only nutritious but also free of germs, pesticides, and other hazards.

THE GENDER ISSUE

We recognize that there's no easy solution to the issue of gender in pronouns. We've elected to alternate the use of he and she instead of using a single gender pronoun or the awkward he/she construction. When a problem is more common in one sex than the other, it is so indicated. Otherwise, you should assume that either gender can be equally affected, even though only one is referred to in the text.

PLEASE NOTE

Although every effort has been made to ensure that the contents of this book are accurate, it must not be treated as a substitute for qualified medical advice. Always consult a qualified medical practitioner. Neither the author nor the publisher can be held responsible for any loss or claim arising out of the use, or misuse, of the suggestions made or the failure to take medical advice.

PART 1

Directory of Common Childhood Symptoms

CHAPTER 1 COMMON SYMPTOMS IN THE FIRST FEW MONTHS

CARING FOR YOUR NEWBORN

Thanks to good ante-natal care, serious illnesses are quite rare in the first months of life. With new technology, it's now possible to diagnose many inborn conditions before birth. In this way, doctors can prepare parents for the special care their baby may need and match them up with the necessary medical resources. In some cases, babies can actually be treated for disorders before birth.

Even healthy infants, however, have days when they don't feel so good. Germs are all around us and infections such as coughs and colds, stomach upsets, and eye problems are not uncommon in young infants. In general, if there are any symptoms such as fever, a cough, or diarrhoea in the first 3 months, your GP will want to see your baby to make sure that there isn't an underlying condition that should be treated.

It's normal to feel a bit overwhelmed by the task of caring for a newborn, especially if you haven't spent much time around babies. Family and friends are usually pleased to be asked for help. In fact, they may give you more advice than you can handle, and some of it may not be completely up-to-date with what we currently know about infants. It's your doctor's main concern to help you build your self-confidence and develop your skills as a parent. Don't hesitate to call on him or her for support. You and your GP have one goal: to see your child grow up healthy and happy. In this, you're a team, and the team leader is your baby.

Although you may feel unsure of yourself at first, your baby won't be shy about telling you what to do. Within just a few days and weeks, you'll be able to recognize the different cries that tell you he or she is hungry, happy, needing a clean nappy, or ready for play. Within months, you'll be cheering his or her attempts to walk and listening to the magical first words. In the following section you'll find a guide to meeting your infant's needs in the first few months. It will also help you to recognize minor symptoms you can deal with alone, as well as the conditions that require your GP's attention. If you're in any doubt – or you just need reassurance – don't hesitate to call your doctor. His or her advice reflects the newest information from research into babies' health and development. It also reflects your doctor's years of experience not just in treating children's ailments, but also in caring for children.

Colic

In General:

All babies cry when they need something. Parents soon learn what their baby's various cries mean: hunger, a soiled nappy, loneliness, among other possibilities. Normal, fussy crying should not be confused with colic: repeated episodes of prolonged, intense crying. These bouts usually occur at about the same time each day, beginning when a baby is 2 to 4 weeks old, and typically last up to 3 or 4 months, although some babies are still colicky at 6 months. Babies with colic often pass a lot of wind; this is perfectly normal. No one knows for sure what causes colic, although many doctors believe it's a stage in the development of the nervous system. About one in five babies develops colic; interestingly, first babies and boys are affected more often than later-born infants or girls.

Consult your doctor to rule out any serious medical cause if:

- Your baby cries recurrently or inconsolably for no obvious reason.

Warning

Colic can be very upsetting, especially for first-time parents. But veteran parents know what you're going through, and your doctor also understands. Don't hesitate to call her when you need to talk about your worries or frustration.

Questions to consider	If answer is	Possible cause is	Action to take
Does your baby cry vigorously at about the same time each day, but calm down after she's had attention?	**YES**	Fussiness.	Keep giving your baby the attention she's asking for. She enjoys your company and will soon find ways to ask for it other than fussy crying.
Is your baby less than 4 months old? Is he generally content? Does he cry regularly and hard for 1 to 3 hours, especially in the late afternoon or evening? Does the baby pass wind, pull up his legs, and wriggle as if in pain?	**YES**	Colicky crying, which normally occurs between 2 weeks and 4 or 5 months of age.	Make sure your baby is properly fed and burped, comfortably clothed, and has a clean nappy. Cuddle your baby and train yourself to put up with the crying, knowing that it will stop on its own within a few weeks. (See Coping with colic, opposite.) If crying seems unusually desperate, contact your doctor, who may wish to examine the child to rule out a medical cause.
Does your breast-fed baby always suffer colic several hours after you eat a dairy product?	**YES**	Sensitivity to cow's milk (uncommon).	Talk to your doctor and, if she agrees, eliminate all dairy products from your diet for 2 weeks. A few children will respond, but most do not. If symptoms do disappear and recur when you reintroduce a dairy product, the child may have a sensitivity. Ask your doctor about modifying your diet.
Does your baby cry a lot at the end of a day involving several new experiences, such as meeting new people?	**YES**	Overstimulation.	None, except for comforting your baby and making sure his needs are met. Some infants are extremely sensitive to new experiences and simply need time to assimilate them.

Questions to consider	If answer is	Possible cause is	Action to take
Is there tension in the family? Is the primary care-giver under an unusual amount of stress?	**YES**	Emotional tension.	Even very young infants sense emotional changes. If a major upheaval is taking place, try to keep your baby's routine as close to normal as possible. Give him extra attention and try to ease your own stress.
Is it unusual for your baby to cry? Did she refuse her last feeding of the day? Does she have a runny nose or sniffles?	**YES**	Ear infection.	Contact your doctor. A baby with an ear infection may appear fine during the day but experience severe pain on lying down or at night. If the diagnosis is confirmed, your baby may require an antibiotic.
Is the crying particularly distressed? Is your baby's abdomen taut and distended? Is he vomiting yellowish-green material or passing blood in the stool?	**YES**	Intestinal blockage or other potentially serious intestinal disorder.	Call your doctor without delay. Do not feed the baby until your doctor has seen him. If the diagnosis is confirmed, emergency treatment will be needed.

Coping with colic

Many babies with colic cry at almost the same time every day, for just about the same duration. A colicky child often cries for 3 to 5 hours a day, beginning in the late afternoon to evening. Very often, such crying stops as suddenly as it began and the baby falls asleep. This difficult phase will pass eventually; colic rarely lasts beyond 4 or 5 months. Consult your doctor to rule out medical causes for the crying, and ask his advice about other measures, such as the following.

- If nursing, check with your doctor about dietary changes. You may want to try cutting out dairy products, caffeine, and foods that cause wind. Colic caused by sensitivity to any of these foods should disappear within a few days.
- Your baby may find it soothing to be held close in a baby sling or swaddled firmly in a blanket. You may need to rock and swaddle your baby for hours at a time. Some doctors suggest placing the baby in an infant swing.
- Offer the baby a dummy; some – particularly breast-fed babies – never accept it, but many enjoy it.
- Lay the baby on his tummy and gently rub his back; the touch is soothing and the pressure on the abdomen may relieve discomfort.
- Quietly sing or hum a repetitive, rhythmical tune.
- A ride in the car is a time-honoured method of calming a crying baby and inducing sleepiness. Alternatives include placing the baby safely in a carrier where he can hear a steady, rhythmic sound such as a clothes dryer. (Never place your baby on the dryer.) Or try playing soothing music.
- If your baby is on a cow's milk formula, ask your doctor to recommend an alternative.
- Try to take regular breaks. If you haven't yet found a dependable baby-sitter, at least alternate evenings with your partner so that one of you can get out of the house for a short break.
- Admit feelings of anger and frustration, but call your doctor or a parents' support group at once if you feel you may lose control or harm your baby. Above all, do not shake your baby: this can cause serious brain damage.

Call your doctor immediately if your baby has diarrhoea and:

- Is 3 months of age or less.
- Has a temperature of 38°C (100.4°F) or higher.
- Is vomiting.
- Is listless or irritable and doesn't want to feed.
- Has signs of dehydration, such as dry mouth, or has not passed urine for 3 hours or more.

In General:

A breast-fed baby's stools are light yellow, soft or even runny in consistency, and often contain small particles that look like seeds. Babies who are formula fed pass stools that are yellow to tan, with a consistency about as firm as peanut butter. By 3 to 6 weeks of age, many breast-fed babies have a bowel movement no more than once or twice a week. This is not a sign of constipation (see p. 48); it's because a diet of breast milk leaves hardly any solid waste. A formula-fed baby usually has at least one bowel movement a day. For diarrhoea in older babies and children, see p. 62.

A greenish tinge to the stools is normal. As long as your baby is feeding and growing normally, there is no cause for concern provided the stools are not whitish and claylike, watery and filled with mucus, or hard and dry.

Warning

A baby can become dehydrated quickly. If your baby is under 3 months old and has a fever (see p. 10) as well as diarrhoea, call your doctor at once. If your baby is over 3 months and has had mild diarrhoea with slight fever for more than a day, check whether he's passing a normal amount of urine and use a thermometer to check his temperature, then call your doctor.

Questions to consider	If answer is	Possible cause is	Action to take
Does your infant pass several stools every day? Are they semisoft and yellow?	**YES**	Normal digestion.	As long as your baby is happy and feeding well, no action is needed. The number of stools will decrease eventually.
Has your infant suddenly started passing more stools than usual? Are they semi-liquid, or is there a watery stain on the nappy? Is she vomiting? Is she feverish or irritable?	**YES**	Diarrhoea; viral gastroenteritis.	Call your doctor, who may examine your child and advise on treatment.

Coping with diarrhoea in an infant

A viral infection causing vomiting and diarrhoea may make your baby irritable for a day or two. If your baby is otherwise healthy, symptoms should clear up on their own. Your doctor will advise you about giving fluids to make up for the fluids and electrolytes (sodium, potassium) lost with the diarrhoea. If you are breast-feeding, your doctor will probably recommend that you keep on breast-feeding as usual. If your baby is formula fed, you may be instructed to give a special drink containing electrolytes and sugar. Don't mix up a homemade solution; chemists carry sachets that can be mixed to provide the right balance of electrolytes for infants.

IN GENERAL:

For the first year, the main food is breast milk, formula, or a combination. (Paediatricians advise solids at 4 to 6 months, or when your baby doubles his birth weight.) Your concern is to establish a regular schedule and make sure your baby is getting enough calories. A baby takes on average 60–90ml (2–3oz) of breast milk or formula every 2 to 4 hours during the first few weeks. Breast-fed babies shouldn't be allowed to sleep through feedings until at least 1 month old. If your bottle-fed newborn misses feedings, you should wake him. By age 1 month, he should be taking at least 120 ml (4 oz) every 4 hours or so, and by 6 months, he'll drink 180–240ml (6–8½oz) four or five times in a 24-hour period. Growth spurts may make your baby hungrier than usual. Even if you can't see a change in the rate of growth, be prepared to let your baby feed more often if he's breast fed, or offer him more at bottle feedings. For feeding problems in older children and adolescents, see pp. 74 and 178.

Consult your doctor if your infant:

- Is losing or failing to gain weight.
- Continues to have wrinkled or yellow skin after the first week.
- Has loose, very watery stools eight or more times a day.
- Vomits forcefully after every feeding.

Warning

Many parents worry needlessly that their infant isn't feeding right, particularly if the baby is their first. If, however, your baby is losing or failing to gain weight, or won't feed, do call your doctor.

QUESTIONS TO CONSIDER	IF ANSWER IS	POSSIBLE CAUSE IS	ACTION TO TAKE
Is your infant sometimes slow to take the breast or nipple? Does she occasionally go back to sleep after a few mouthfuls?	YES	Infant not yet really hungry; sleepy infant.	Stroke your baby's cheek and mouth next to the breast or bottle to stimulate the rooting reflex and make her seek the nipple. If your baby isn't hungry, wait a few minutes.
Does your infant get too frantic and upset to feed?	YES	Infant's temperament; over-hungry infant; colic (see p. 6).	Have everything ready before your baby becomes overly upset. Feed her in a quiet place. Your baby will outgrow colic.
Does your baby vomit, or posset, after most feedings? Is he gaining weight normally?	YES	Normal behaviour; gastroesophageal reflux (normal).	Your baby will outgrow posseting. Protect yourself with a towel and keep the baby calm after feedings. (Also see p. 16.)
Does your baby vomit after every feeding? Is he losing or failing to gain weight?	YES	Pyloric stenosis; digestive blockage; oesophageal reflux.	Call your doctor.
Are the stools watery, bloody, or full of mucus? Is he passing eight or more in a day?	YES	Infectious diarrhoea; food sensitivity or allergy.	Call your doctor.

A dummy to keep your infant happy

Dummies should never be used to replace or delay feedings. If you give a dummy to a hungry baby, he may get so upset that he can't feed. Properly used, dummies don't cause any medical or psychological problems. If you're buying a dummy, look for a one-piece model with a soft nipple in the right size for your baby's age. Clean it by boiling or washing in the dishwasher. Never tie a dummy around your baby's neck or give a bottle nipple to take the place of a dummy.

Fever in Infants Under 3 Months

Pyrexia

In General:

Babies who are breast fed are partly protected against many infections by antibodies in their mothers' milk; formula-fed infants don't enjoy the same level of immunity. Even with the best defences, however, germs manage to slip through. Fever, an increase in body temperature, is often a sign that the body is fighting off an infection.

Normal human body temperature ranges within about 1 degree Fahrenheit on either side of the average of 37°C (98.6°F). Few babies get through infancy without at least a mild infection or two, signalled by an increase in body temperature. With an infant under 3 months, you should contact your doctor immediately if the rectal temperature is higher than 38°C (100.4°F). When your baby is 3 months or older, contact your doctor if the temperature rises above 38.3°C (101°F), or the baby has other symptoms as well.

Prolonged fever can lead to dehydration from excessive loss of water through sweating. The danger is compounded if your baby is also vomiting or has diarrhoea. In addition, a baby may have a febrile (fever-related) convulsion if his temperature rises very rapidly. (See Convulsions, p. 50.) In children between 6 months and 5 years old, a febrile seizure may not indicate a serious condition. But tremors and spasms in a young infant may be serious and should be evaluated by your doctor.

☎

Call your doctor immediately if:

- Your baby under 3 months has a rectal temperature higher than 38°C (100.4°F).
- Your baby also has symptoms such as difficulty breathing, listlessness, diarrhoea, or vomiting.

Warning

Never give aspirin to reduce your infant's fever. The use of aspirin has been linked to an increased risk of Reye syndrome, a rare but serious disease, associated with viral infections, that affects the brain and liver. Although acetaminophen can help reduce fever and relieve discomfort, you should never give acetaminophen or any other medication to a baby under 3 months without your doctor's advice. Be careful not to exceed the recommended dose by giving a child cold medication containing acetaminophen.

Questions to Consider	If Answer Is	Possible Cause Is	Action to Take
Is your baby's temperature over 38°C (100.4°F)? Is he 3 months or less?	**YES**	Infection or other condition that may require treatment.	Contact your doctor.
Does your baby's face look flushed? Is he restless and sweaty, although he doesn't seem ill? Is his hair damp? Does he have a heat rash?	**YES**	Overheating.	Check to make sure your baby is not overdressed. Make sure his cot is not next to a radiator. Don't tuck your baby tightly under covers. Keep the temperature of his room no higher than about 20–21°C (68–70°F).
Is your baby's rectal temperature 38°C (100.4°F) or higher? Does she have fever along with other symptoms such as a runny nose, noisy breathing, rash, or diarrhoea? Does she seem fretful or uncomfortable?	**YES**	Infection or other condition that may require treatment.	Contact your doctor. The doctor will want to examine your baby to rule out serious infection or disease.

Questions to consider	If answer is	Possible cause is	Action to take
Did your baby recently have a high temperature for 3 to 5 days? Does he now have a spotty pink rash on his trunk? Did the rash appear as his temperature went back to normal?	**YES**	Roseola infantum, a contagious viral illness.	Contact your doctor, who will recommend ways to control the temperature and advise you to call again if your baby's condition doesn't improve or the fever persists.

Taking your baby's temperature

You can measure a baby's temperature by using a rectal thermometer. To read a mercury thermometer: hold it between your thumb and index finger, and slowly roll the tube back and forth until you can see the end of the mercury column, which corresponds to your baby's temperature.

To measure the rectal temperature:

- Wash the bulb with soap and water and rinse it under running water.
- Shake the thermometer until the mercury is below 35°C (96°F).
- Rub a small amount of petroleum jelly on the bulb.
- Lay your baby on your lap or a firm surface.
- Firmly press with one hand over your baby's lower back just above the buttocks.
- With your other hand, gently insert the lubricated thermometer 1–3cm (½–1in) into the anus. Hold it steady between your index and middle fingers for 2 minutes. Talk to the baby to calm and distract her.
- If the mercury shows more than 38°C (100.4°F), your baby has a fever. Check again in 30 minutes and, if her temperature is still high, contact your doctor for advice.
- Taking your baby's temperature can also be done by putting the thermometer under her arm, or using a forehead strip thermometer. These are not as accurate but will give a reasonable guide to whether your baby is feverish or not. The newer electronic thermometers that you put in the baby's ear are expensive, but do seem accurate.

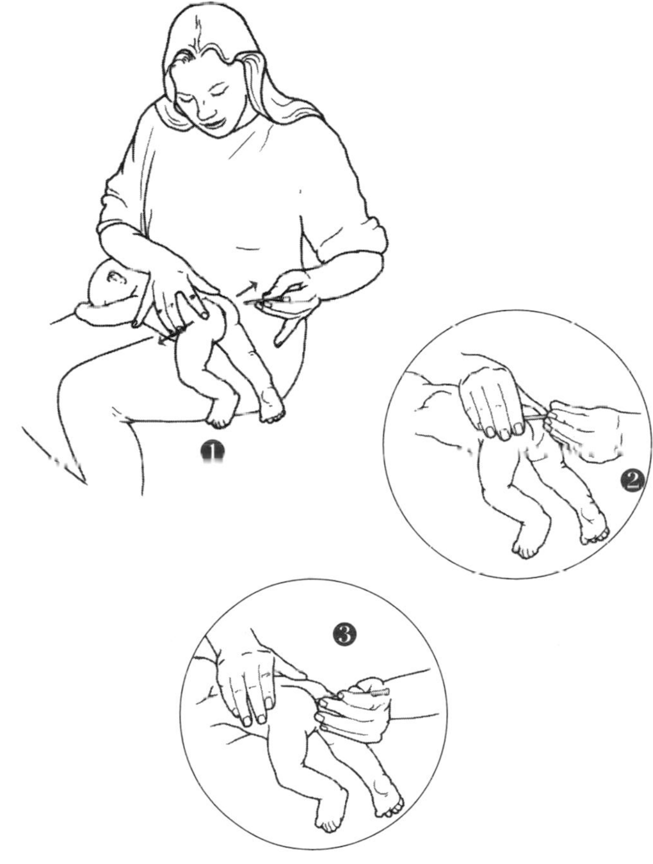

To take a rectal temperature, steady your baby by pressing with one hand just above his buttocks ❶. With the other hand, insert the lubricated thermometer 1–3 cm (½–1 in) inside the anus ❷. Gently hold the thermometer in place for 2 minutes, then remove it and read the temperature ❸.

In General:

Babies' skin is protected before birth by a cheesy coating, called vernix, which is produced toward the end of pregnancy. Once the vernix is washed off, the skin may peel a little as it is exposed to air. This is normal and doesn't require treatment. Many babies have birthmarks that gradually fade away without treatment, although some may grow larger before they disappear and some birthmarks are permanent. Your GP will advise whether a birthmark should be treated or left alone. Infants may develop a variety of rashes in their first months. Like birthmarks, they generally disappear without treatment. But if your baby has a persistent or widespread rash, bring it to your doctor's attention.

Contact your doctor if your infant has:

- A persistent or widespread rash.
- An enlarging birthmark.

Warning

Use plain water and cotton wool or a fresh flannel for cleaning your baby. It's not necessary to use commercial wet-wipes. If you use these products, choose those made for babies; adult versions contain alcohol, which may dry and irritate the skin.

A baby normally doesn't need powders, oils, and lotions to keep the skin smooth, no matter what advertisements for baby products may claim. If your baby's skin seems very dry, rub a little nonperfumed baby lotion on the dry patches. Don't use baby oil, which doesn't lubricate as well as lotion. Use only soaps and skin-care products that are made specially for babies; regular products may contain perfumes, dyes, alcohol, and other chemicals that can cause irritation.

Infants don't need daily baths, although most enjoy a chance to splash in the water once they get used to it. Many paediatricians feel that bathing two or three times a week is enough for the first year. More frequent baths may dry out the skin, especially during the winter. If your baby feels dry all over, cut his baths down to once or twice a week. Keep your baby clean by washing all traces of food from his face and hands, and wash the nappy area thoroughly during changes.

Questions to consider	If answer is	Possible cause is	Action to take
Does your newborn have one or more pinkish, brown, red, or purple patches anywhere on her body?	**YES**	Birthmarks, which may be either vascular (formed of blood vessels) or pigmented; some are both vascular and pigmented.	Pink or brown angiomas and flat red stains (stork bites) usually disappear by 18 months. Bright red hemangiomas (strawberry marks) first grow rapidly then gradually disappear by about 5 to 7 years. A port-wine stain may be permanent. Ask your doctor whether treatment is advisable and, if so, when it should be done. Cosmetics can be used to disguise disfiguring marks.
Does your newborn have a large bluish-grey mark like a bruise on her back?	**YES**	Mongolian spot.	This mark is common, especially among babies of Asian or African ancestry. It will disappear, probably before the child reaches 5 years.
Does your new baby have lots of little yellow-white spots on her nose, upper lip, cheeks, and forehead?	**YES**	Sebaceous hyperplasia; milia (tiny whiteheads); miliaria (prickly heat).	The first two conditions are due to enlarged oil glands, require no treatment, and will disappear. Prickly heat will clear up without treatment; avoid using plastic pants and don't overdress your infant.

Questions to consider	If answer is	Possible cause is	Action to take
Is your newborn getting blackheads, whiteheads, or other acne-like blemishes?	**YES**	Neonatal acne.	Acne is common in newborn babies, possibly due to the mother's hormones. It should clear up without treatment, but if it persists, talk to your pediatrician.
Has your baby developed greasy, yellow-brown patches on his scalp and behind his ears?	**YES**	Cradle cap (seborrheic dermatitis; see Hair Loss, p. 84).	Wash the scalp often with a mild shampoo and pat dry; rubbing with baby oil or petroleum jelly before washing may soften the crusts. Your health visitor may recommend a cream.
Does your baby have a red, spotty rash in the nappy area?	**YES**	Nappy rash; infection caused by yeast or bacteria; seborrhoea; psoriasis (rare).	Change wet or soiled nappies promptly. Clean the baby with plain water, pat dry, and apply a powder containing cornstarch (cornflour). Expose the nappy area to air as much as possible and avoid plastic or rubber pants. Petroleum jelly or a zinc oxide cream can protect the skin. If the rash doesn't improve, contact your doctor.
Does your infant have red, scaly patches on the cheeks, nappy area, or elsewhere?	**YES**	Eczema.	Consult your doctor. If the eczema is severe and your pediatrician suspects allergy to milk, dietary changes may be recommended. (See Allergic Reactions, p. 26.)
Has your infant developed fluid-filled blisters anywhere on her body?	**YES**	Bullous impetigo, a staphylococcal infection.	Call your doctor. This is a potentially serious problem and requires prompt medical treatment.

Coping with nappy rash

Many babies have a mild rash in the nappy area at some time. The most common cause is leaving a nappy on too long. Chemicals that form in the wet or soiled nappy irritate the skin, making it vulnerable to infection. The rash usually appears as redness or bumps on skin surfaces in direct contact with a wet or soiled nappy: the lower abdomen, buttocks, genitals, and folds of the thighs. If promptly attended to, it usually improves in 3 or 4 days. It's important to treat nappy rash, because damaged skin is more easily irritated by contact with urine and stool.

Nappy rash is more likely if babies are not changed frequently. It is also common in babies who have very frequent stools. Babies also tend to get nappy rashes when they are being treated with antibiotics, which kill friendly bacteria and allow an overgrowth of yeasts normally found on the skin.

Try to reduce your baby's risk of nappy rash by changing the nappy as soon as possible after bowel movements. Clean the nappy area with plain water and cotton wool or a soft cloth after movements. Change wet nappies to keep the skin from being exposed to moisture and chemicals in the urine. Let your baby go without a nappy whenever you can. If you use plastic pants or disposable nappies that close tightly around the thighs and abdomen, make sure they are loose enough so that air can circulate inside the nappy.

If your baby gets a nappy rash, apply a lotion or ointment and change the nappy frequently. Consult your doctor if you don't see an improvement in 2 to 3 days.

In General:

Very young babies sleep when their stomachs are full and wake up when it's time for a feed. Even at this stage, however, you can begin to teach your infant that daytime is for play and nighttime is for sleeping. During nighttime feeds, keep lights dim, speak quietly, and don't take longer than necessary for changing nappies. Put your baby right back to bed after feeding, changing, and a quiet cuddle.

By the time a baby reaches 5 or 6kg (12–13lb), her stomach can hold enough to tide her through the night. In fact, by 3 months most babies are sleeping 6 to 8 hours without waking most nights. Don't be upset when the pattern changes, however; sleep can be broken by colds and other illnesses, separation anxiety (see Fears, p. 72), and many other factors. Even after you've established a routine, your baby may get mixed up by oversleeping during the day and needing less sleep at night. Your baby will return to her old sleep patterns if you are patient and keep to the schedule.

Ending your baby's day with a bath and changing her into sleep clothes, and following a regular going-to-bed routine also help divide the hours into waking and sleeping. If you set a regular schedule, you'll find it easier to cope with occasional exceptions to the rule.

If your baby is waking up more than once a night at 6 months, something may be disturbing her. If she's still sleeping in your room, she may sense your presence and should be moved to another room nearby. If her bed is very small, she may be ready to move to a full-sized cot. If her room is dark, leaving a nightlight on may reassure her that she's in familiar surroundings.

Babies sometimes need a little help to get back to sleep, particularly in the first few months. Newborns get to sleep more easily in a soothing environment. A dummy is helpful for many infants. Listening to soft music can help. Once your baby is drowsy, place her in her cot while she's still awake. (For further hints on calming a restless baby, see Crying/Colic, p. 6.) While babies can often sleep through a surprisingly high level of steady noise, such as the sounds of street traffic or older siblings playing, a sudden, different sound – crinkling paper or a key in a lock – wakes them up at once.

By about 1 year, your increasingly active child may find it hard to wind down at bedtime. This is when a regular evening routine of story, songs, and a quiet game is essential. Don't expect your baby to fall asleep during the routine; instead, settle her into her cot so she learns to fall asleep on her own. Tuck her in, say your goodnights, and leave the room. She may cry for a moment but will soon calm down and fall asleep. If she's still crying after about 5 minutes, go in and comfort her, let her know you're nearby, but don't stay longer than a minute or two. Repeat this sequence several times if necessary, each time at a slightly longer interval. Be consistent, but not inflexible.

Consult your doctor if:

- Your infant is waking at night and has fever.
- Your baby sleeps almost all the time and is never fully alert.

Warning

Don't rush to your baby every time you hear a sound. He may be fussing or even crying during a phase of very light sleep. This is normal for some infants as they learn to resettle back to sleep. Of course, if his crying tells you he's hungry or in pain, or wants his diaper changed, give him the attention he needs and then put him back to bed.

Questions to consider	If answer is	Possible cause is	Action to take
Does your baby twitch, jerk, and move his eyes when asleep? Does he sleep with his eyes partly open?	**YES**	Normal infant sleep behaviour.	None. The movements are probably occurring during rapid eye movement (REM) sleep, when the baby is dreaming. In time, he will close his eyes when asleep.
Is your baby 3 months old but not sleeping through the night? Is she feeding well and growing normally?	**YES**	Normal behaviour.	Your baby will settle eventually. Try to establish a bedtime routine, and delay her bedtime slightly if the waking upsets you.
Did your baby cry as if in pain when you laid him in his cot? Is he feverish? Does he have other symptoms?	**YES**	Illness such as a respiratory or ear infection. (See Fever in Infants Under 3 Months, p. 10.)	Contact your doctor.
Does your baby breathe noisily whether asleep or awake?	**YES**	Normal softness of airway tissues (laryngotracheal malacia).	If your baby is feeding, sleeping, and growing normally, the noisy breathing just shows that the tissues are not yet firmed up. She will outgrow this noisy breathing by about 18 months. Bring it to your GP's attention.
Is your infant's breathing laboured? Does he seem to be having trouble breathing?	**YES**	Respiratory distress. (See Breathing Difficulty/Breathlessness, p. 44.)	Call your doctor right away or go directly to the hospital emergency department.
Has your child become more wakeful at night during the latter half of his first year?	**YES**	Separation anxiety. (See Fears, p. 72.)	Discuss your concerns with your doctor.

Positioning your baby for sleep

For years paediatricians advised parents to lay infants on their stomachs for sleeping. This, they thought, could save a baby from choking if he spat up or vomited. Now, however, studies suggest that the sudden infant death syndrome (SIDS) occurs less often in babies who sleep on their backs. **All the experts advise, therefore, that parents place healthy infants on their backs.** Exceptions to this practice include premature babies; those with facial malformations that could cause an airway blockage in a child lying on his back; babies who are vomiting, who spit up a lot, or have gastroesophageal reflux; and others as advised by their doctors.

There are probably many reasons for SIDS and sleep position may be only a minor one. Still, doctors feel that if there is a possible link, it makes sense to try to avoid it. Once a baby can roll over and find a comfortable position for himself (this generally happens between 4 and 7 months), he's usually past the highest-risk time for SIDS.

Spitting Up

Regurgitation

IN GENERAL:

Immaturity of the muscles in the digestive tract is the major reason most babies spit up after meals. It happens because the cardiac, or cardioesophageal, sphincter (the ring that seals off the stomach from the oesophagus), like all the baby's muscles, takes time to gain full working strength. If the baby's stomach is full or her position is abruptly changed after a feed, the stomach contents press the sphincter open and flood back through the oesophagus. In contrast to vomiting (see p. 160), spitting up may not involve forceful muscle contractions, brings up only small amounts of milk, and doesn't distress the baby or make her uncomfortable.

Many babies spit up after gulping down air with their milk or formula. The best way to prevent this is to feed the baby before she gets ravenous and hold her at an angle that prevents air from entering her mouth while she feeds. Gently burp the baby at intervals during feeds (see Tips to reduce spitting up, p. 17). Limit active play after meals. If spitting up is excessive, some paediatricians advise thickening the formula with a small amount of rice cereal (1 to 3 teaspoons per 30ml [1oz] of formula). Your doctor or health visitor may also suggest keeping the baby upright after eating. Spitting up usually stops once the baby learns to pull herself into a sitting position, though a few babies continue to spit up until they are weaned to a cup or can walk. Until it stops, get in the habit of protecting yourself with a towel or nappy during feedings and burpings.

Consult your doctor if:

- Your baby vomits forcefully after every feed.
- Your baby is losing or failing to gain weight.
- Your baby brings up blood in the vomit.

Warning

Don't persist with feeding once your baby has turned away from the bottle. She knows how much her stomach can handle, and the extra you urge her to take may only cause her to spit up.

QUESTIONS TO CONSIDER	IF ANSWER IS	POSSIBLE CAUSE IS	ACTION TO TAKE
Does your baby spit up a little after most feeds?	YES	Gastroesophageal reflux (normal if mild).	None: The spitting up will grow less frequent and stop as the baby's muscles mature.
Does your baby gulp his feeds? Does he seem to have a lot of wind?	YES	Swallowing air (aerophagia).	Make sure your baby is positioned properly. (See Tips to reduce spitting up, opposite; also see Feeding Problems in Infants, p. 9.)
Does your baby spit up when you bounce him or play after meals?	YES	Overstimulation.	Keep mealtimes calm and limit active play for about 30 minutes afterwards.
Has your baby's spitting up changed to vomiting, with muscle contractions? Does it happen after every feed? Does the vomit shoot out with force?	YES	Pyloric stenosis or another condition requiring diagnosis and treatment.	Consult your doctor, who will examine the baby to determine the reason for vomiting.

QUESTIONS TO CONSIDER	IF ANSWER IS	POSSIBLE CAUSE IS	ACTION TO TAKE
Is your baby not gaining weight as you think she should?	**YES**	Failure to thrive.	Consult your doctor promptly. Your baby may need only simple measures, but your doctor should examine her to rule out serious disorders.
Is there blood in the material your baby is spitting or vomiting?	**YES**	Oesophagitis or another condition requiring diagnosis and treatment.	Contact your doctor straightaway for an examination.

Tips to reduce spitting up

It's almost impossible to prevent spitting up, but it helps if your feeding techniques keep your baby from swallowing air unnecessarily. The following tips may help you to reduce the amount of food spat up and the frequency of episodes.

- Feed your baby before he gets famished.
- Keep feeding times calm, quiet, and unhurried.
- Burp your baby every 3 to 4 minutes, or when he pauses or changes over from one breast to the other.
- Your breast-fed baby will be frustrated and upset if he's not getting a good flow of milk. You can help by positioning him correctly. Hold the baby so his whole body – not just his head – faces yours. Hold the breast with the thumb above the areola (the pink area around the nipple) and your fingers and palm beneath it. Or use a scissors grip if it's more comfortable. Gently press the breast and guide it into the baby's mouth so he can grasp the entire nipple.
- Feed your baby in a comfortable sitting position and keep him upright on your lap or in his pushchair or infant seat for about 20 minutes after feeds.
- Don't jiggle your baby or start a vigorous game right after a feeding.
- If he has a bottle, make sure the nipple is in good condition and the hole is the right size (when you turn the bottle upside down, a few drops should come out and then stop).
- Your health visitor may suggest that you thicken the formula with a small amount of cereal.
- If your baby spits up a lot, protect his undersheet with a towel or nappy and raise the head of the cot with blocks to keep his head higher than his stomach. Place him on his side in the cot with his feet against the bottom bumper. A sheet or blanket tucked over him will keep him from rolling sideways.

CHAPTER 2 COMMON SYMPTOMS IN BABIES AND YOUNG CHILDREN

REARING A HEALTHY YOUNGSTER

Once babies are past the settling-in period of the first few months, they come into increasingly frequent contact with people and objects that spark their curiosity and stimulate development. Exciting as parents find this new phase, they also find it worrying, as a widening circle of contacts also means exposure to diseases and hazardous situations.

Even though you take all possible precautions to protect your child from illness and harm, there are those inevitable occasions when even the most healthy child develops symptoms. Some may signal acute but only temporary discomfort, such as with the common cold; others may point to a more serious illness that demands your doctor's immediate attention. The charts on the following pages cover the most common symptoms seen from infancy to pre-adolescence. The charts are designed to help you tell when your youngster's symptoms are likely to clear up on their own and when you should seek your doctor's attention. If your child's symptoms don't quite fit the picture that's given or you have any doubts about what to do, don't hesitate to get your doctor's advice.

Abdominal Pain, Acute

IN GENERAL:
Children have abdominal pain for any number of physical and emotional reasons. Luckily, most stomachaches disappear on their own, without special treatment. But parents should be familiar with the symptoms that indicate unusual, possibly serious causes, making it all the easier to deal with more common, minor conditions.

Call your GP immediately if:

- Your baby under age 1 shows signs suggesting abdominal pain (unusual crying, legs pulled up towards abdomen).
- Your child has continuous pain for 3 hours or longer.
- Your child has pain along with swelling in the groin or testicles.
- Your child still has pain 3 hours after vomiting or diarrhoea.
- Your child vomits greenish-yellow material or passes blood in the stool.

Warning

Do not force a child with abdominal pain to eat, but make sure he has plenty of clear fluids to drink if he wishes. Don't give a pain reliever until your doctor has seen the child and says it's all right to do so.

QUESTIONS TO CONSIDER	IF ANSWER IS	POSSIBLE CAUSE IS	ACTION TO TAKE
Does your child have diarrhea and/or vomiting?	YES	Gastroenteritis.	If the child is under 6 months, continue breast-feeding or formula. In an older child, give electrolyte drinks and small servings of a normal diet. If symptoms do not improve in 48 hours, contact your GP.
Does your child frequently complain of pain, with no symptoms between bouts? Is she at least 4 years old?	YES	Nonspecific abdominal pain, often related to stress. (See Abdominal Pain, Chronic or Recurrent, p. 22.)	Let the child rest with a hot water bottle and offer fluids. Watch for danger signals (see box above). Talk to your GP, who will examine the child to rule out disease and discuss possible pain triggers.
Is your child unwilling to let you gently press on his abdomen?	YES	Gastroenteritis or, if the pain persists longer than 3 hours, early appendicitis.	If symptoms improve, give clear liquids and a normal diet as soon as the child can tolerate food. If diarrhoea develops, treat as for gastroenteritis, above. If pain lasts more than 3 hours, contact your GP.
Has your child had continuous pain for at least 3 hours? Did it begin near the navel and migrate towards the lower right abdomen?	YES	Appendicitis.	Call your doctor; give nothing to eat or drink until after the doctor's examination. If your doctor suspects appendicitis or another serious condition, your child will be given tests and may be hospitalized.

QUESTIONS TO CONSIDER	IF ANSWER IS	POSSIBLE CAUSE IS	ACTION TO TAKE
Does your child over 3 years also have a sore throat with other symptoms such as a headache?	**YES**	Viral infection or streptococcal throat infection (strep throat).	Contact your GP to examine the child and recommend treatment. Give your child drinks he enjoys and paracetamol to relieve pain and discomfort.
Does your child have a tender swelling in the groin or testicles?	**YES**	Strangulated hernia; torsion (twisting) of the testicle.	Call your doctor immediately. The child may be hospitalized for treatment.
Does your child have at least two of the following: temperature over 38.3°C (101°F); bed-wetting (in a child previously dry); urination with pain, frequency, or odour?	**YES**	Urinary tract infection.	Consult your GP, who may order diagnostic tests and prescribe an antibiotic.
Has your child vomited greenish-yellow material?	**YES**	Intestinal obstruction.	Call your GP at once. Give nothing to eat or drink until after the doctor's examination.

Treatment of appendicitis

Appendicitis is an infection or inflammation of the appendix, a worm-shaped pouch near the junction of the large and small intestines. When a child's abdominal pain and other symptoms and tests indicate appendicitis, an operation should be performed as soon as possible. If the inflamed appendix is not removed it may burst, causing peritonitis, a dangerous infection that spreads throughout the abdomen. After surgery, children almost always recover quickly with no aftereffects.

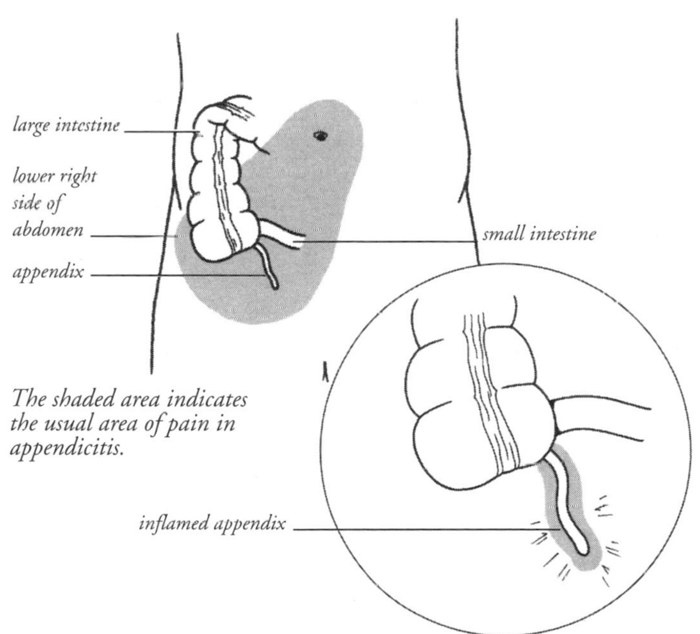

The shaded area indicates the usual area of pain in appendicitis.

In General:

Recurrent abdominal pain is common but not often serious in children. Often, stomachaches disappear within an hour or two. In many cases, no physical cause is found and the symptom is described as 'functional' pain: that is, nonspecific pain most often related to stress. The pattern and site of symptoms may yield clues to the reason for the recurrent pain: anxiety related to school, for example, or emotional upset due to problems at home. Provided the child's growth and physical examination are normal, the pain is not limited to a specific site, and there are no associated symptoms, a stomachache is unlikely to signal a serious condition that would require immediate treatment. Even when no cause is found, however, the pain is real and the child's distress requires attention.

Consult your GP if:

- Your child has very severe, unrelenting pain.
- Pain awakens your child from sleep.
- A child 4 years old or younger has recurrent abdominal pain.
- Your child has a decreased appetite and weight loss.
- Your child has severe vomiting with abdominal pain.
- Your child has blood in the stool, urine, or vomit.

Warning

Although recurrent abdominal pain can be upsetting, exhaustive testing and treatment efforts are not always helpful and may only increase the child's anxiety.

All children with recurrent abdominal pain should have their urine examined to rule out a urine infection.

Questions to consider	If answer is	Possible cause is	Action to take
Has your child had fewer bowel movements than usual (for him) over the past 2 or 3 days?	**YES**	Constipation.	If your child is generally well, increase his fluid and fibre intake. If his bowels still don't move, contact your GP, who may prescribe a stool softener. (See Constipation, p. 48.)
Does pain occur at times of stress, such as school tests or problems at home?	**YES**	Functional pain.	Consult your GP, who will examine the child, order tests if necessary, and discuss pain triggers, which may be physical, emotional, or dietary.
Does the child also have bloating, cramping, and diarrhoea? Does she get rashes or swelling? Do attacks follow certain foods—even hours or days later?	**YES**	Food allergy.	Talk to your doctor who will examine your child and may suggest keeping a food diary, eliminating then reintroducing certain foods, or other measures to identify and avoid the offending food. (See Allergic Reactions, p. 26.)
Does pain occur when the child drinks milk or eats ice cream? Do bouts include bloating, wind, cramps, and diarrhoea?	**YES**	Lactase deficiency/ lactose intolerance (sometimes seen after about age 4 in children of African or Asian ancestry).	If your doctor agrees, use fortified soy or rice substitutes for dairy products for 1 to 2 weeks, then reintroduce milk to see if symptoms recur. (A breath test can also identify lactase deficiency.)

Questions to consider	If answer is	Possible cause is	Action to take
Does your child complain of vague abdominal pain? Does your family live in an older home that has peeling paint or is being renovated?	**YES**	Lead poisoning (common in urban areas and in regions with older housing).	Consult your GP, who will order blood tests to determine the lead level in your child's blood. Your child may require treatment and measures must be taken to remove the source of lead.
Are bouts of pain accompanied by bloating, wind, cramps, and diarrhoea? Do you live where fresh water may be contaminated or has the child been on holiday in such an area?	**YES**	Parasitic infection, possibly giardiasis.	Consult your doctor, who may order tests for giardia and other parasites. If results are positive, medication will be prescribed.
If your child has bloating, wind, and diarrhoea, has she recently had large quantities of apples or juice, or had sugarless sweets or gum?	**YES**	Excessive consumption of fructose or sorbitol.	Reduce your child's intake of apples and fruit juice; withhold sweets and gum. If symptoms do not improve in 2 days, check with your doctor.
Does your child have frequent headaches, or nausea with or without vomiting? Does sleep help to stop a bout of pain? Are pain attacks preceded by visual symptoms (blurring, blind spots, flashes of light)? Do any family members have migraine?	**YES**	Migraine with associated nausea and/or vomiting (uncommon in children).	Help your child to rest in a quiet, darkened room. Consult your GP, who may recommend antimigraine treatment or medication for severe nausea and vomiting.
Are pain attacks always the same and accompanied by at least five bouts of vomiting?	**YES**	Cyclical vomiting disorder (rare in children).	Consult your doctor. Some children with this rare condition improve with antimigraine therapy.

Coping with recurrent stomachaches

Even when no physical cause can be found for recurrent stomachaches, the pain is real and your child is in discomfort. What's more, youngsters who get recurrent stomachaches for no apparent reason are just as likely as others to develop a serious abdominal condition involving pain. Don't ignore such stomachaches, and call your GP if your child develops stomachache symptoms that are different from usual.

Abdominal Swelling

Abdominal distention

In General:

Toddlers typically look as if they have a 'pot belly', with a large, protruding abdomen balanced by a sway back – an inward curving of the lower back. This is perfectly normal. By your child's third birthday, however, she will probably have a longer, leaner look marked by a flatter stomach, straighter back, and longer, slimmer legs. If you feel that there is something wrong with your child's posture, or worry that she's not growing normally, check with your GP.

Call your GP immediately if:

- The abdominal swelling is hard or painful.
- Your child has diarrhoea, vomiting, or severe constipation.
- Your child's temperature is higher than 38.3°C (101°F).

Warning:

Swelling of the abdomen can indicate a problem in the digestive tract or other organs. The cause may be a buildup of fluid or wind, or an intestinal obstruction.

Questions to consider	If answer is	Possible cause is	Action to take
Is your child constipated but otherwise well?	**YES**	Constipation.	Make sure your child is getting enough fluids and fibre. If the problem persists, consult your doctor. (See Constipation, p. 48.)
Did swelling and very severe pain come on suddenly?	**YES**	Intestinal obstruction.	Call your doctor, who will examine your child, order tests, and start treatment to remove the obstruction.
Are the stools pale, bulky, and unusually foul smelling? Does your child often pass wind? Does she have a persistent cough? Is she underweight? Does her skin taste salty?	**YES**	Malabsorption problem, such as coeliac disease; cystic fibrosis.	Consult your doctor, who will examine your child and order tests. Depending on the results, the doctor may recommend a treatment progamme and refer you to a dietitian for guidance in adapting your child's diet.
Has your child recently had a streptococcal infection such as a sore throat or impetigo? Is his urine 'smoky' or reddish-brown? Is his face swollen? Does he have a headache and/or fever?	**YES**	Post-streptococcal glomerulonephritis (kidney inflammation).	Call your doctor immediately. This kidney condition can follow a streptococcal infection and may lead to chronic kidney disease if not treated promptly.
In addition to abdominal swelling, does your child have generalized swelling, especially around his eyes and face? Is his urine normal in appearance but scant?	**YES**	Nephrotic syndrome.	Consult your doctor at once. This kidney condition (more common in boys between 1 and 6 years old) may become chronic and requires prompt diagnosis and treatment.

Questions to consider	If answer is	Possible cause is	Action to take
Is the swelling especially prominent in the upper abdomen? Does your child also have unexplained bruising or fever? Has she lost weight?	**YES**	Uncommon blood disorder such as leukaemia.	Consult your doctor straightaway.

Swelling around the navel

If your baby's navel looks as if it's pushing outward when he cries, he may have an umbilical hernia. In this condition, a small weak spot lets tissue bulge outward through the muscular abdominal wall when there is pressure inside the abdomen. An umbilical hernia is not serious and usually closes up by the time a child is between 3 and 4 years old. When the condition doesn't heal itself, your GP may advise a consultation with a surgeon. Abdominal binders, once wrapped around every infant's navel, are no longer recommended.

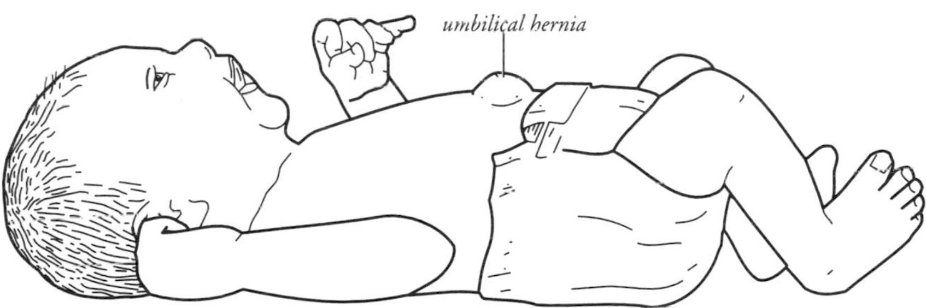

An umbilical hernia is a small weak spot that lets tissue bulge out through the muscular abdominal wall. The hernia is usually more apparent when the baby cries. This fairly common condition is not serious and usually heals on its own by the time the child is 3 to 4 years old. The rare cases that do not heal spontaneously can be treated with surgery.

Allergic Reactions

Hypersensitivity

In General:

The body's immune system is on constant alert against threats from the environment. When a foreign substance tries to break through the body's defences, the immune system fights back with inflammation, irritation, and symptoms affecting sensitive areas such as the skin, nose, eyes, throat, lungs, and digestive tract. Sometimes the immune system overreacts by trying to defend the body against substances that are harmless or even beneficial, and the result is an allergic reaction.

Allergies tend to run in families; if one or both parents have allergies, the odds are high that their children will also develop them. However, youngsters may not be allergic to the same substances as their parents.

Many allergens (allergy-causing substances) can be identified because a reaction always follows exposure to the substance. Skin tests can be useful for diagnosing allergies, although they are not 100 percent reliable. In addition, special blood tests may be done.

There is no cure for allergies, but flare-ups can often be prevented by simply avoiding the offending substance. When contact can't be avoided, medication can help to control symptoms. In very severe cases, your doctor may recommend allergy shots – a series of desensitizing injections in which tiny amounts of the problem substance are given to make your child less sensitive to it.

Call 999 or your doctor immediately if your child has:

- Difficulty in breathing or swallowing, or other symptoms of a severe allergic reaction (called anaphylaxis) such as widespread swelling, pale skin, sweating, rapid or difficult breathing, drowsiness, or confusion.

Warning

Do not use over-the-counter products to treat your child's rash, runny nose, or respiratory symptoms. Commercial nasal sprays can cause worse congestion, which may be more uncomfortable and harder to treat than the original allergy. Antihistamine creams and lotions may increase your child's sensitivity. Use medications only as instructed by your doctor.

Questions to consider	If answer is	Possible cause is	Action to take
Does your child have a runny nose with clear discharge, itchy eyes, tearing, and sneezing? Are symptoms worse during pollen seasons?	**YES**	Hay fever (allergic rhinitis).	Consult your GP, who may prescribe medication to relieve acute symptoms and recommend measures to lessen exposure to offending substances.
Does your child have a flaky red rash with scaling and blistering? Is the rash mainly on her limbs and face? Do other family members have eczema?	**YES**	Eczema (nonallergic atopic dermatitis).	If the rash is mild, no medical treatment is necessary. Use a mild, unscented soap, limit the time spent in baths, and apply an unscented moisturizing cream after bathing. Avoid woollen clothing next to the skin.
Is your child's breathing fast and noisy? Is he wheezing and coughing? Does he have hay fever or eczema? Is there asthma in the family?	**YES**	Asthma, perhaps triggered by allergies.	Consult your GP, who will examine the child and prescribe treatment to improve symptoms and prevent attacks. Sensitivity testing may be necessary to find the asthma trigger, and your doctor may recommend changes in your home and lifestyle.

Questions to consider	If answer is	Possible cause is	Action to take
Is the rash made up of bright red, raised spots with paler centres? Do the spots vary in size and location?	**YES**	Hives, usually due to an allergic reaction to infection, medication, heat, cold, or foods.	Most hives disappear without treatment. Apply a cold compress to ease itching and swelling. Consult your GP if you suspect a drug reaction, if your child has repeated attacks, or a rash lasts more than 4 hours.
Are your child's eyes reddened, with tearing, itching, and puffiness?	**YES**	Allergic conjunctivitis.	Consult your GP for treatment to relieve the acute discomfort. Avoid known irritants.
Does your child have a red rash with scaling and blistering confined to one part of the body?	**YES**	Allergic contact dermatitis.	Avoid exposing affected area to possible allergens (such as detergents). If the rash does not improve in a few days, consult your GP.
Does your child have recurrent nausea and vomiting, cramps and/or diarrhoea, headache, and/or hives, but no fever?	**YES**	Food allergy.	Consult your GP and report any suspect food. Sensitivity testing may identify allergens and guide you in avoiding the problem foodstuff.

Food allergies vs. sensitivities

True food allergies are rare; more often a child has an intolerance to a particular ingredient. People with lactose intolerance, for example, lack an enzyme needed to digest milk sugar; those with coeliac disease cannot tolerate gluten, a protein in grains, especially wheat. The resulting symptoms – diarrhoea, bloating, wind – are similar to allergic reactions but don't involve the immune system. A paediatrician can test your child for food intolerance or allergy.

A food diary can often identify foods that cause symptoms. Keep a daily record of all foods and beverages, with the time they're consumed, and note down any symptoms and when they occur (see sample). The pattern of symptoms may point to the offending food. Eliminate a suspect food for a week or so, then reintroduce it. If your child gets symptoms again, avoid that food in the future.

Sample Diary

Food	Time	Symptoms	Time
Milk/Rice cereal	8am		
Orange juice			
Cheese	10:30am		
Crackers			
Peanut butter sandwich	12pm	Itching mouth	12:40 pm
Milk and Apple		Slight rash	
Yoghurt	2pm		
Apple juice			
Chicken	6pm		
Baked potato			
Salad			
Carrots			
Poached pear			
Orange juice	8pm	Itching	8:30pm
Peanut butter cookie		Rash	

Peanuts are the likely allergen. Try eliminating them from the diet for 7 to 10 days, then reintroduce them to see if symptoms recur.

Appetite Loss

Anorexia

IN GENERAL:

Although many parents worry whether their children are eating enough (or too much), the fact is most children eat what they need to make up for energy spent in growth and play. It's perfectly normal for children's appetites to vary, just as those of adults do. Your child may ask for second helpings one day and turn his nose up at food the next.

Young children's food fads can drive parents wild: a 2-year-old, for example, may suddenly refuse all foods of a certain colour, or insist that no food touch another on the plate. But when parents get upset, children quickly learn that food can be used to get their own way. If parents take these whims in stride, children eventually lose interest in food as a means of control.

So long as they have access to nourishing foods, children won't starve themselves and they rarely lose weight. An exception is the older child or teenager with the eating disorder called anorexia nervosa. (See Eating Disorders, p. 178.)

Consult your doctor if your child:

- Has a marked appetite loss for more than a week.
- Refuses fluids.
- Has lost weight or failed to gain over a 3-month to 4-month period.

Warning

Children should drink plenty of fluids, including several cups of milk a day. But don't go to extremes. Some youngsters fill up on liquids and have little appetite for solid foods.

QUESTIONS TO CONSIDER	IF ANSWER IS	POSSIBLE CAUSE IS	ACTION TO TAKE
Is your child a healthy 1-year-old to 2-year-old with normal growth and energy?	YES	Normal change in appetite due to slowing of growth rate.	None. A decrease in appetite is normal at this age. However, be sure to provide a varied diet based on the Food Guide Pyramid. (See p. 180.)
Does your child have a sore throat, cough, runny nose, and fever?	YES	Upper respiratory tract infection (viral).	Provide cold drinks, ice cream, or yoghurt to soothe inflammation. Give paracetamol to relieve discomfort.
Does your child have swollen glands in the neck? Is he feverish? Does he have a worsening sore throat? Have further symptoms, such as difficulty in swallowing, developed?	YES	Streptococcal throat infection; infectious mononucleosis (glandular fever).	Contact your GP, who will examine your child and prescribe appropriate treatment.
Does your child have diarrhoea?	YES	Gastroenteritis.	If the diarrhoea is mild, continue a normal diet. If it is severe, give rehydrating fluids. (See Diarrhoea, p. 62.) Call your GP if vomiting persists more than 12 hours, or if diarrhoea is bloody or lasts more than 48 hours.

Questions to consider	If answer is	Possible cause is	Action to take
Has your child been urinating frequently? Is urination painful or urgent? Does she have a stomachache?	**YES**	Urinary tract infection.	Consult your GP, who will test the urine and prescribe an antibiotic, if such treatment is appropriate.
Is your child passing large volumes of urine? Has he lost weight? Does he seem unusually tired?	**YES**	Diabetes mellitus.	Consult your GP without delay; if diagnostic tests indicate diabetes, insulin injections and other measures to control the disease must be started.
Does your child have pain that began around the navel and has moved to the lower right abdomen? Is there nausea or vomiting?	**YES**	Acute appendicitis.	Consult your doctor without delay. (See Abdominal Pain, Acute, p. 20.)
Has your child been unusually pale, lethargic, or irritable over a period of weeks?	**YES**	Systemic illness.	Consult your GP, who will examine your child for anaemia, lead poisoning, or other illness.

Fostering good eating habits

Eating habits that are laid down early in life often become a lifelong pattern. Many adults bear the consequences of being urged to clean their plates when they weren't hungry, or being bribed with food treats for good behaviour. In Britain, as well as the United States, obesity is the result of overeating often coupled with underactivity. Many experts note that people are eating less now than 100 years ago, but weigh more, because of their sedentary lifestyle. In any event, obesity is a far more common and a more serious threat to health than being underweight.

Trust your children's instincts: left to themselves, youngsters will eat as much as they need to keep up their energy stores. Encourage your children's dawning independence – and make allowances for their natural likes and dislikes – by ensuring that they have a moderate array of appealing foods to choose from. Children know how much they need: it's up to the parents to provide wholesome foods for healthy eating.

In General:

Problems affecting children's backs are most often due to injuries from sport or play, falls, or unusual strain. The most frequent cause is a pulled muscle, strained ligament, or bruising resulting in pain and stiffness. Back symptoms usually disappear within a week, without special treatment.

While regular exercise is beneficial for all youngsters, intensive training may lead to over-use injuries with back pain in some young athletes. Dancers and gymnasts, for example, are particularly prone to develop back pain resulting from over-use.

Severe curvature of the spine or scoliosis (see opposite) is a possible cause of back pain, especially in adolescent girls. Your doctor or health visitor evaluates your child's posture during childhood to make sure her back is straight and she is growing normally.

☎

Consult your GP if your child with back pain is under 10 years old or has:

- Persistent or increasing pain.
- Fever or weight loss.
- Difficulty in moving any limb.
- Numbness or tingling in a limb.
- Loss of bladder or bowel control.
- A change in gait or posture.

Warning

Back pain in a young child who has not been injured is not normal and needs to be evaluated by your GP.

Questions to consider	If answer is	Possible cause is	Action to take
Has your child recently been involved in sport or vigorous play? Did she have a minor fall or other injury?	**YES**	Muscle pull, strained ligament, bruise.	Apply a cold compress to the injury straightaway; a warm bath may be comforting later. Give paracetamol or ibuprofen for pain relief.
Did your child fall from a considerable height?	**YES**	Spinal injury.	Call 999 at once. Do not try to move your child unless his life is in danger. If he has to be moved, improvise a carrying board. (See Fractures, p. 217.)
Following an apparently minor back injury, has your child had difficulty in moving, numbness or tingling in a limb, or loss of bladder or bowel control?	**YES**	Spinal injury.	Call your doctor or take your child to the nearest hospital emergency department.
Is your child complaining of a sharp, one-sided pain in the middle of her back? Does she have painful or frequent urination? Does she have a fever? Is she nauseated?	**YES**	Acute kidney infection.	Consult your GP without delay. Try to collect a urine specimen first.
Does your child have back pain that awakens him from a sound sleep at night?	**YES**	Diskitis (inflammation of a spinal disc); infection; tumour.	Consult your GP, who will examine your child, order tests or x-rays, and recommend referral to another specialist, if necessary.

Curvature of the spine

About 7 percent of adolescent girls have curvature of the spine (scoliosis) to some degree. Scoliosis occurs in boys almost as often as girls, but girls generally have more severe curvature and require treatment more often. School Medical Officers now have screening programmes to detect scoliosis in youngsters as they approach puberty and before their bone growth is complete. If any abnormality is detected, your school health authority will contact you and advise you to consult your GP. For mild curvature, close observation by your doctor may be all that's recommended. More severe, progressive scoliosis may require wearing a special brace or surgery to straighten the spine.

Scientific studies have not shown any benefit from manipulation therapy in youngsters with scoliosis.

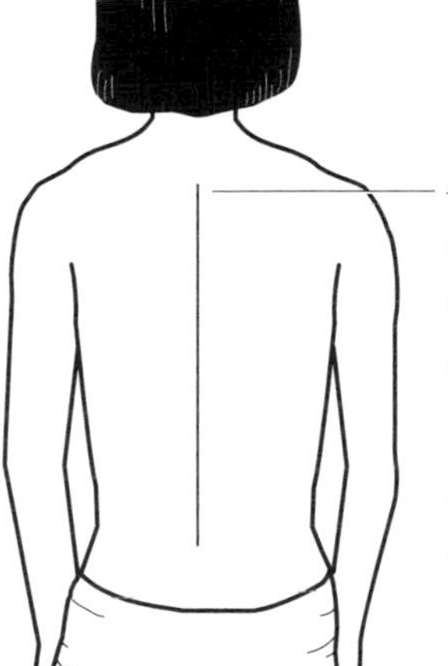

Normal

- *Head centred over mid-buttocks.*
- *Shoulders level.*
- *Shoulder blades level and equally prominent.*
- *Hips level and symmetrical.*
- *Equal distance between arms and body.*

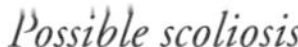

Possible scoliosis

- *Upper back, lower back, or possibly both, asymmetrical.*

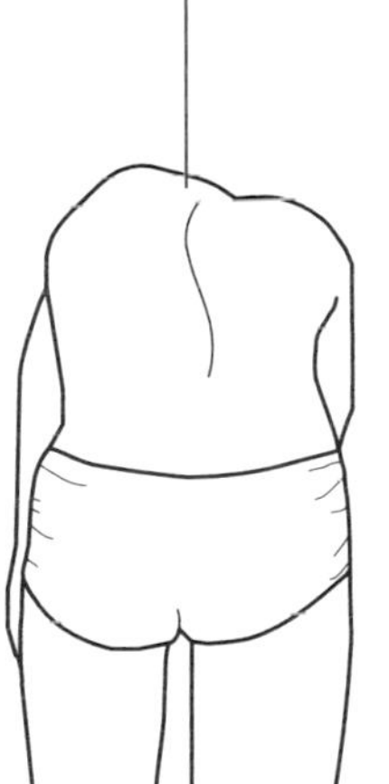

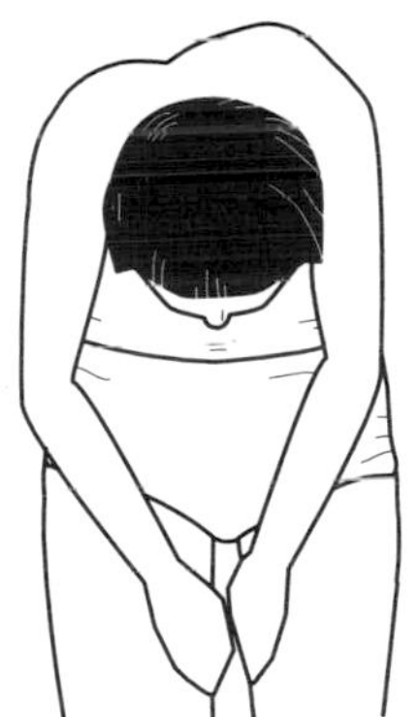

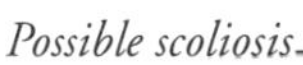

Possible scoliosis

- *Head over to one side of mid-buttocks.*
- *One shoulder higher.*
- *One shoulder blade higher, possibly more prominent.*
- *One hip more prominent.*
- *Unequal distance between arms and body.*

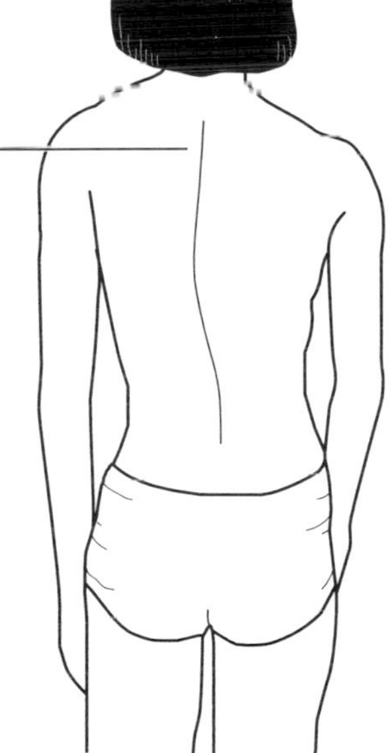

Bed-wetting

Nocturnal enuresis

In General

Although children vary widely in the order and timing at which they achieve daytime bladder control and nighttime dryness, most are fully toilet trained between the ages of 3 and 4, with control over nighttime urination coming about 6 months to a year after daytime control. But many – up to 15 percent – continue to wet the bed regularly until age 5 or even later. Bed-wetting is more common among boys than girls; in many cases the fathers had a similar problem as children, leading researchers to suspect a genetic tendency. In any event, most youngsters outgrow bed-wetting by puberty.

Consult your GP if your child:

- Continues bed-wetting at night beyond age 5.
- Resumes regular nighttime bed-wetting after months of dryness.
- Has bladder control problems both day and night.
- Has other symptoms, such as excessive thirst, pain or burning during urination, or daytime wetting.

Warning

Be wary of claims for bed-wetting treatments in mail-order advertisements. Your GP is your reliable source for information; don't enroll in or pay for any bed-wetting treatment without your doctor's advice.

Questions to consider	If answer is	Possible cause is	Action to take
Is your child less than 3 years old?	**YES**	Immature bladder control or arousal mechanism.	The mechanisms for controlling bladder and arousal are still developing. Your child will achieve control as these mechanisms mature.
Is your child under age 5? Does he wear a nappy at night and/or still wet the bed?	**YES**	Immature bladder size or arousal mechanism.	In many children, nighttime dryness may lag behind daytime control. The situation is not a cause for concern and will eventually resolve itself.
Is your child older than 6 years and still wetting the bed?	**YES**	Continuing immaturity of nocturnal arousal (nocturnal enuresis).	Consult your GP, who will evaluate your child's condition and family history. Your doctor may recommend treatment based on a nighttime alarm, behaviour modification, counselling, and/or medication.
Has your normally dry child wet the bed during a time of stress (e.g., starting school, parental discord)?	**YES**	Emotional stress.	Reassure your child, and protect the mattress with a waterproof sheet. If bed-wetting lasts for longer than 2 weeks, or if the source of stress is not clear, consult your GP.
Has bed-wetting recurred in a previously dry child? Does the child complain of burning? Is she urinating frequently during the day?	**YES**	Urinary tract infection.	Consult your GP, who may order tests and prescribe an antibiotic, if one is appropriate.

QUESTIONS TO CONSIDER	IF ANSWER IS	POSSIBLE CAUSE IS	ACTION TO TAKE
In addition to bed-wetting, does your child also pass large volumes of urine during the day? Has he lost weight? Does he seem unusually tired?	**YES**	Diabetes mellitus.	Consult your GP at once and take a urine specimen, if possible.

Steps to toilet training

Children gain control of bladder and bowel function when they are physically ready. Parents cannot hasten the process, but they can bolster children's confidence and encourage their efforts. Pushing a child into toilet training before she is ready may only prolong the process. Toilet training isn't likely to succeed until your child is past the negativism and resistance often seen in the early toddler months. A child must want to take on the independence that comes with this major step forward. This stage usually occurs between 18 and 24 months, but it's quite normal for it to happen a bit later.

When your child is ready to start, toilet training should go fairly smoothly as long as you both stay relaxed about it. Praise your toddler for her efforts and don't bother to mention her mistakes or accidents. Showing displeasure will add an element of tension that won't help and may hinder progress.

1. Let your toddler become familiar with a potty chair or the toilet fitted with a toddler seat, but don't expect her to use it for some time. Look for signs that your child is uncomfortable when wetting or soiling the nappy during the day. Once your child is able to control urination and bowel movements for several hours, suggest – but don't insist – that she use the potty chair or toilet from time to time.
2. Encourage your child to use the potty chair or toilet, but don't get upset when accidents occur. Phase out nappies until she is wearing them only at night.
3. When your child is confident with the potty chair, fit a child's seat and stepstool to the toilet and let her become familiar with the new arrangement. She can alternate use of the potty chair and toilet until eventually she is using the toilet exclusively.
4. A dry nappy several mornings in a row usually signals that your child is ready to sleep without nappies. Be prepared for frequent accidents, protect the mattress with a plastic undersheet, and use training nappies. If your child resists the change or wets the bed every night, she is not ready. It's better to continue nappies and let your child try again when she feels the time is right than to allow tension and distress to complicate the process. Many children are helped to stay dry if parents remind them to urinate one final time before lights out. And although restricting fluids in the evening doesn't prevent bed-wetting, it's not helpful to let your child have a big drink just before bedtime.

In General:

Children express themselves through behaviour long before they can talk. Behaviour is formed partly out of a child's temperament and his ability to adapt. It is modified by the parents' responses, the family situation, and stresses and changes. Good discipline teaches a child how to express his feelings and to behave properly.

Children learn to behave largely by copying others and watching how adults and other children resolve their differences. Parents provide a good example when they treat their family and outsiders with kindness and civility. But parents are also showing a way to behave when they act aggressively, allow destructiveness, or praise macho and sexist attitudes as well as violence on television and in films.

Behaviour that is acceptable at one developmental stage may cause concern at others. For example, temper tantrums (see p. 148) are normal during the 'terrible twos' but worrisome at school age. What is never acceptable is behaviour that can harm the child, the family, and others, including animals and property. The child who is acting up may be sending out a cry for help. Often overlooked, however, is the overly good child whose self-control and eagerness to please may also be signs of trouble.

'Normal' behaviour also varies according to family customs. Some cultural groups, for example, let children be outspoken in a way that others find unbearable. Some children don't learn self-control because their parents fail to set limits. At the very least, children should be taught to respect the rights and feelings of others. Give your child specific guidelines on how to behave. But don't make unreasonable demands and place him in situations he's not ready to handle. Don't be in a hurry to label your child's behaviour. Labels tend to become self-fulfilling prophecies. What is important is the overall pattern of behaviour, not an occasional lapse when the child is tired or overexcited.

☎

Consult your GP if your child is behaving in any of the following patterns:

- Acts younger than others of the same age.
- Is defiant and does not respond to reasonable requests and discipline.
- Often overreacts to events and cannot be calmed down.
- Acts without regard to safety.
- Threatens others, is cruel to animals, plays with fire, or harms property.
- Has changed for the worse, with mood swings, poor school performance, loss of friends, alcohol or drug use, and lack of self-esteem.

Warning

The earlier a behaviour problem is recognized and dealt with, the greater the likelihood of success. Without help, a youngster with a behaviour problem may eventually develop a conduct disorder and emotional problems.

Questions to consider	If answer is	Possible cause is	Action to take
Is your child usually disobedient? Is she defiant when you correct her?	YES	Testing behaviour; temperamental, school, or family difficulties; unreasonable expectations.	When both of you are calm, agree on a plan of action to change behaviour in specific areas. For a school-age child, set up a scoring system. If a 2-month trial doesn't work, see your doctor.
Is your child aggressive at home? Or have you had complaints of bullying from his kindergarten or school?	YES	Lack of self-control; attention-seeking; stress; sibling rivalry; jealousy.	Children should be able to control their aggressive impulses by the time they are in kindergarten. Your GP may advise therapy and parent–effectiveness training.

Questions to consider	If answer is	Possible cause is	Action to take
Is your child being bullied at school? Is he anxious and insecure? Does he lack social skills?	**YES**	Social, emotional, and/or developmental factors.	Your GP may refer your child to a therapist. Victims of bullying tend to stay that way unless they get help to find new ways of thinking and acting.
Is your child almost too well behaved? Is she shy? Does she avoid children and seek adult company instead?	**YES**	Normal behaviour; anxious child; shy child.	Encourage your child to take part in hobbies or sports that let her mix with other children. If she has anxiety attacks with rapid breathing, consult your doctor.
Does your child frequently use profanity? Does he swear at people or call them names?	**YES**	Lack of self-control; mimicking adult behaviour or media; disrespect for others.	Let your child know that while a mild oath may do no harm under extreme provocation, foul words and swearing at others are not tolerated. Set a good example.
Does your child have money or possessions he can't account for? Are you worried that he may have stolen or shoplifted goods?	**YES**	Unacceptable but not abnormal phase of development; stress; peer pressure; need for attention.	Ask your child where he got the goods. If he stole them, insist he return them with an apology and go with him, if necessary. Let him know that stealing is never tolerated. If it seems to be a pattern or you find a hoard of stolen goods, your child may need urgent help. Consult your doctor.
Have you found your school-age child to be lying?	**YES**	Awareness of having done something wrong; fear of punishment or of disappointing parents; peer behaviour.	Tell your child that lying isn't acceptable and he'll be in less trouble if he tells the truth. Change your behaviour if you are setting a double standard with white lies and partial truths. If lying is chronic, or the child can't tell fact from fiction, see your doctor.

Physical punishment: a self-defeating approach to discipline

Spanking may allow a parent to let off steam, but it doesn't teach a child the right way to behave. What's more, it is humiliating and emotionally harmful, and it can lead to physical injury. Worst of all, spanking teaches youngsters that violence is an acceptable way to communicate.

Nearly every expert on child development strongly opposes hitting children. Sometimes a parent loses control and spontaneously spanks a child while under acute stress, such as when the child acts impulsively and risks injury. Once the parent has calmed down, she should explain what provoked the spanking and why she felt angry enough to strike the child. She should apologize for her loss of control. This may help the child understand and accept the spanking.

Bites and Stings

In General:

Animal bites may appear minor, but they carry a high risk of infection. In contrast, most insect bites and stings cause minor redness, irritation, and itching that soon disappear without special treatment. In some people, however, insect venom causes an allergic reaction ranging from mild to life-threatening in severity. It is important to remove an insect stinger quickly and completely. Bites or stings may become infected from scratching the itch. And a few insects can transmit disease; for example, deer ticks can carry Lyme disease. Make sure your children know what dangerous insects, plants, and animals are common in your area.

Consult your GP straightaway if your child:

- Is bitten by a snake, wild animal, or unknown dog or other animal.
- Gets a rash or hives away from the original bite or sting.
- Develops a rash and other symptoms following a tick bite.
- Develops signs of infection (red streaks, warmth, increased swelling) around a bite.

Warning

Call 999 immediately if signs of a severe allergic reaction, known as anaphylaxis, develop following an insect bite or sting. Symptoms include swelling of the mouth, tongue, and throat; clammy skin and paleness; weakness and/or confusion; and difficulty breathing.

Questions to consider	If answer is	Possible cause is	Action to take
Does your child have minor pain, swelling, redness, and itching from a sting or bite?	YES	Minor bite or sting such as from mosquitoes, flies, or ants.	Apply a cold compress to reduce discomfort (for a child under 2, use a cold, wet cloth but not an ice pack).
Was your child stung by an insect? Is the site red, itchy, swollen, and sore?	YES	Bee, hornet, or wasp sting.	If you can see the sting, use a dull blade to scrape it out. Wash the area with soap and water. Apply an ice pack or cold compress.
Is your child showing signs of a severe reaction, such as weakness, pallor, and shortness of breath? Is there a rash or widespread swelling?	YES	Severe, generalized allergic reaction.	If your child has swelling around the mouth or other signs of anaphylaxis, call 999 immediately. If there is no pulse, start CPR immediately after calling for help. (See p. 204.)
Does your child have a mark resembling a target: a dark central blotch surrounded by a light halo and a red ring?	YES	Lyme disease caused by tick bite (which may have occurred days earlier).	Consult your doctor, who will examine your child and prescribe antibiotics if Lyme disease is diagnosed.
Has your child's skin been punctured by an animal or human bite?	YES	Bite with risk of infection, including tetanus or rabies.	Wash the bite with soap and water and call your doctor immediately for help in preventing infection. Your child may need a tetanus booster. Capture the animal if you can do so without risk (or keep dead animal) for rabies testing. (See Animal Bites, p. 209.)

Questions to consider	If answer is	Possible cause is	Action to take
Was your child stung while swimming in salt water?	**YES**	Jellyfish venom.	Apply a cold compress. If the child is short of breath or faint, or you suspect a sting by a Portuguese man o' war, call 999; meanwhile, use clothing or sand to brush tentacles from skin.
Did your child come in contact with nettles or another 'stinging' plant?	**YES**	Allergy-type reaction to plant toxin.	The hivelike rash of nettles disappears without special treatment. If your child touched poison ivy or oak, remove his clothing and wash exposed skin with soap and water. Wash the clothing. Keep your child from scratching the area. If the rash is severe, affects the face or genitals, or infection develops, call your doctor promptly.
Was your child bitten by a snake?	**YES**	Snake venom.	Call 999 or take your child to the emergency department at once. Do not apply ice or a tourniquet; use a splint to keep the bitten area immobile.

Keeping bugs at bay

- Apply insect repellent to children's clothing, not the skin. Read the label to make sure an insect repellent is safe for this purpose.
- Oil of citronella and peppermint are natural insect repellents that can be diluted with vegetable oil and applied to clothing.
- If mosquitoes are common where you live, cover your baby's cot with mosquito netting.
- Before venturing outside where there may be ticks, dress your child in light-coloured clothing with long sleeves and trousers. Apply an insect repellent to the clothing. On returning home, look for ticks and use tweezers to remove them completely.
- If you are going on a camping holiday abroad, find out about any local troublesome insects, such as those shown below.

The deer tick carries Lyme disease; the brown dog tick and the wood tick carry Rocky Mountain spotted fever. (These renderings are greatly enlarged. The deer tick is only about the size of a poppy seed.)

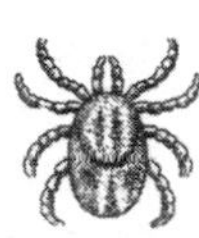

deer tick

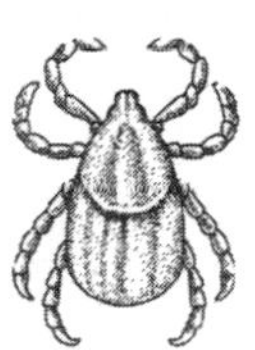

dog tick

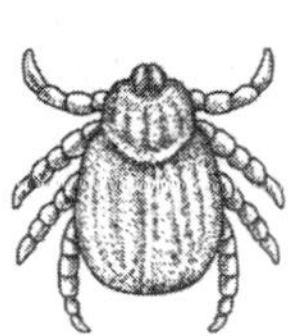

wood tick

Use tweezers to remove a tick, taking care to pull out the entire insect.

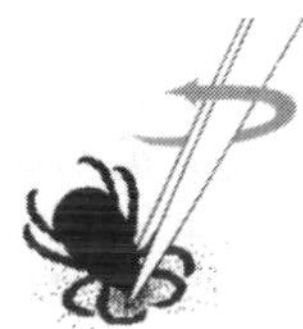

Bleeding and Bruising

Haemorrhage and ecchymosis

In General:

In a healthy child, blood clots within a few minutes to form a protective cover over wounds. Parents are often alarmed when blood gushes from children's head wounds, but even superficial head wounds can bleed a lot because the scalp has a particularly rich supply of blood vessels. The bleeding usually slows and stops in a few minutes, but large wounds may require first aid or medical attention. (See Cuts and Scrapes, p. 213.)

Bruising is a leakage of blood into tissue just under the skin. Even healthy children often get bruises from minor falls and bumps when they first become mobile and later as they test their bodies in sports and play. Children between the ages of about 11 months and 4 years stumble so often that their shins usually have a few black and blue marks. But extensive bruising or bruises in odd places – shoulders, face, buttocks, or back – may be caused by more severe injury, whether accidental or intentional, or by any of several uncommon disorders that interfere with blood clotting.

Consult your doctor if your child has:

- Unexplained bruising or bruising in unusual sites.
- Blood in the stool or urine.
- Prolonged bleeding from trivial cuts.
- Unusual pallor, fatigue, and other symptoms along with easy bruising.

Warning

Persistent bleeding or bruises in unexpected places should be seen by your doctor. Don't overlook the possibility of abuse, especially if your child doesn't want to tell you how he got the bruises.

Questions to consider	If answer is	Possible cause is	Action to take
Are bruises mainly on the shins? Is your child healthy and energetic?	**YES**	Normal wear and tear from minor bumps and falls.	None. This is a healthy, active child.
Is your child having nose-bleeds? Is she generally healthy?	**YES**	Childhood nose-bleeds (epistaxis, see p. 116).	Apply firm, continuous pressure to the soft part of the nose. Have your child sit leaning forward until the bleeding stops. If your child's nose bleeds often and profusely, discuss preventive measures with your GP.
Is your child feverish? Does she have a headache? Is she weak and generally unwell?	**YES**	Bacterial, viral, or parasitic infection.	Consult your GP, who will examine the child and order tests to determine the cause and recommend treatment.
Is your child bleeding from the rectum? Is there blood in the stool?	**YES**	Anal fissure; gastroenteritis; intussusception; juvenile polyps.	Consult your GP; further tests may be necessary.
Does your child have multiple 'pin-dot' bruises (petechiae) or large, expanding bruises?	**YES**	Blood disorder, such as idiopathic thrombocytopenic purpura.	Consult your GP, who will order appropriate tests and may refer the child to a pediatric haematologist.

QUESTIONS TO CONSIDER	IF ANSWER IS	POSSIBLE CAUSE IS	ACTION TO TAKE
Does your child have expanding bruises with fever and vomiting? Is he sleepy, dazed, or irritable?	**YES**	Serious bacterial infection.	Call your GP immediately.
Has your child developed pin-dot bruises and vomiting while taking a medication such as an antibiotic?	**YES**	Reaction to medication.	Call your GP without delay; an alternative medication may need to be prescribed.
Does your child have unexplained bruises on his legs and ankles? Does he have a stomachache? Are his joints swollen and tender?	**YES**	Allergic disorder; Henoch-Schönlein purpura.	Call your GP, who will examine your child and order diagnostic tests.
Has bleeding from a minor cut and/or from mucous membranes persisted for hours or days?	**YES**	Clotting factor deficiency, such as haemophilia or von Willebrand disease.	Consult your GP for diagnostic tests and management. (See Better treatment for haemophilia, below.)
Does your child return from childcare or a baby-sitter with an unusual number of bruises, or with oddly shaped bruises? Is the child fearful or withdrawn?	**YES**	Child abuse.	Consult your GP immediately; if abuse is confirmed, the proper authorities should be notified and steps taken to protect the child.
Does your child bruise easily? Is she pale, lethargic, and/or irritable?	**YES**	A generalized disorder, which may include leukaemia.	Consult your GP.

Better treatment for haemophilia

Haemophilia is a rare, inherited disease, passed from mother to son, in which there is a deficiency of a clotting factor. When a person lacks a clotting factor – one of several naturally occurring substances that help the blood to form clots – minor cuts and bumps can cause severe, even life-threatening bleeding. Although most people with haemophilia are male, a few very rare bleeding disorders also affect females.

Haemophilia is usually diagnosed when a baby is very young and, fortunately, most cases can be controlled by treatment with the missing clotting factor. Concentrated clotting factors are obtained from donor blood. New ways of processing this blood, which is taken from a large number of donors, have practically eliminated the risk of passing on blood-borne diseases such as hepatitis and AIDS. Today, most children with haemophilia can enjoy an active life and grow into healthy adults.

Bluish Skin

Cyanosis

In General:

A bluish tinge to the skin shows that the underlying tissues are not getting enough oxygen. Blue colour in just one part, such as a hand or foot, may mean that blood flow has been reduced, such as by tight clothing or a bandage. Exposure to the cold can cause the lips, fingers, or toes to turn blue, and the skin returns to its normal colour when it's warmed.

Very young babies often develop a blue-white ring around the mouth during feeding. This is perfectly normal and disappears when the baby is burped. However, if blue discoloration covers a large part of the body, it may be a sign that the child is starved for oxygen and requires medical attention right away.

Call your GP immediately if your child has bluish discoloration of:

- The entire body.
- The lips and tongue, together with noisy breathing.
- The face, with fever.

Warning

If your child turns blue and cannot breathe, speak, or cough, call 999 immediately and follow procedures under First Aid/Choking. (See p. 201.)

Questions to consider	If answer is	Possible cause is	Action to take
Has your child been outdoors in the cold? Or has she been swimming or playing in water for an extended period? Is she shivering?	**YES**	Reaction to cold temperature (hypothermia).	Dry your child and wrap her in a blanket or move her to a warm room. If she is very cold, put her in a tub of tepid water. Prevent hypothermia by dressing children according to the temperature.
Does your child have a barking, 'croupy' cough? Is his breathing laboured and noisy?	**YES**	Croup.	Call your doctor or go to the nearest hospital emergency department. (See Dealing with croup, p. 53.)
Is your child blue around the mouth? Is she wheezing?	**YES**	Respiratory problem, possibly asthma.	Call your doctor, or 999, at once. (Also see Allergic Reactions, p. 26, and Breathing Difficulty/Breathlessness, p. 44.)
Does your infant's skin look blue? Has he had a worsening cold and cough for the last day or two? Is he breathing rapidly and with difficulty? Is he refusing to eat? Is he irritable and generally unwell?	**YES**	Bronchiolitis (also see Breathing Difficulty/Breathlessness, p. 44).	Call your doctor at once. If the diagnosis of bronchiolitis is confirmed, your baby needs prompt treatment and will be hospitalized for a few days.
Did your child cry, hold his breath, and pass out? Did he quickly come to?	**YES**	Breath-holding spell.	Consult your GP, who will examine the child to rule out physical problems and recommend ways to deal with upsets and tantrums. (See Dealing with breath-holding, opposite, and Temper Tantrums, p. 148.)

Questions to consider	If answer is	Possible cause is	Action to take
Does your toddler or older child look bluish, especially around the lips? Is she feverish? Does she feel poorly? Has she recently had symptoms of a cold or other viral illness, such as chickenpox? Is she breathing rapidly?	**YES**	Bronchopneumonia.	Call your doctor immediately. He will examine the child and may prescribe treatment or advise admission to hospital.
Did your child turn blue while exercising? Are her nails, lips, tongue, and mucous membranes blue?	**YES**	Heart, lung, and/or circulatory disorder.	Call your doctor, who will examine your child and may refer her to a specialist for evaluation.
Has your child passed out and lost bladder control? Has she previously had a seizure?	**YES**	Seizure disorder (epilepsy, see Convulsions, p. 50).	Consult your GP, who will order tests and may prescribe an anticonvulsant medication.

Dealing with breath-holding

Parents are often more frightened by a breath-holding episode than the child is himself. Here's what happens: the child screams and cries so hard – usually during a temper tantrum but also when he's frightened or in pain – that he can't catch his breath and inhale. His face may go from scarlet to a greyish blue; some youngsters fall to the floor and seem to pass out or go into a convulsion. This looks alarming, but resist the temptation to restrain your child or force him to breathe; it's physically impossible for even the most determined and angry toddler to hold his breath long enough to cause any harm. If the youngster loses consciousness, his natural reflexes take over and he soon breathes normally again.

Even so, if your child faints or has a convulsion during a breath-holding episode, call your GP. She may want to examine the child to make sure there is not a physical cause for the loss of consciousness or seizure. If your GP suspects an emotional problem, she may refer you to a mental health professional. Most episodes, however, are harmless and the child eventually finds more constructive ways to vent his anger. In the meantime, don't overreact to breath-holding. Stay calm, make sure your child is safe, but resist the temptation to play up the incident or give in to his demands. Such responses simply set the stage for future incidents. (For further guidelines, see Temper Tantrums, p. 148.)

Bow Legs, Knock Knees, Pigeon Toes

Genu varum, genu valgum, tibial torsion

In General:

A baby's typical bow legs and pigeon toes gradually straighten out over the first 3 years. Few toddlers have really straight legs, however, and as the child begins to walk, the inward curve of the lower leg often turns to mild knock knees between ages 2 and 3. The curvature corrects itself by about 10 years; braces and corrective shoes are rarely helpful. Most children have straight legs by adolescence, although bow legs, knock knees, in-toeing, or out-toeing in adulthood run in some families. Severe curvature may be corrected by surgery.

Consult your doctor if you notice any of the following:

- Extreme curvature of any limb.
- Curvature of a limb on one side.
- Bow legs getting worse after age 3.
- Severe knock knees after age 11.
- Bow legs and extremely short stature for the child's age.

Warning

Make sure your children wear properly fitted shoes and get plenty of exercise.

Questions to consider	If answer is	Possible cause is	Action to take
Do your child's legs look bowed? Is he under age 3?	**YES**	Bow legs (genu varum).	The bowed appearance is normal. The legs usually become straight by age 3 years.
Are the lower legs turned inward and bowed? Do the feet point in? Is your child between 12 and 24 months?	**YES**	A turning of the shinbone (internal tibial torsion).	This condition is normal. It may appear very marked at 18 to 24 months but usually corrects spontaneously by age 3.
Is your child unable to make his ankles meet when standing with his knees together?	**YES**	Knock knees (genu valgum).	If the condition is very severe, or if it interferes with the child's walking or running, consult your doctor.
Does your child have bowing in just one leg? Is your child over age 2 severely bowed?	**YES**	Blount disease.	Consult your doctor.
Is your child older than 10? Do his feet still turn in when running?	**YES**	Thigh bone turning inward (femoral anteversion).	Check with your doctor.
Has bowing developed after a fracture?	**YES**	Injury to growth plate; poor healing.	Consult your doctor.

Preventing rickets

Once a leading cause of deformities, rickets has become less common with better nutrition. Staple foods are now supplemented with vitamin D, which is needed for bone formation. Children still at risk for rickets include those with absorption disorders or on long-term anticonvulsant treatment, and older infants and toddlers who are exclusively breast fed and do not get adequate nutrition. Sunlight is an excellent source of vitamin D. Youngsters should play outdoors, with appropriate sun protection, whenever possible.

Gynaecomastia

In General:

Newborn babies occasionally have breast swelling. Sometimes their breasts even secrete small amounts of milk. This happens because some of the mother's oestrogen is passed on to her baby while he is in the womb. The baby's breasts will reduce in size as the effect of the mother's hormones fades during the first few weeks of life.

Girls and boys who are very overweight often look as if their breasts are developing. In fact, the enlargement is just due to accumulated fat in the upper chest and not to breast development. For breast development during puberty, including breast swelling in teenage boys, see Sexual Maturation, p. 128.

☎

Consult your doctor if:

- Your child has an isolated lump outside the areola (the central pink area) rather than a general swelling.
- The swelling is inflamed and tender, and your child has fever.

Warning

A tender breast swelling, especially if it's red, in a child of any age may indicate an infection. The child must be seen by a doctor and treated promptly with an antibiotic.

Questions to consider	If answer is	Possible cause is	Action to take
Is the swelling a generalized enlargement of the breasts in your otherwise healthy newborn baby?	YES	Effect of mother's hormones.	None. The swelling will subside as the hormonal effects fade over several weeks.
Is one of your baby's breasts red or swollen? Is the baby in the first months of life?	YES	Breast infection or abscess.	Consult your doctor who will examine the baby. Antibiotic treatment and/or hospitalization may be necessary.
Does your child age 6 years or younger have enlarged breasts?	YES	Premature breast development (thelarche).	Consult your doctor, who will evaluate your child's health and development and may perform blood tests for hormone levels.
Have you noticed breast swelling in your daughter under age 8 or your son under age 10?	YES	Accidental exposure to hormones; or, in a girl, premature breast development.	Consult your doctor. Your child may have taken a family member's hormone medication, such as contraceptive pills.

Premature breast growth

Occasionally, a young child's breasts begin to enlarge when there are no other signs of sexual development. This condition – called premature thelarche (breast growth) – is rare, but when it occurs, the child is usually under 3 years old. The cause may be unknown, although in some cases the child may be producing certain hormones too early. It's important to distinguish true breast enlargement from excess fat tissue.

A paediatrician should examine a child with premature thelarche to make sure she is not going through precocious puberty. The breasts usually return to normal within a year or two, but they may remain enlarged until the child enters puberty at the normal age.

Breathing Difficulty/Breathlessness

Dyspnoea

In General:

Shortness of breath (dyspnoea) or difficulty in breathing often means that a child needs medical attention. Feeling short of breath occurs in many conditions, from respiratory diseases such as asthma and pneumonia to less common disorders such as defects in the lung or heart failure resulting in fluid buildup in the lungs. The problem also may be caused by a blockage or infection in the airways of the lungs. In some cases, anxiety may cause a child to hyperventilate (breathe too fast), which leads to a change in the body's chemistry that, in turn, spurs more overbreathing.

Warning

Don't put off seeking emergency treatment if your child's breathing gets increasingly laboured, if he's not making sounds or speaking, or is turning blue. These are signs that the respiratory tract is blocked and your child is in danger of suffocating. (See Choking, p. 201.)

Consult your doctor if your child:

- Has severe shortness of breath.
- Makes a whistling or barking noise when breathing in.
- Wheezes on breathing out or in.

And has any of the following:

- Fever and chills; vomiting.
- Chest pain.
- Thick, discoloured, or bloody sputum.
- Bluish skin and tongue.
- Unusual drowsiness.
- Inability to swallow or speak.
- Drooling.
- An odd sitting posture.

Questions to consider	If answer is	Possible cause is	Action to take
Does your child have a stuffy nose? Does he also have a sore throat and cough? Is there a mild fever?	**YES**	Common cold. (Also see Cough, p. 52.)	Encourage rest; offer fluids to thin secretions; give paracetamol. Call your doctor if symptoms worsen or last a week. If your baby has a stuffy nose, ask whether you should use nasal suction.
Does your child have a barking cough, hoarseness, low fever, and/or chest discomfort? Are symptoms worse at night? Has he recently had a viral infection?	**YES**	Croup, known medically as laryngotracheobronchitis (inflammation of the larynx, trachea, or bronchi).	Consult your doctor. Give paracetamol to reduce discomfort. Use of a cold vaporizer at night may help. (See Dealing with croup, p. 53.) If breathing is laboured or your child begins to turn blue, go to the nearest hospital emergency department or call 999.
Has your child suddenly started gasping? Is her face turning blue? Is she unable to speak or make normal sounds?	**YES**	Choking on a foreign object or food.	This is an emergency: give help for choking or the Heimlich manoeuvre and have someone else call 999. (See Choking, p. 201.)
Does your child wheeze and cough, especially at night or with exercise?	**YES**	Asthma.	Consult your doctor, who will examine the child to confirm the diagnosis, and recommend ways to control the disease.
Is your child having an asthma attack, with bluish skin and difficulty speaking? Is she confused or agitated?	**YES**	Acute, severe asthma attack.	If your child has bronchodilator medication, try it immediately. Go to the nearest hospital emergency department or call 999 at once.

Dyspnoea

QUESTIONS TO CONSIDER	IF ANSWER IS	POSSIBLE CAUSE IS	ACTION TO TAKE
Is your child sitting up, gasping noisily, with mouth wide open and chin pushed down? Are her skin and nails bluish? Does she have a high fever?	**YES**	Epiglottitis (swelling of the tissue that protects the windpipe from foreign objects).	This is a medical emergency. Call 999 straightaway or take the child to the nearest emergency department. Epiglottitis, a now-rare infection that usually occurs only in children aged 3 and older, can be treated with antibiotics.
Is your baby breathing fast and hard? Has he had a cold and cough for a day or two? Is he refusing to eat? Is he irritable and unwell?	**YES**	Bronchiolitis.	Call your doctor at once for an examination. If the diagnosis of bronchiolitis is confirmed, your baby needs prompt treatment and may be admitted to the hospital for a few days.
Is your child breathing fast and noisily, with a cough and chest pain? Is she feverish? Has she recently had a respiratory illness?	**YES**	Pneumonia.	Call your doctor; pneumonia can frequently be managed at home with rest and medication as prescribed by your GP. Some children need oxygen either at home or in hospital.
Has your young child developed noisy breathing over hours or days? Is he coughing, with or without fever?	**YES**	Aspiration pneumonia due to an inhaled object or food.	Call your doctor, who will order x-rays and, if necessary, arrange treatment.
Is your child suddenly having trouble breathing? Is her skin clammy? Pulse racing? Is there widespread swelling? Is she allergic? Has she been stung by an insect?	**YES**	Anaphylaxis (severe allergic reaction).	Call 999 straightaway or get your child to the nearest hospital emergency department. This is a medical emergency. Your child needs urgent attention.
Is your pre-adolescent or teenager having difficulty breathing? Is she light-headed? Does she have numbness or tingling in the hands and feet?	**YES**	Hyperventilation (overbreathing) due to anxiety (also see p. 174).	Try to identify and eliminate causes of anxiety. Your doctor may want to examine your child to rule out physical conditions that produce symptoms similar to anxiety, and will recommend a treatment plan.

Keeping asthma under control

Asthma affects one in five children in Britain. Most cases are mild, but some youngsters suffer frequent flare-ups. Even severe cases, however, can usually be controlled by avoiding factors that trigger attacks.

Asthma occurs when muscle spasms and inflammation in the bronchial tubes prevent air from flowing into and out of the lungs. Attacks are often set off by viral infections, allergies, exercise, cold air, and smoke. The incidence is rising, and experts believe exposure to various allergens and an indoor lifestyle may play a role among urban youngsters. Although stress can also trigger attacks, asthma is a lung disorder, not an emotional problem.

It's important to identify your child's asthma triggers. Your GP may recommend skin tests to identify allergens or a diary to see what activities are related to attacks. Most doctors advise a combined approach – avoidance of triggers, preventive medication, and lifestyle changes – to control asthma.

In General:

Intermittent chest pain is not uncommon in children, and is not usually caused by a serious disorder. The most common cause is chest muscle strain – typically when a child increases physical activity or takes up a new sport. Chest pain may also be caused by muscle tension stemming from emotional stress at school or home, or just from the child's own inner anxiety. Pain in the chest wall may be due to inflammation, termed costochondritis. This condition can be treated with an anti-inflammatory medication such as ibuprofen. Heart and lung conditions that could cause chest pain need to be checked for and, if found to be present, treated appropriately. Serious but unusual causes of chest pain in children include infectious diseases such as pneumonia, problems in the digestive tract such as an inflamed oesophagus (oesophagitis) or ulcers, hyperventilation in older children, and collapsed lung (pneumothorax).

Consult your doctor immediately if your child:

- Has persistent or unusually severe chest pain, even when resting.
- Complains of unusual thumping or racing sensations in the chest.
- Has difficulty breathing.

Warning

If your child has chest pain that persists and gets worse during exercise, see your doctor. Chest pain that develops after an injury warrants prompt medical attention to rule out a broken rib, collapsed lung, and other injuries.

Questions to consider	If answer is	Possible cause is	Action to take
Is your child growing at a normal rate? Is his appetite good? Is he breathing normally? Has he recently changed his athletic activity or taken up a new sport? Has he had an injury?	**YES**	Muscle strain; bruise; inflammation of the chest wall (costochondritis).	Give ibuprofen or paracetamol for pain relief. Consult your doctor if the pain does not improve in 2 to 3 days.
Does your child feel pain while resting, but not for longer than 1 to 2 minutes at a time? Is his health generally good? Is he having any academic or social difficulties at school? Is there unusual tension at home? Is your child a worrier?	**YES**	Nonspecific chest pain.	Consult your GP, who will examine the child to rule out any serious causes. If none is found, the physician will reassure your youngster. Sensitive questioning may identify sources of anxiety. Concentrating on a hobby may divert your child's attention from his physical symptoms. Your GP may suggest treatment.
Does your child have a cough or respiratory illness? Is her temperature elevated (38.3°C [101°F] or higher)?	**YES**	Pneumonia or another infectious disease.	Consult your GP, who will examine the child. Treatment may be necessary. Your GP will advise on pain relief and prescribe other medications as appropriate.

QUESTIONS TO CONSIDER	IF ANSWER IS	POSSIBLE CAUSE IS	ACTION TO TAKE
Does your child sometimes awake from sleep with pain in the chest or upper abdomen? Is he growing normally? Does he complain of heartburn or a sour taste in the mouth? Does he sometimes vomit?	**YES**	Digestive disorder, such as gastro-esophageal reflux, oesophagitis, or peptic ulcer.	Consult your GP, who may prescribe medication. Cut out caffeine (such as in colas or chocolate). Raising the head of your child's bed may help to prevent night-time reflux of acidic stomach contents into the oesophagus.
Does your child complain of a pounding heart or irregular changes in heart rhythm (other than normal increases with exercise)? Do the changes last longer than 1 or 2 minutes? Does she get chest pain when exercising? Is the child dizzy, light-headed, or faint? Does she appear pale, ill, or sweaty during these episodes?	**YES**	Heart disorder (unusual).	Call your doctor without delay. Your child may require an extensive examination and diagnostic tests to rule out serious causes and identify the source of chest pain.
In addition to chest pain at rest, does your child have swelling and tenderness of the joints? Is there a rash on her face or body?	**YES**	Auto-immune disorder such as juvenile rheumatoid arthritis or lupus	Consult your GP, who will examine the child and refer her, if necessary, for evaluation by a specialist.

Collapsed lung as a cause of chest pain

Occasionally, collapsed lung, or spontaneous pneumothorax, causes sharp chest pain and acute shortness of breath in a child, although it is more common in men between the ages of 20 and 40. Children with chronic disorders, such as cystic fibrosis, are most often affected, but spontaneous pneumothorax can also occur in healthy children – usually thin teenage boys – for no apparent reason.

Spontaneous pneumothorax occurs when a small patch of lung tissue ruptures, allowing air to leak out and accumulate between the lung and the chest wall. If the leak is small, the child has pain but no other symptoms. In this case, no treatment is needed: the leak will seal itself and the free air will gradually be absorbed. If, however, a large accumulation of air causes part of the lung to collapse, the child may have sharp chest pain; a dry, hacking cough; and difficulty breathing. Treatment may involve a minor procedure to draw off the air, but in most cases children recover under medical observation.

Constipation

In General:

Many parents mistakenly think that a child who doesn't have a daily bowel movement is constipated. The fact is, children's bowel patterns vary widely: some children have several bowel movements daily, while others may go 2 or 3 days, then pass a stool of normal consistency. (Such infrequent bowel movements are especially common in breast-fed babies.) In contrast, true constipation is marked by the passage of a hard, dry stool that may require straining and even cause pain.

Don't be alarmed if your baby gets red in the face, grimaces, squawks, twists, and grunts during his bowel movements. This is perfectly normal. If the stool is soft, the baby is not constipated or in pain.

Children's diets should include plenty of fluids and high-fibre foods such as fruits, vegetables, and whole-grain products. Regular exercise and a regular toilet schedule can help to set good bowel habits for life.

☎

Consult your doctor if your child:

- Complains of painful bowel movements.
- Passes hard, dry stools.
- Has abdominal pain that is relieved by bowel movements.
- Has blood in or on stools.
- Is leaking fluid between bowel movements.

Warning

Do not use laxatives or enemas to treat your child's constipation without consulting your GP: unwarranted use of laxatives can disrupt normal bowel function.

Questions to consider	If answer is	Possible cause is	Action to take
Has your breast-fed infant of 4 to 6 months changed her bowel pattern, passing fewer, harder stools?	**YES**	Mild constipation during transition to solid foods, or child's own bowel rhythm.	Some breast-fed babies get mildly constipated when solid foods are introduced but soon return to normal. If the stool is hard, your GP or health visitor may suggest a change in your baby's diet.
Is your formula-fed infant passing hard, dry stools?	**YES**	Composition of formula.	Consult your GP, who may recommend stool-softening measures.
Does your child have a normal bowel movement at least every 3 days? Is she otherwise healthy and in no discomfort?	**YES**	The child's own bowel rhythm.	Make sure your child gets plenty of fluids and high-fibre foods, including fruits and vegetables.
Has your baby been weaned from breast milk or formula to cow's milk?	**YES**	The switch to cow's milk and dairy products, which may have a binding effect.	Limit cow's milk to 475–710ml (17–25oz) per day. Ask your health visitor for dietary suggestions, such as giving prune juice.
Has your child become constipated since you started toilet training?	**YES**	Your child is not yet ready to be trained.	Hold off on toilet training for now; try again when your child takes the initiative and is no longer constipated.

Questions to consider	If answer is	Possible cause is	Action to take
Is your child complaining of discomfort because he cannot move his bowels? Are the stools small, dry pellets?	**YES**	Constipation, which may have many causes, including not enough fibre and fluid in the diet, or stress.	Consult your GP, who will help with a course of treatment. Increase the fibre and liquids in your child's diet. Encourage the child to eat fresh fruits and vegetables and take part in regular physical activity. Try to eliminate sources of stress.
Does your child complain of pain during or after a bowel movement? Is there blood on or in the stool? Is there a rash around the anus?	**YES**	Anal fissure; skin inflammation in the anal area (perianal dermatitis).	Consult your GP, who will examine the child and advise treatment. Use of a stool softener may be recommended.
Is your constipated child vomiting greenish-yellow material? Is the abdomen distended? (Also see Abdominal Swelling, p. 24.)	**YES**	Intestinal obstruction.	Call your GP immediately. Give nothing to eat or drink until the doctor has examined your child. If the diagnosis is confirmed, your child may be hospitalized for treatment.
Is your baby passing infrequent, hard stools? Does he cry with pain when his bowels move?	**YES**	Tight anal sphincter.	Consult your GP, who will examine the baby and may recommend treatment.
Has your young baby passed only a few, hard stools since birth, despite being given a stool softener? Is her abdomen distended?	**YES**	Hirschsprung disease, an uncommon inborn absence of the nerves needed for bowel movements.	Consult your GP who will examine the baby to determine whether retained stool is distending the abdomen while the rectum is empty. If Hirschsprung disease is diagnosed, it can be treated with surgery.

Anxiety and stool withholding

Conflicting emotions about independence and control often emerge when toilet training is introduced, and some youngsters express these feelings through reluctance to move their bowels on the potty or toilet. They respond to parents' toilet-training efforts by withholding stool, with the result that retained faeces become dry and compacted, and bowel movements are painful. A vicious cycle of stool withholding and pain can lead to severe anxiety and a situation in which the family's attention is focused on the child's bowel movements. Occasionally, liquid waste leaks out around the compacted faeces and parents mistake this soiling for diarrhoea.

The doctor approaches this problem with a stepwise programme of bowel retraining, which usually involves administration of a stool softener and a regular toilet schedule. Increasing fibre in the child's diet with more fruits, vegetables, and cereals may be helpful. The child should also be encouraged to drink plenty of water, juices, and other fluids, especially in hot weather and after exercise. Regular physical activity also promotes smooth bowel function (also see p. 143).

Convulsions

Seizure disorder

IN GENERAL:

A convulsion or seizure is a change of consciousness caused by a surge in the brain's electrical impulses. A few children have convulsions when their temperature rises rapidly. Most outgrow these benign febrile seizures and have no long-term effects; indeed, most who have one febrile seizure never have another. Because serious infections may also cause seizures, however, always call your doctor when a feverish child has a seizure.

Recurrent seizures are termed epilepsy. The cause is not always clear and the child must be evaluated. Epilepsy can generally be controlled with medication, and there are certain epileptic syndromes (such as simple absences or petit mal) that children outgrow.

Call your doctor immediately if a convulsing child:

- Remains unconscious for more than 2 minutes.
- Has difficulty breathing for more than 1 minute.

Warning

If your child has epilepsy, explain first aid measures to teachers and care-givers. Ask your GP about precautions for potentially dangerous activities. A child with epilepsy should not be left unsupervised in a bath or swimming pool.

QUESTIONS TO CONSIDER	IF ANSWER IS	POSSIBLE CAUSE IS	ACTION TO TAKE
Is your child twitching, unconscious, and feverish? Is he irritable and unwell?	YES	Febrile convulsion associated with an infectious disease.	Call your GP at once. Give a susceptible child paracetamol and sponge with cool – not cold – water.
Does your child switch off, not speaking or hearing, for several seconds at a time? Is she unaware of the incident?	YES	Absence seizures (petit mal).	Your GP may refer the child to a neurologist. Petit mal can be controlled with medication, and children eventually outgrow it.
Did your child lose consciousness for a minute or longer? Did she twitch? Did she lose control of her bladder, bite her tongue, or vomit?	YES	Generalized seizure (grand mal epilepsy); partial (focal) seizure.	Your GP will examine the child, order diagnostic tests, and provide a referral to a neurologist if advisable. Most epilepsy can be controlled with medication.
Does your infant of 6 months or older have repeated symmetrical contractions of the neck, trunk, and limbs when drowsy?	YES	Infantile spasms.	Consult your GP, who will examine your baby and may refer him for a specialist evaluation.
Did your child have a seizure while on anticonvulsant medication?	YES	Need to adjust dosage.	Your GP will order tests and possibly change the medication.

Conditions that resemble seizures

Several conditions may be mistaken for convulsions because they involve jerking movements and alterations in consciousness. They include night terrors (see Fears, p. 72) and breath-holding spells (see Bluish Skin, p. 40). Children with asthma sometimes have paroxysmal coughing that causes fainting spells resembling seizures. Your GP will differentiate these conditions from seizures.

Dyscoordination

In General:

Children develop coordination and dexterity at different rates. While a few children are naturally graceful and agile, others never outgrow clumsiness. Toddlers have to acquire gross motor skills for crawling and walking before they develop fine motor control. Many adolescents go through an awkward phase as they adjust to the changes and growth spurt of puberty.

Children can be helped to improve coordination with crafts and sports. Encourage your children to take part in recreational activities at a level they find physically and emotionally rewarding.

Consult your doctor if:

- Your coordinated child becomes clumsy.
- Your child develops clumsiness with headaches, vomiting, or vision problems.
- Your child becomes increasingly clumsy.

Warning

If clumsiness is making your child self-conscious or keeping him out of activities, consult your doctor. She may recommend physical, movement, or occupational therapy to improve coordination.

Questions to consider	If answer is	Possible cause is	Action to take
Is your clumsy child under age 3?	**YES**	Normal motor development.	Discuss your concerns with your doctor. Play games to develop coordination and hone fine motor skills.
Is your school-age child clumsy? Does the clumsiness get worse under stress?	**YES**	Slow development.	Your doctor will examine the child to rule out physical problems and may recommend further evaluation and therapy.
Does your school-age child find it hard to tell right from left or to recognize words, letters, and numbers?	**YES**	Developmental problems (central processing disorder).	Your doctor will examine the child and, if necessary, refer him for psychological and educational evaluation.
Is your child taking a prescribed medication?	**YES**	Medication side effect.	Your doctor will determine whether the medication can cause clumsiness, and modify dosage or order tests.
Has your child developed a tendency to stumble or muscle weakness? Does he have headaches or vomiting?	**YES**	Disorder of the muscles or nervous system.	Call your doctor without delay to arrange an examination. She will refer your child to a specialist, if necessary.

Clumsiness and hyperactivity

Impulsive, fidgety, uncontrollable: if this sounds like your child, see your doctor. In many cases, these and certain other behaviour features point to attention deficit hyperactivity disorder (ADHD, see p. 93), especially if a close relative (parent or sibling) had similar difficulties in childhood. Only specialists can diagnose ADHD and recommend the treatment needed. If your family is under stress because your child is clumsy, restless, and unpredictable, get professional help.

Cough

In General:

Coughing is the body's way of keeping the airways clear. During a cold or other minor illness, coughs and other symptoms gradually go away, but in more serious conditions such as asthma or whooping cough, the cough is unrelenting and can tire the child out. Medical help may be needed to cure the underlying cause, open the airways, clear away secretions, and help the child get the rest he needs to recuperate.

Consult your doctor immediately if a child with a cough also:

- Has noisy, rapid, difficult breathing.
- Develops a fever (temperature of 38.3°C [101°F]).
- Is sluggish or drowsy.
- Has bluish discoloration around the lips, mouth, and fingernails.
- Refuses to drink.

Warning

Don't give children over-the-counter cough medicines without consulting your doctor. Cough suppressants are not recommended unless coughing is interfering with sleep.

Questions to consider	If answer is	Possible cause is	Action to take
Does your child have a runny nose and/or a sore throat?	**YES**	Common cold.	Offer clear fluids to help thin the secretions. Apply salve to soothe irritated lips and nostrils. Cold symptoms should clear up in about a week. (Also see Breathing Difficulty/Breathlessness, p. 44, and Runny/Stuffy Nose, p. 126.)
Does your child wake at night with a barking cough and difficulty breathing? Is he under age 5? Has he recently had a cold?	**YES**	Croup.	Ease your child's breathing in a steamy bathroom. (See Dealing with croup, opposite.)
Has your baby under 12 months been coughing hard for at least 2 hours? Has she recently had a cold or sniffles?	**YES**	Bronchiolitis, a viral lung infection that sometimes follows a cold.	Call your doctor for advice and care. The infection usually clears up within a week. (See Breathing Difficulty/Breathlessness, p. 44.)
Is your child's temperature over 38°C (100.4°F)? Does she have a runny nose, sore throat, and cough? Joint and muscle pains? Does she feel generally unwell?	**YES**	Influenza.	Make sure your child drinks enough; give paracetamol to lower the temperature and ease discomfort. Call your GP if symptoms do not improve within 2 days, the child develops a rash or breathing difficulty (see p. 44), or seems sicker.
Does your child cough and sneeze throughout the day but rarely at night? Does he have a constantly runny nose with clear discharge?	**YES**	Hay fever (allergic rhinitis) or inflammation of the airway (tracheobronchitis).	Consult your GP, who may recommend a medication. (See Allergic Reactions, p. 26.)

Questions to consider	If answer is	Possible cause is	Action to take
Has your child had a persistent cough and a yellowish nasal discharge for 10 days or more following a cold?	**YES**	Sinusitis.	Consult your GP, who will examine the child and prescribe an antibiotic if a sinus infection is confirmed. (See Treating sinusitis, p. 127.)
Does your child have a persistent daytime cough with no other symptoms? Is there tension at home? Is the child bottling up anxieties?	**YES**	Psychogenic cough or tic.	Try to identify and remove sources of anxiety. Consult with your child's teachers if school difficulties are causing emotional problems. Ask your doctor whether counselling might help.
Does your child have a persistent cough and throat irritation? Is there a source of air pollution nearby? Does anyone in the household smoke?	**YES**	Environmental irritant.	Ask your GP how to lessen irritant exposure. Investigate methods of filtering household air or minimizing the effects of pollutants. Encourage family members to stop smoking. (At the very least, bar smoking inside your house or apartment.)
Is coughing worse at night? Does your child cough when exercising or in cold air? Does he wheeze? Do family members have asthma or allergies?	**YES**	Asthma.	Your GP will examine your child and evaluate his lung function. If asthma is confirmed, your child will need treatment and measures to lessen exposure to asthma triggers. (See Breathing Difficulty/Breathlessness, p. 44.)
Has your young child suddenly started coughing without other symptoms? Could she be choking on a small object or piece of food?	**YES**	Foreign object in the airway.	If the child can't speak and is turning blue, start help for choking (see Choking, p. 201) and call 999. Otherwise, call your GP at once. The child needs treatment to remove the object and prevent complications.
Does your child have a chronic cough and frequent colds? Is her sputum hard to cough up? Does she seem to be growing slowly? Are her stools copious, greasy, and foul smelling? Does her sweat taste salty?	**YES**	Cystic fibrosis.	Your GP will examine the child and order tests. This inherited disorder is usually diagnosed in babies, but a cough and poor growth, among other symptoms, may point to cystic fibrosis in an older child. If the diagnosis is confirmed, lifelong treatment and a special diet will be needed.

Dealing with croup

Croup attacks usually ease when the child breathes in a steamy bathroom or next to a window opened to let in cool air. Medical treatment may be necessary, however, if symptoms are severe or prolonged. Children should not be exposed to secondhand tobacco smoke, particularly if prone to croup. A cool mist humidifier in the bedroom can often prevent croup attacks, especially if the air is dry.

Boys get croup more often than girls. Attacks often follow a viral infection, such as the common cold or influenza, so antibiotics are rarely helpful. Children generally outgrow croup by about age 5.

Crossed Eyes/Wandering Eye

Strabismus

IN GENERAL:

A baby's eyes normally tend to wander intermittently during the first few months of life. Soon, however, the child learns to use both eyes together and is able to coordinate eye movements between 3 and 6 months of age.

If the eyes continue to wander at times, cross, or move in different directions after early infancy, the child may have an eye muscle imbalance, termed strabismus (misaligned eyes), that makes it impossible for both eyes to focus on a single object at once.

Occasionally, a child may appear to have crossed eyes because a wide nasal bridge and broad skin folds distort the appearance of the eye alignment. This is known as pseudo-strabismus. As the face matures and the bridge of the nose becomes narrower, the eyes look normal. A child whose eyes are crossed needs medical attention, as this problem is not outgrown.

Consult your doctor if:

- Your baby's eyes appear crossed or don't move together after the age of 4 months.
- Your child always holds her head in an abnormal or tilted position.
- Your child squints.
- A drooping eyelid makes one eye appear much smaller than the other.
- Your child often closes one eye.
- Your child's eyes are 'bouncing' or shaking.

Warning

If strabismus is not diagnosed and treated early, the child will use one eye at the expense of the other, risking a loss of vision in the unused eye.

QUESTIONS TO CONSIDER	IF ANSWER IS	POSSIBLE CAUSE IS	ACTION TO TAKE
Is your child 6 months or older? Do his eyes still move independently, at least part of the time? Does one eye look out or in while the other focuses? Are both eyes turned in?	**YES**	Strabismus (crossed or misaligned eyes).	Consult your GP, who will examine your child and recommend referral to an eye specialist (ophthalmologist) for complete evaluation and treatment.
Does one eye appear much smaller than the other because of a drooping lid? Does the drooping lid appear to interfere with vision? Does your child lift his chin or face to see?	**YES**	Ptosis (drooping lid).	Consult your GP, who will determine whether referral to a specialist is advisable. Severe ptosis may interfere with vision development and should be treated.
Does your child always close one eye while reading or focusing on close tasks? Does he hold books up close? Does he cover one eye when looking at more distant objects? Does the less used eye have any tendency to wander? Is there a family history of lazy eye?	**YES**	Amblyopia (lazy eye).	Consult your GP. If amblyopia persists after about age 5 to 6 years, the vision in the unused eye may be permanently damaged. (See Correcting eye problems, opposite.)

Questions to consider	If answer is	Possible cause is	Action to take
Has a child whose eyes were previously normal suddenly developed crossed eyes or a wandering eye? Have the eyes started to 'bounce' or 'wiggle'?	**YES**	Visual or nerve disorder.	Consult your GP without delay; your child may need to be evaluated by a neurologist or ophthalmologist to determine the cause of his eye problem.

Correcting eye problems

Eye problems in children must be treated early because certain conditions can no longer be corrected once the visual-motor system is fully developed by mid-adolescence. That's why your doctor checks your child's eyes at every regular visit for evidence of eye disease, as well as to make sure that both eyes are working together. Formal vision testing is often done when the child is aged 3 years – old enough to follow directions and describe what she sees. If you have a family history of serious eye disorders, lazy eye or crossed eyes, or are concerned about specific problems, your GP will perform an examination and refer even a very young infant for more extensive testing by an eye specialist (ophthalmologist).

Youngsters born prematurely are more likely than others to develop eye problems, including crossed eyes (strabismus). In some cases, strabismus is caused by disease or injury of the eye or brain. Treatment usually involves spectacles, eyedrops, exercises, and/or surgery. Surgery, if needed, can usually be performed between 6 and 18 months of age, or later in some cases. Many children still need spectacles and patching, at least for a while, after undergoing corrective surgery.

Treatment of lazy eye (amblyopia) may involve consistent use of spectacles, wearing a patch over the stronger eye, and possibly eyedrops to improve the vision in the amblyopic eye.

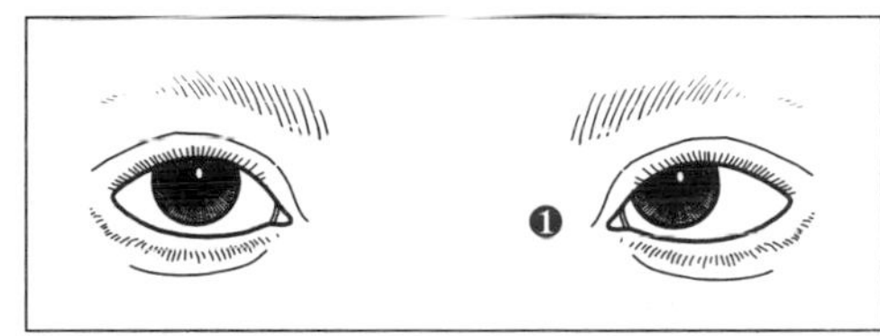

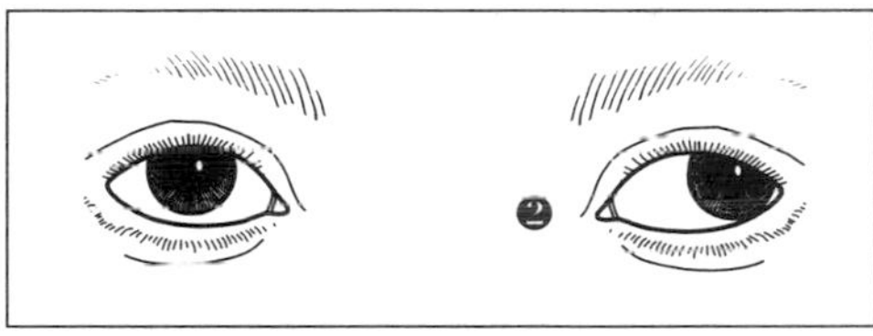

When one eye is 'lazy' and not tracking correctly, as shown here in the child's left eye, it may move ❶ inward or ❷ outward.
A young child with this condition may need to wear spectacles and/or a patch to correct a lazy eye. Glasses, exercise, or surgery can help correct the misalignment.

Call your child's dentist immediately if a permanent tooth has been knocked loose. A tooth can often be reimplanted if:

- You immediately rinse it under running tap water but do not touch the root, then place it in milk for transport to the dentist.
- The dentist is able to treat the child within 30 minutes of the injury.

In General:

Healthy teeth are essential to an attractive appearance, clear speech, and proper nutrition. The primary teeth must be well cared for if the permanent teeth are to be sound and well positioned. A baby's teeth should be cleaned regularly with a cotton bud or damp gauze. Toddlers should be taught to brush as soon as they can handle a toothbrush, although it may be a while until they can master flossing. In fact, most children need close supervision and help with brushing and flossing until they are about 8 years old. But even long afterwards, parents may have to remind youngsters to brush their teeth every night and morning until it becomes second nature.

Sugar directly damages the teeth; sugars that linger on the teeth – such as sticky dried fruits or sugars produced from starchy cereal residues in the mouth – are especially injurious. Children's diets should emphasize calcium to build strong teeth, as well as noncariogenic (foods that do not produce tooth decay) snacks such as raw vegetables, which also exercise the gums and jaw.

Regular dental checkups should begin when a child is about 3 years old, or earlier if your GP has noted problems. Many dentists prefer that youngsters become familiar with the dentist's office even before they start checkups. A toddler, for example, can try out the chair when he accompanies his parents on their dental visits. Dentists use an array of approaches, including sealants and fluoride treatments, to prevent tooth decay. Orthodontic treatment, when necessary, is most effective while the bones are young and pliable. It can help to promote lifelong dental health.

Don't ignore a child's complaint of mouth pain (see p. 112). While some minor causes of discomfort clear up by themselves, severe or nagging pain may signal a serious problem that could have lasting effects on your child's health and appearance if left untreated.

Warning

Never put a child to bed with a bottle of milk, formula, juice, or similar sweet drinks. Prolonged contact with their sugar can cause serious dental decay, called 'nursing bottle caries'. If a child cannot settle down without a bottle, fill it with plain water. Similarly, never dip a dummy in honey or other sweet foods.

Questions to consider	If answer is	Possible cause is	Action to take
Is your baby drooling more than usual? Does he keep his fist or finger constantly in his mouth?	**YES**	Teething, a normal developmental stage.	Comfort your baby and ease the soreness by rubbing his gums with your finger (see Coping with drooling and biting, opposite). If he is unusually upset or has a temperature over 38°C (100.4°F), call your GP; the symptoms may be due to another condition.

Questions to consider	If answer is	Possible cause is	Action to take
Does your child have a recurrent, throbbing tooth pain? Is the tooth sensitive to heat and cold?	**YES**	Tooth decay (caries).	Make an appointment with your child's dentist as soon as possible. Treatment may require a filling.
Does a recently filled tooth hurt when your child bites on it? Does the tooth feel as though it doesn't fit properly?	**YES**	Temporary sensitivity following treatment.	Sensitivity lingering after a filling will eventually subside. If the tooth doesn't feel right, consult your dentist, who may adjust the filling for a better fit.
Are your child's gums red and swollen? Do they bleed easily on brushing?	**YES**	Gingivitis; gum (periodontal) disease (adolescents are especially susceptible).	Consult your GP, who will refer you to the child's dentist if treatment is needed for gum disease.
Does your child grind his teeth while asleep? Does he complain of jaw pain on awakening?	**YES**	Bruxism (tooth grinding), usually due to stress.	Consult your child's dentist. Tooth grinding may damage the teeth or gums; a nighttime mouth guard may help to break the habit.
Does a child older than 6 years still suck her thumb? Are you concerned that thumb-sucking may distort her permanent teeth?	**YES**	Thumb-sucking habit.	If she sucks her thumb briefly to get to sleep, no treatment is needed. If the habit is more severe, ask your doctor or dentist for advice about dealing with thumb-sucking.
Does your child have steady pain? Does the tooth feel loose, high, or different? Does it ache when your child eats sweets or cold foods?	**YES**	Abscessed tooth; cracked tooth; decay under a filling.	Call your dentist immediately. Give paracetamol to relieve discomfort until the dentist can determine whether the tooth can be saved or extraction is necessary.
Has a primary tooth apparently been knocked out? Is the tooth nowhere to be found?	**YES**	Tooth intrusion.	Call your dentist immediately. Occasionally, a tooth is forced back into the gum. Intruded teeth often re-erupt spontaneously and remain healthy until shed at the appropriate time.

Coping with drooling and biting

A baby entering the teething phase usually drools more and may keep several fingers or a fist constantly in his mouth. Contrary to popular belief, fever, diarrhoea, and other symptoms are not caused by teething. If your baby has these symptoms, consult your GP. A fussy, teething baby may be comforted by chewing on a teething ring or a hard, unsweetened teething biscuit. Don't use frozen teething toys; the extreme cold may injure the mouth tissues and cause more pain. The pain relievers you rub on the gums are not necessary or helpful; with the extra drooling, they are washed out of the mouth in a few minutes.

In General:

Growth and development tend to follow a general pattern, but every child develops at his own pace, depending on heredity and other factors. The age at which major milestones, such as walking and talking, are reached varies from one child to another, and so long as your child is reaching his milestones within the acceptable time range (see Developmental Milestones for the First 3 Years, p. 60), his progress is probably quite normal.

About 3 out of every 100 children, however, have a hereditary or inborn condition that may interfere with development, while in others, severe illness or injury leads to developmental problems. Occasionally, a child will suffer a temporary setback after a serious illness and rebound once he recovers his health. Other problems are less clear-cut or appear only when a child begins school and has trouble keeping up with classmates.

In a large number of hereditary or congenital defects the cause can be identified; new techniques can detect many such problems before birth, so that parents are better prepared to deal with the extra care their child may need from the very beginning. In some cases, developmental delay overlaps with a chronic medical condition. Early detection and treatment can lessen the impact and give the child a better quality of life.

A child whose development seems slow should have a complete medical and developmental examination. If your doctor is concerned that your child is not developing normally, he will advise an evaluation, possibly including a consultation with a developmental specialist. Properly conducted tests show not only a child's problems but also his particular strengths and abilities. In many communities, evaluations are provided without charge or at minimal cost. Your local education authority, health department, or social services agency can provide information about services offered in your area.

Depending on the results of tests, your paediatrician can recommend a plan for physical, speech, and occupational therapy, as well as psychological counselling, if necessary. Special education may also be required. With the support of teachers and therapists, parents can set realistic goals and help their child develop his abilities.

Even experts find it difficult to make long-range predictions about development from tests conducted when a child is 1 or 2 years old. Children born with the same condition – Down's syndrome, for example – vary widely in their degree of developmental delay. A series of tests over time provides a broader and more accurate picture than a single assessment. And studies have confirmed that regardless of any disability detected during the early years, the environment in which a child is reared is a very important factor in helping him reach his potential. Loving encouragement can often yield surprising results.

Consult your doctor if your child:

- Was making progress but is losing skills such as sucking, talking, or walking.
- Is not attaining the skills outlined in Developmental Milestones for the First 3 Years, p. 60.

Warning

Although it can be difficult, parents must encourage their child to deal with disability on his own terms: overprotectiveness inhibits the child and limits his opportunities. Some children with vision or hearing loss become 'pseudoretarded' because they are misdiagnosed. Too often, prematurely labelling a child as retarded has turned out to be a self-fulfilling prophecy.

QUESTIONS TO CONSIDER	IF ANSWER IS	POSSIBLE CAUSE IS	ACTION TO TAKE
At 2 months: does your baby feel unusually stiff or floppy? Does his head fall backward if you pull him up while he's lying flat? At 6 months: does your baby always reach with only one hand while keeping the other in a fist? At 10 months or older: does your baby crawl lopsidedly, pushing with the leg and arm on one side while dragging the opposite limbs? Does he move about but not crawl on all fours?	**YES**	Developmental delay; cerebral palsy (while sometimes caused by illness during pregnancy, cerebral palsy may also follow a severe illness or injury during infancy).	Consult your doctor, who will examine the child and determine whether he should be seen by a specialist.
Was your child making normal progress, but now seems to be losing one or more skills? Is she making fewer efforts to speak? Does she resist physical contact? Does she seem to live in her own world?	**YES**	Developmental delay; autism; metabolic disorder.	Talk to your doctor, who will evaluate the child and provide a referral to a specialist, if advisable.
Is your child showing signs of increasing clumsiness and difficulty walking?	**YES**	Neurologic and/or muscular disorder.	Consult your doctor, who will examine the child and refer you to a specialist, if needed. (See Coordination Problems, p. 51.)
Does your child seem to be unusually late in talking? Does she understand what is said to her? Does she speak at least 5 words clearly? Is she over age 2?	**YES**	Reluctance to speak (if the child pronounces words clearly, there is probably not a speech disorder).	Check with your doctor, who will give your child a full evaluation, including hearing tests and, if appropriate, refer her for further testing.
Is your late talker also behind schedule in walking and other motor skills? Is he over 2? Does he say fewer than 5 words? Are the words unclear?	**YES**	Delayed development; hearing defect; lack of stimulation.	Talk to your doctor, who will examine the child with special attention to hearing; your child may need to be referred to a specialist.
Is your child having difficulty at school? Is he having problems reading or with numbers? Does he have trouble keeping up with classmates in learning and social development?	**YES**	Delayed development; learning problems (see p. 106); emotional stress.	Consult with teachers to determine the extent of the problem. Your GP will examine the child to rule out physical problems and recommend a treatment plan.

Continued on next page

DEVELOPMENTAL MILESTONES FOR THE FIRST 3 YEARS

3 MONTHS	*Raises head and chest, arms out, from prone position; reaches for (but usually misses) objects; waves at toys; has some head control when raised to sitting position; smiles, giggles; listens to voices; responds to music; says 'aagh' and 'ngah'.*
6 MONTHS	*Rolls over; lifts head; may sit for a short time; may support most of weight when helped to stand; bounces actively; grasps objects; starting to transfer objects from one hand to the other (6 to 8 months); babbles and makes linked-up vowel sounds; responds to change in surroundings; recognizes parents, prefers mother.*
9 MONTHS	*Sits unsupported with back straight; pulls up to standing position; begins to crawl; starting to pick up objects with thumb and forefinger (9 to 11 months); plays pat-a-cake, peek-a-boo; can find hidden toy and tries to retrieve dropped objects; may say 'mama' and 'dada'; responds to name; waves.*
12 MONTHS	*Walks with help; picks up small objects; may say a few words; plays simple ball games.*
15 MONTHS	*Walks alone; crawls upstairs; stacks two blocks; makes lines with crayon; can place smaller objects inside larger ones; may be able to name familiar objects and have a vocabulary of several words; can follow simple commands.*
18 MONTHS	*Runs stiffly; sits on chair; climbs stairs; stacks three blocks; scribbles; identifies body parts, pictures; feeds self; asks for help; kisses parents; may complain when nappy is soiled.*
24 MONTHS	*Runs well; walks up and down stairs one step at a time; opens doors; climbs; stacks six blocks; scribbles circles; folds paper; links three words; handles spoon; listens to stories; helps in undressing; has a 25- to 50-word vocabulary.*
30 MONTHS	*Jumps; stacks eight blocks; draws vertical and horizontal strokes; tries to draw circles; knows full name, refers to self with pronoun 'I'; helps tidy up; engages in pretend play.*
36 MONTHS	*Rides tricycle; alternates feet when walking up and down stairs; uses blocks to build bridges; copies a circle; counts three objects; repeats three words of a sentence; plays simple games with other children; helps in dressing; washes hands.*

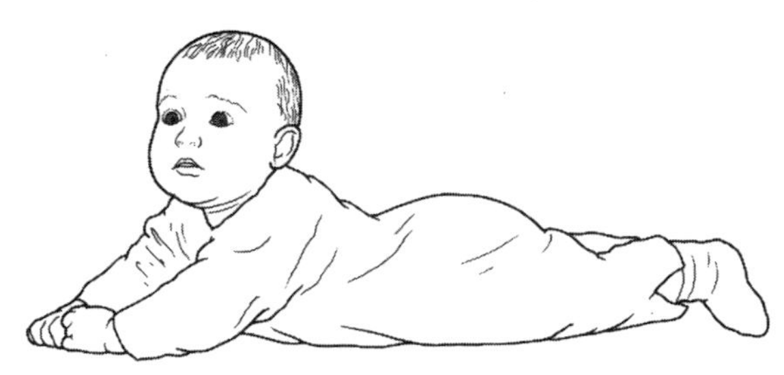

At 3 months, raises head and chest.

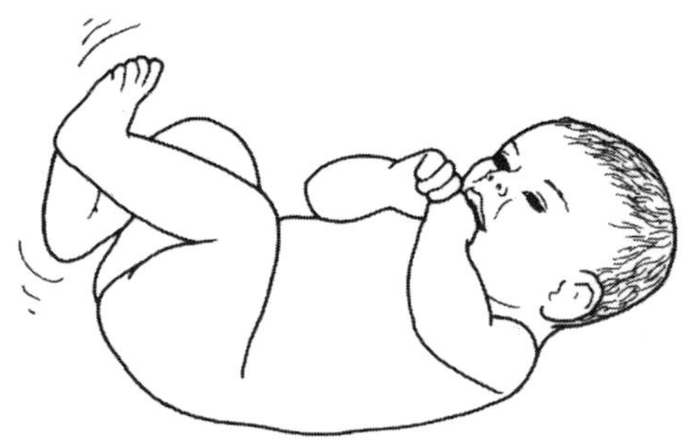

At 6 months, rolls over.

Helping children to develop intelligence

The results of studies still in progress are confirming what parents have long known: the more you talk to your child, the brighter he or she is likely to be. The researchers are not just reinventing the wheel, however; their studies are valuable because they show that physical stimulation plays a big role in moulding intelligence and creativity. In other words, the right kind of loving care helps the brain to grow right.

Two crucial facts have emerged. First, spoken language seems to be the most important stimulus for brain development in the period from birth to 3 years, but especially in the first year. In fact, some researchers claim they can relate the actual number of words an infant hears each day to later intelligence, success in learning, and the ability to get on with others. Second, infants need to hear the words from parents or care-givers who are actively involved in looking after them. Chatter from radio and television doesn't have the same effect.

Before birth, the brain's wiring system of nerve cells is laid down according to the genetic pattern we inherit. The way a mother takes care of her health and nutrition is important in making sure this foundation is sound. Some researchers think that the mind starts developing even while the baby is in the womb. Babies may recognize their mothers' voices at birth, and some doctors encourage parents to talk to the developing foetus and play music to help the brain cells develop.

After birth, genes and environmental factors work together. Starting at the moment of birth and continuing nonstop throughout the first year, the brain is literally moulded by the inflow to the senses. Sights, sounds, smells, touch, and most importantly, language and eye contact drive the nerve cells to organize into networks that help us to be smart, inventive, creative, and adaptable for the rest of our lives.

Researchers warn that their results don't mean that parents should try to make superkids by subjecting babies to a day-and-night barrage of stimulating activities. On the contrary, it's probably dangerous to overstimulate infants and it's wrong to push a child to overachieve at any age. What's important is to provide a nurturing, secure environment where your child can reach his potential on his own terms, and take proper credit for his achievements.

The brain is ready for different kinds of stimulation at various ages. Youngsters thrive when they get stimulation their brains are adapted to handle. But most important of all, they need to talk, play, and interact with their parents and care-givers at every age.

Birth to 1 month Babies are more alert and less stressed if they get low-level stimulation such as gentle talking. Because the baby's brain has trouble filtering out extraneous sounds, child development experts recommend that you turn off distracting noises such as radios, televisions, or appliances when talking to your infant.

Months 1-3 The networks of nerve cells controlling vision are laid down at this time. Your baby also begins to differentiate sound patterns such as the tone and pitch of your voice. Showing high-contrast pictures and objects and speaking to your baby help these networks to form.

Months 3-5 Your baby is learning primarily by seeing at this stage. Moving objects capture her attention. Talk to her and show her increasingly complex pictures corresponding to real objects, such as in brightly illustrated infant storybooks.

Months 6-7 Your baby is beginning to learn about cause and effect: what things do, how things work. Talk about actions as you do them. For example, turn the knob and open the door, or turn on the cold tap and feel the water.

Months 7-8 Now your baby can connect relatively distant sounds to something he knows. When the doorbell rings, say it must be a visitor, or if you hear a car in the driveway, Mummy or Daddy must be home.

Months 9-12 Your baby is ready to put some of his learning into practice, coordinating his sensory and motor skills. Help him to turn on a light switch or tap.

Months 13-18 The whole system is speeding up and growing more complex. Follow your youngster's cues as he starts to speak and explore the world with his motor skills and let him take risks under your supervision.

In General:

From time to time, all children get bouts of diarrhoea, passing frequent, watery stools. This symptom can signal a range of conditions, from a toddler's overconsumption of fruit juice to a mild viral infection, a bacterial or parasitic infection, or food poisoning.

In most cases, acute diarrhoea clears up on its own as the underlying condition clears up. Until then, however, it's important to make sure your child has enough fluids to prevent dehydration and returns to a normal diet as soon as possible. A temporary loss of appetite is not harmful in a well nourished child. Usually, children are ready to eat again once symptoms clear up.

Outbreaks of infectious diarrhoea are common among youngsters attending childcare centres, particularly centres caring for children who are not yet toilet trained. Children should be taught to wash their hands with soap and water every time they use the potty or lavatory. Chronic diarrhoea should always be investigated, as it may be a symptom of a serious disorder. Without treatment, chronic diarrhoea may deprive the child of nutrients and lead to malnutrition.

☎

Call your doctor immediately if diarrhoea is accompanied by signs of dehydration, such as:

- Infrequent urination.
- Dark urine.
- Sunken eyes.
- Refusal to drink.
- Dry, sticky lips and mouth.
- Lethargy, decreased activity.

Warning

Over-the-counter antidiarrhoeal medications are not recommended for children age 2 or under, and should be used only on a doctor's advice in older children. These medications may cause fluid and salt to remain in the intestine, which appears to stop the diarrhoea but, in fact, may make it harder to recognize dehydration. This may further injure the intestine.

Questions to consider	If answer is	Possible cause is	Action to take
Has your child abruptly developed diarrhoea with abdominal cramps, vomiting, and mild fever?	YES	Viral gastroenteritis.	If the child is an infant, consult your doctor at once. For an older child, follow the guidelines in Coping with diarrhoea (see opposite). Call your GP if diarrhoea lasts longer than 48 hours, or vomiting continues more than 12 hours.
Does your child have severe diarrhoea with or without vomiting? Is there blood in the stool? Is he feverish?	YES	Infectious diarrhoea (*Escherichia coli*, salmonella, shigella).	Consult your doctor promptly. Follow guidelines for rehydration (see Coping with diarrhoea, opposite).
Has your toddler had diarrhoea longer than 2 days? Does he have several loose bowel movements every day? Is he otherwise healthy and gaining weight? Does he drink a lot of juice, sweet drinks, and water?	YES	Nonspecific diarrhoea; toddler diarrhoea; too much juice.	Consult your doctor, who will examine the child to rule out serious conditions and may suggest dietary changes, such as cutting down on your child's consumption of juices and sweet drinks.

QUESTIONS TO CONSIDER	IF ANSWER IS	POSSIBLE CAUSE IS	ACTION TO TAKE
Does your child have vomiting and diarrhoea with cramps, and/or headache and fever? Is there blood in the stool? Do others in the household have similar symptoms?	**YES**	Bacterial food poisoning.	Call your GP. Treatment will depend on the type and severity of food poisoning.
Does your toddler or young child have diarrhoea, with bloating and/or nausea? Is the child in a group child-care setting or school?	**YES**	Parasitic infection, such as giardiasis, especially if the child attends group care.	Call your GP, who will examine the child, order diagnostic tests as required, and prescribe treatment.
Did your child get diarrhoea during or just after antibiotic treatment?	**YES**	Medication side effect.	Call your GP. If your child needs an antibiotic, the doctor will prescribe an alternative and advise on diet.
Does your otherwise healthy school-age child have alternating diarrhoea and constipation? Do bouts occur at times of stress? Is there intermittent abdominal pain, nausea, bloating, or wind?	**YES**	Irritable bowel syndrome (IBS).	Consult your GP, who will examine the child to rule out serious disorders. If IBS is confirmed, treatment may involve an increase in dietary fibre or an antispasmodic medication for cramps, as well as reassurance that the condition is common but not serious.
Are your child's stools bulky and foul smelling? Are symptoms worse after eating certain foods? Is he growing and gaining weight slowly?	**YES**	Malabsorption disorder.	Consult your GP without delay for diagnostic tests and treatment, if required.
Is your child passing bloody stools? Is there pain in the abdomen and joints? Has she lost her appetite? Is she nauseated and fatigued?	**YES**	Inflammatory bowel disease such as ulcerative colitis or Crohn disease.	Consult your GP without delay; diagnostic tests and appropriate treatment are necessary.

Coping with diarrhoea

Water and salt lost in diarrhoea must be replenished to prevent dehydration. For rehydration, use only commercially available electrolyte solutions. Don't use sports drinks: their sugar content can make the diarrhoea worse. As your child begins to feel better, resume a normal diet.

Even if your child is vomiting, ask your GP to recommend a commercially available electrolyte drink to keep up the body's normal water and salt levels until the vomiting has stopped. If vomiting persists or nothing is staying down, consult your doctor.

If the diarrhoea is not severe and the vomiting has stopped, let your child eat a normal diet in moderation. There is no need to limit food or drinks once your child is feeling better.

Dizziness

Vertigo

In General:

When children say they feel dizzy, they usually mean that they feel light-headed, such as with the unsteady feeling that sometimes accompanies a fever. A person with vertigo, on the other hand, has the sensation that the room is spinning around or his body is veering out of control. It's not uncommon for healthy children, and particularly adolescents, to feel momentarily unsteady as a result of a minor change in blood flow when they stand abruptly after squatting or sitting. Unless the child actually faints this is of no consequence. The self-induced dizziness that results from spinning around or running in circles is also no cause for concern.

Some children get dizzy and nauseated when riding in a car. Children's dizziness, however, rarely means true vertigo, which involves an unpleasant sensation of spinning and disorientation.

Consult your doctor if:

- Your normally coordinated child develops a staggering, 'drunken' gait.
- Your child complains of dizziness and loses his balance or cannot walk a straight line.
- Your child has dizziness and recurrent headache that is worse on lying down.

Warning

True vertigo is unusual in children. A child with vertigo and ringing or buzzing in the ears should always be seen by a doctor.

Questions to consider	If answer is	Possible cause is	Action to take
Is your child unwell and feverish, with a temperature over 37.8°C (100°F)?	YES	Light-headedness due to illness.	Give paracetamol to reduce fever and discomfort. If symptoms become worse or don't clear up in 1 to 2 days, consult your doctor.
Has your child had an isolated episode of feeling dizzy or faint?	YES	Faintness due to heat, hunger, anxiety, or other stress.	Have your child rest in a cool place. Offer a drink containing sugar, a light snack, and cold water. If your child is still faint after 30 minutes, call your GP (See Fainting, p. 181.)
Is your child suddenly complaining that the room is spinning around? Is he losing his balance? Does he have ringing in the ears (tinnitus)?	YES	A viral infection of the inner ear (labyrinthitis).	Consult your doctor, who will examine the child to rule out other disorders and confirm the diagnosis. The viral infection usually clears up within a week without treatment; the doctor may prescribe medication to reduce the symptoms.
Is your child unsteady after a recent viral illness, such as chickenpox?	YES	Weakness and loss of muscle coordination (postviral cerebellar ataxia).	Consult your GP for a more extensive evaluation.
Does your child get dizzy and nauseated while riding in a car, lift, or boat?	YES	Motion sickness.	Ask your doctor what measures you should take to prevent motion sickness.

Questions to consider	If answer is	Possible cause is	Action to take
Is your child complaining of dizziness following a fall or head injury?	**YES**	Head injury.	Call your doctor without delay; your child may need x-rays and other tests.
Does your child complain of dizziness and disorientation? Does she have frequent, repeated, momentary lapses of attention?	**YES**	Petit mal seizures or absence seizures (epilepsy).	Consult your doctor. (See Convulsions, p. 50.)
Does your child have headaches that are worse on lying down? Does he have difficulty balancing or walking a straight line? Is he nauseated or vomiting?	**YES**	Unusual condition, such as tumour requiring diagnosis and treatment.	Consult your doctor. Although rare in children, these conditions can occur and require prompt treatment. (See Headache, p. 86.)
Does your toddler or older child topple over when sitting or standing still? Or does he lose his balance if he closes his eyes while standing? Does he usually miss when he reaches for objects? Does he miss if you ask him to touch his nose with his finger?	**YES**	In rare cases, neuromuscular disorder (ataxia).	Consult your doctor, who will examine the child and determine whether he should be seen by a specialist.

Keeping a sense of balance

Our ability to remain upright depends on a delicate interplay between the nerves and muscles involved in hearing, sight, and touch. Through our sense of hearing we learn to place ourselves in relation to sounds. And our limbs and muscles are equipped with sense organs that help us gauge our position relative to our surroundings. A disturbance in any part of the balance mechanism may cause dizziness, vertigo, and nausea.

Dizziness usually goes away once the stimulus that caused it stops. True vertigo, on the other hand, is often an ongoing condition caused by a disorder of the inner ear. People with vertigo sometimes have tinnitus as well; this ringing or buzzing sound is caused by a related disturbance in the nerve we use to perceive sound.

Drooling

Salivation

In General:

Drooling and blowing bubbles give pleasure to babies during the phase of development when their satisfaction is centred on the mouth. This becomes especially apparent at 3 to 6 months of age. The increased flow of saliva that often heralds the appearance of a new tooth seems to soothe the baby's tender gums. If, however, your child appears to be drooling excessively and looks ill, drooling may be a sign that he is having trouble swallowing and requires medical attention.

Call 999 or take your child to the nearest hospital emergency department:

- If a child with a sore throat or cold symptoms starts drooling, breathing hard and noisily, and gasping for breath with mouth wide open. This may be epiglottitis, a now infrequent but serious medical emergency.

Warning

If a child is suddenly drooling, can't speak, and is having difficulty breathing, he may be choking on food or a foreign object. Call 999 and follow first aid procedures on choking (see p. 201) while you're waiting for help.

Questions to consider	If answer is	Possible cause is	Action to take
Is your baby between 3 and 6 months old? Is he a little fussy? Does he seem to want to chew and bite on firm objects, including your fingers?	**YES**	Normal drooling.	Comfort your baby and give him a pacifier or a smooth teething ring to chew on. (See Dental Problems, p. 56.)
Does your child have fever of 38.3°C (101°F) or higher, headache, and sore throat? Has she lost her appetite? Does she have pain on swallowing? Are the glands in her neck swollen?	**YES**	Viral infection of the throat or mouth; streptococcal throat infection; tonsillitis.	Consult your GP, who will examine the child and advise appropriate treatment. If the doctor agrees, give paracetamol to reduce fever.
Does your child have spots or ulcerations inside her mouth? Does she find them painful?	**YES**	Viral stomatitis.	Call your GP, who will advise appropriate treatment.
Is your drooling child straining and gasping for air, with his mouth wide open? Does he have a severe sore throat?	**YES**	Epiglottitis, inflammation of the flap of tissue that prevents food and liquids from entering the windpipe (trachea).	Call 999 or take your child to the nearest hospital emergency department. This condition is serious and could cause the child to stop breathing. Once a grave threat, it has become less common since the introduction of the HIb vaccine for children.

Questions to consider	If answer is	Possible cause is	Action to take
Is your child's face turning blue? Is he speechless, spluttering, and trying to cough?	**YES**	Choking.	This is an emergency. Have someone else call 999 while you start the Heimlich manoeuvre (see p. 203) or the procedure for a baby under 1 year (see Choking, p. 201). If your child stops breathing and has no pulse, start CPR and keep it up until help arrives (see p. 204).
Has your child passed out? Are his limbs and muscles jerking uncontrollably? Is he also drooling?	**YES**	Seizure.	During the seizure, make sure your child is safe from objects that could injure him (see Convulsions, p. 50). Don't leave the child, but call your doctor as soon as possible and follow his instructions.

Role of saliva

Drooling fulfils several important functions. The saliva softens and moistens food once solids are part of the diet, keeps the mouth moist and makes it easier to swallow, washes away food residues, and protects the teeth. Saliva also contains ptyalin, a digestive enzyme that changes starch into sugar (young babies lack this enzyme, which is why in earlier times, mothers chewed most starchy foods before feeding them to their offspring). A natural antacid in saliva neutralizes stomach acid and aids digestion. Saliva also protects against tooth decay.

Saliva is produced in the salivary glands. The submandibular gland lies under the jaw, the sublingual gland is under the tongue, and the parotid is close to the ear.

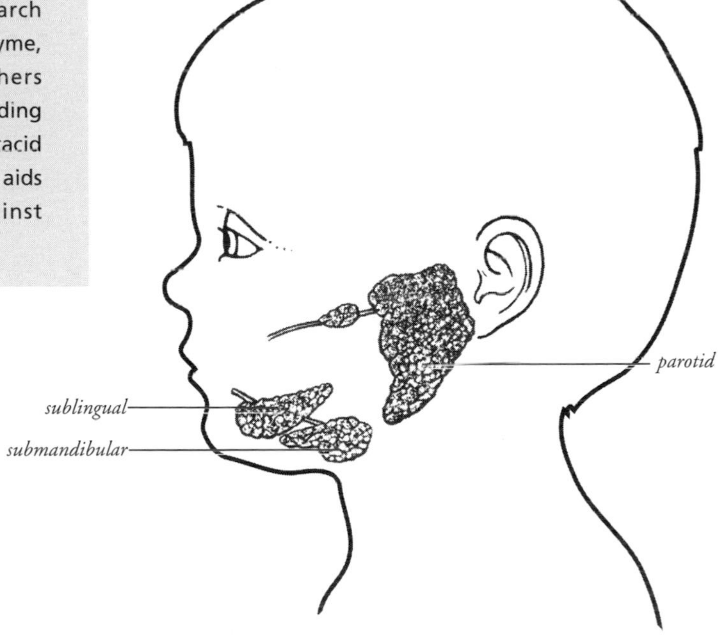

Earache/Ear Infection

Otalgia/Otitis

In General:

Ear infections are common in young children: most toddlers have had at least one bout by age 2. Ear problems are so common in this age group because children are exposed to a host of germs before their immune systems are mature enough to resist infections. In addition, children's tiny Eustachian tubes (the canals linking the middle ear and pharynx) allow infectious material to remain in or travel up to the middle ear space. Luckily, children tend to outgrow these illnesses as their susceptibility decreases and their Eustachian tubes mature.

In infants and young children who have not yet learned to talk, an upper respiratory infection usually precedes the telltale signs of ear infection, including nighttime crying and daytime irritability, fever (a temperature of 38°C [100.4°F], or higher), and loss of appetite. A baby with an ear infection will often cry in distress when feeding as his ear pressure changes with the sucking motion. A slightly older child may rub or pull at his ear. And once your child can talk, he will tell you if his ear hurts.

Ear infections are often treated with antibiotics. Don't hesitate to consult your GP if you suspect your child may have an ear infection, but antibiotics are not always essential.

Consult your doctor if your child has earache along with any of the following symptoms:

- Discharge from the ear.
- Swelling around the ear.
- Headache.
- Fever of 39°C (102°F) or higher.
- Dizziness.
- Hearing loss.

Warning

Never leave a baby alone to finish a bottle while lying on his back. Formula or other liquid can occasionally travel up the Eustachian tube, creating ideal conditions for bacterial growth in the middle ear.

Children who are exposed to second-hand tobacco smoke have an increased risk of developing health problems, including ear infections.

Questions to consider	If answer is	Possible cause is	Action to take
Does your child have a cold, with runny nose, cough, mild fever, or conjunctivitis? Is there a discharge from the ear? Is she having ear pain?	**YES**	Middle ear infection (otitis media).	Consult your GP, who will examine your child and advise appropriate treatment.
Is your child complaining of pain, itching, or fullness in the ear? Does pulling on the earlobe make the pain worse? Is there a discharge? Has the child been swimming a lot? Or does he often dip his head under the bathwater?	**YES**	Swimmer's ear (otitis externa).	Consult your GP, who will examine the child and prescribe appropriate treatment. Eardrops may be needed. Ask whether you need to take any other measures to prevent a recurrence.
Is your child's outer ear red and swollen?	**YES**	Insect sting or bite; impetigo (a bacterial infection).	Check with your GP. A cold compress will help to relieve discomfort in case of an insect sting. If your child has impetigo, antibiotic treatment will be necessary.

QUESTIONS TO CONSIDER	IF ANSWER IS	POSSIBLE CAUSE IS	ACTION TO TAKE
Is your child between about 18 months and 4 years old? Is he complaining of ear pain, without other symptoms such as runny nose or sore throat? Has he been playing with small objects or paper? Can you see something stuck in the ear canal?	**YES**	Foreign body in the ear.	Don't try to dig out the object; you may injure the ear. Call your GP, who will examine the ear with a magnifying device and special lights, which make a foreign object easier to see and extract. It may be necessary to refer your child to a specialist for help with this.
Does your child have the feeling that something is moving around inside her ear? Can she hear buzzing? Is there any pain?	**YES.**	Insect in ear.	Most insects eventually find their way out; if not, consult your doctor, who will confirm if an insect is in the ear and, if it is present, remove it.
Has your child's ear been injured in an accident? Is it bleeding, cut, and/or bruised?	**YES**	Injury with cuts and bruising.	Clean the outside of the ear gently with plain water and lightly tape or bandage a sterile pad over the wound. Then call your doctor, who will want to examine the child to make sure that there is no injury to the internal tissues that needs attention.
Is your child's ear sticking out at an angle? Is the area behind the ear tender and painful?	**YES**	Mastoiditis.	Call your doctor at once for an examination and treatment.

Treating ear infections

Concerns about the overuse of antibiotics and the corresponding rise in bacterial resistance are leading some doctors to revise their treatment of middle ear infections (otitis media). Although antibiotics remain the mainstay of treatment, your doctor may recommend a wait-and-see approach if an ear infection is mild and your child is otherwise healthy and not in severe pain. The aim is to reserve antibiotics for serious conditions in which powerful medication is really needed, and to cut down on nonessential treatments that may promote the growth of resistant bacteria.

A warm pad over the ear and a dose of paracetamol may help to make the child more comfortable while her immune system fights off the infection. Of course, if there's any sign that the infection is not going to go away on its own, your doctor will prescribe an antibiotic. These medications usually have to be taken for 24 to 48 hours before you can see any effects.

In the past, large numbers of young children with frequent middle ear infections underwent surgery to implant a small plastic tube (grommet) in the ear to promote drainage. This procedure is still widely done, but the indications have been refined. Before the insertion of a tube, a course of preventive antibiotic is often recommended. The tendency to suffer recurrent ear infections diminishes as the child matures.

In General:

Common eye problems in childhood include infection, such as sties and pinkeye (conjunctivitis), and irritation caused by a foreign body or allergy. Eye infections after the newborn period are seldom serious as long as they're treated promptly.

Injuries to the eye or lid should always be seen by a doctor, and a child with a potentially serious injury should be taken straight to the nearest hospital emergency department. If you can't remove a foreign body by washing out with water, seek your doctor's help straightaway. For problems affecting the way the eyes work, see Crossed Eyes/Wandering Eye (p. 54) and Vision Problems (p. 158).

Consult your doctor if your child has:

- Redness, swelling, and eye discharge lasting more than 24 hours.
- Persistent eye pain.
- Unusual sensitivity to light.
- Excessive tearing.
- Frequent blinking.
- Decreased or blurred vision.

Warning

Some eye infections are highly contagious. Wash your hands before and after touching the area around an infected eye. Don't directly touch the eye or the discharge from it. Don't let the tip of an eye dropper or ointment tube touch the infected area. Keep a child with discharging conjunctivitis home from school or childcare until 24 hours after starting treatment. Launder the youngster's towel and flannel after each use.

Questions to consider	If answer is	Possible cause is	Action to take
Is your baby's eye watering? Is there a discharge? Is there a bulge under the eyelid near the nose?	YES	Blocked tear duct.	Your doctor will make sure the eyes are not infected. Blocked tear ducts usually open on their own during the first few months of life, but your GP may recommend massaging the area.
Does your child feel pain when she blinks? Does it feel as if there's something in her eye?	YES	Foreign body in the eye.	Wash out the eye with lukewarm water; if this doesn't help, consult your doctor.
Are there streaks or spots of blood in the whites of your child's eyes? Are the eyes otherwise free of pain or irritation?	YES	Subconjunctival haemorrhage.	These streaks look alarming but are not serious. They may follow coughing, sneezing, or a mild injury. If streaks increase or do not clear up within a week, call your doctor.
Are your child's eyes pinkish, irritated, and swollen? Does she have symptoms of an upper respiratory infection?	YES	Conjunctivitis, possibly due to a viral infection such as the common cold.	Consult your doctor, who will determine if treatment is needed.

QUESTIONS TO CONSIDER	IF ANSWER IS	POSSIBLE CAUSE IS	ACTION TO TAKE
Are your child's eyes red, tearing, and itchy? Does he have a runny nose and sneezing? Do allergies run in your family?	**YES**	Allergic conjunctivitis.	Consult your doctor, who may recommend treatment to relieve symptoms and other measures to reduce exposure to allergens. (See Allergic Reactions, p. 26.)
Are your child's eyes red? Is there a discharge, or are his eyes crusted shut in the morning?	**YES**	Pinkeye (bacterial conjunctivitis).	Your doctor will examine the child and prescribe treatment, if necessary. (See Warning.)
Is there a tender, red swelling on the edge of your child's eyelid? Any discharge or crusting?	**YES**	Sty (hordeolum).	Your doctor will examine the child, prescribe an antibiotic if necessary, and recommend other measures if advisable.
Does your child have a non-tender or slightly tender swelling within the eyelid?	**YES**	Inflamed meibomian gland (chalazion).	Try a warm compress several times a day. If swelling persists, consult your doctor.
Are your child's eyelids red and scaly? Are they crusted when he wakes up? Does he complain of burning or grittiness?	**YES**	Blepharitis (inflammation of the eyelid margins).	Consult your doctor, who will examine the child and prescribe any necessary measures to clean the lashes.
Has your child had an injury to the eye area? Is there bruising, bleeding, or swelling?	**YES**	Eye injury.	Consult your doctor; any injury to the sensitive eye area should be examined.
Are your child's eyelids swollen, red, and tender? Is it hard to open his eyes? Are they tearing? Does he have a fever? Is he generally unwell?	**YES**	Periorbital cellulitis (deep infection of the tissue around the eye).	Consult your doctor at once. Left untreated, this infection may cause serious, long-lasting damage. Your child may need to be hospitalized for intensive treatment.
Is your child's eye sensitive to light? Has she had joint pain or a rash? Has her eye been injured?	**YES**	Iritis (deep inflammation, not infection).	Your GP will examine your child and refer you to a specialist, if necessary.

Fireworks injuries: serious but preventable

Fireworks are among the most common causes of serious, preventable eye injuries. Most injuries occur around Bonfire Night. Most often those injured are bystanders, including children. Fireworks injuries are usually permanent and can cause partial or complete blindness.

The sale of fireworks is strictly controlled in the UK, and it is wise never to let children handle fireworks, except sparklers if they are old enough. Enjoy fireworks from a safe distance only at public displays conducted by professionals.

Fears

Phobias

IN GENERAL:

All healthy children have fears and worries; indeed, well defined fears mark different developmental stages. A baby as young as 5 months, for example, may become wary in the presence of a strange face. The vivid imagination of the pre-schooler is expressed in fears of the dark or monsters that have little to do – at least directly – with daily life. In normal school-age children, imaginary threats are replaced by more realistic fears such as bodily harm. In general, healthy fears stop children from taking unnecessary risks.

Children who are shy and withdrawn are more likely to develop marked fears than those who are outgoing. Girls are more likely than boys to develop the severe, irrational fears called phobias. Certain fears may grow out of parents' needs. After a divorce or the death of a spouse, for example, a parent may unwittingly encourage a child's separation anxiety out of a desire for companionship. And if parents are overprotective or fearful themselves, they may foster timidity and hamper a youngster's attempts to stretch his abilities.

Consult your doctor if your child's fears are:

- Interfering with family activities.
- Creating problems in making friends.
- Creating an excuse for not going to school.
- Disrupting normal sleep habits.
- Resulting in compulsive behaviour.

Warning

Although most childhood fears are not a reason for concern, some should alert parents to probe for a serious cause. A sudden, intense fear of a previously trusted person, for example, may stem from abuse. Don't dismiss seemingly irrational fears as just another phase; it may be a good idea to look for an underlying cause.

QUESTIONS TO CONSIDER	IF ANSWER IS	POSSIBLE CAUSE IS	ACTION TO TAKE
Is your 5- or 6-month-old less outgoing than before? Is she fretful when she sees a strange face? Does she cry when you leave the room?	YES	Normal development; stranger anxiety.	Your baby by now is strongly attached to you and her other regular care-givers. Make a special effort to reassure her among new people or surroundings. Children generally outgrow stranger anxiety by about age 1.
Does your toddler scream when he recognizes a familiar baby-sitter? Does he sob and try to hold you back as you leave the house?	YES	Separation anxiety; attention seeking.	Don't prolong your goodbyes; give the baby-sitter instructions away from your child. Have the baby-sitter engage your toddler's attention with a book or game. Assure your child that you'll be back soon and then leave quickly.
Does your baby often wake up and call for you at night? Is he between about 10 and 18 months old?	YES	Normal separation anxiety (which generally reaches a peak in this age group).	Quietly comfort your child and change his nappies if necessary. Put him back in his bed and stay until he is calm. Children usually settle down with reassurance. Nightly waking may continue for weeks or months.
Is your toddler or pre-schooler terrified by common events, such as thunder or noisy appliances?	YES	Normal fearfulness.	The fears will fade with time. Run noisy appliances during naptime or in a room away from your child. During storms, hold your child and talk calmly to show you're not afraid.

QUESTIONS TO CONSIDER	IF ANSWER IS	POSSIBLE CAUSE IS	ACTION TO TAKE
Does your pre-schooler refuse to get into the bath-tub or sit on the toilet?	**YES**	A still-developing sense of size and strength.	If your child is afraid of being flushed down the drain, he may prefer showers or sponge-baths. Let him use a child's toilet seat or a potty until he's more confident. Help him develop a sense of his size and strength.
Is your child abnormally fear-ful and withdrawn around people or in unfamiliar situations?	**YES**	Shyness (avoidant disorder).	Prepare for new experiences by talking about them, but be careful not to make your child apprehensive. Let your child take her time getting used to new situations.
Does your child adopt extreme delaying tactics or throw tantrums at bedtime?	**YES**	Fear of the dark; separation anxiety; fatigue; overstimulation.	Follow the same bedtime routine every night. Avoid rough play and overstimulation. Place nightlights to orient your child.
Does your pre-schooler scream about an hour after falling asleep? Is he unresponsive although his eyes are open?	**YES**	Night terrors (also see Convulsions, p. 50).	Quietly reassure your child. He won't respond; he's not awake. The terror may last half an hour or more, but eventually your child will settle back to sleep, and have no recall of the incident in the morning.
Does your pre-schooler wake up in the night, afraid and crying?	**YES**	Nightmare.	A pre-schooler may not understand the difference between dreams and real life. Reassure the child the dream wasn't real. Stay with her until she's calm.
Is your child refusing to go to school? Does she complain of severe but vague symptoms (headache, nausea, dizziness) to avoid school?	**YES**	School phobia (see below); separation anxiety; bullying and other school factors.	Your GP will rule out a physical cause and may recommend counselling. Consult your child's teachers to identify problems. Insist that your child attend school, but try to find solutions to specific problems.
Has your child developed fears or phobias after witnessing a violent event?	**YES**	Post-traumatic stress disorder.	Consult your doctor, who will evaluate the child's condition and may recommend counselling. (Also see Anxiety, p. 174.)

School reluctance/phobia

About 1 or 2 out of every 100 children become reluctant to go to school. Studies have shown that most are depressed, many have separation anxiety, and about half have both depression and anxiety. Some are overdependent, while others are adept at manipulating their parents. Either consciously or unconsciously, parents may foster reluctance.

School phobia usually appears between the first and fourth year, after an absence from school because of vacation or illness. A few children develop school phobia when they transfer from home schooling to school.

Children with school phobia need help before it undermines their education and socialization. Your GP may offer a plan or refer you to a family therapy centre. Treatment involves not only the child but also the school and the parents. Young children usually respond to a consistent approach. Treatment of adolescents may require a longer effort. Returning to school is a critical part of treatment.

Consult your GP if your child is:

- Losing or failing to gain weight.
- Gaining too much weight.

IN GENERAL:

When a child has a healthy attitude to food, eating is a natural response to hunger and meals are pleasant social occasions. The eating patterns we establish in our early years can influence our health and habits for a lifetime.

Sooner or later, most children go through a phase of fussy eating. (See Appetite Loss, p. 28). During this often nerve-wracking time, they seem to refuse every food that's put in front of them and resist efforts to persuade them to eat. At the opposite extreme are children who appear to lack any appetite control. Luckily, in most cases these minor feeding problems quickly pass. Severe feeding problems, however, can affect health.

According to health and diet experts, most feeding problems can be resolved if parents provide an appealing selection of healthy meals and snacks, and let children have as much or as little as they want.

Children need certain rules and boundaries in eating as in other aspects of their lives. When feeding is irregular and unreliable, it may make youngsters worry that they're not going to be taken care of. In contrast, some mothers use food as a pacifier, urging children to eat to ease any upset. Constant snacking not only upsets normal appetite controls, but can also lead to unwanted weight gain and poor eating habits.

Warning

If the dinner table is turning into a battleground, or you are worried that feeding problems may interfere with your child's growth, it's time to seek professional help. Talk over your concerns with your doctor or health specialist.

QUESTIONS TO CONSIDER	IF ANSWER IS	POSSIBLE CAUSE IS	ACTION TO TAKE
Is your baby under 6 months? Is she always restless and irritable? Is she breast fed? Is she failing to gain weight even though she empties the breast?	**YES**	Insufficient calorie intake.	Consult your doctor, who will examine your child and may recommend changes in her diet and/or your feeding method. (Also see Feeding Problems in Infants, p. 9).
Does your baby vomit after most feeds? Do you persist in feeding after your child has turned away? Have you been adding cereal to the bottle? Is your baby otherwise healthy?	**YES**	Overfeeding.	When your child avoids the bottle, he's telling you he has had enough. Babies take just as much as they need and may vomit if they're forced to drink more (vomiting is not the same as Spitting Up, p. 16). If vomiting continues even when less milk or formula is consumed, consult your GP or health visitor.

QUESTIONS TO CONSIDER	IF ANSWER IS	POSSIBLE CAUSE IS	ACTION TO TAKE
Does your baby refuse solid foods, even though your health visitor says it's time he had the extra calories? Is he about 4 to 6 months old?	**YES**	Normal transition to solid foods.	Be patient, and continue breast- or bottle-feeding. Stop solids if attempts at solid feeding are upsetting the baby and you. When you try again, alternate milk and solids so the baby associates a feeling of satisfaction with the sensation of spoon-feeding.
Does your 1-year-old leave most of the food on her plate? Is she drinking less? Is she otherwise happy and energetic?	**YES**	Normal appetite decrease as the growth rate slows down.	Give smaller portions, with second helpings only if your child asks for them. This slowing down of the appetite is a normal stage in development, not a feeding problem.
Is your school-age child still eating like a picky toddler?	**YES**	Unsatisfactory eating habits.	Keep your child on a regular (but not rigid) schedule for meals and sleep. Avoid overstimulating games and entertainment around mealtime and bedtime. Avoid excessive snacking, especially in the hour or two before meals.
Is your child always eating? Does he hoard food? Or is he constantly snacking between meals? Is his weight noticeably more than it should be for his height and build?	**YES**	Anxiety; stress; overeating; poor impulse control.	Discuss your concerns with your doctor. Prepare regular meals and snacks, with normal portions of foods moderate in calories (but not 'diet' foods). Encourage exercise and activities to take your youngster's mind off food.

A common-sense approach to feeding your child

Your child will eat right if you keep to the following guidelines:

- Respect your child's likes and dislikes.
- Offer modest servings, with second helpings if your child asks for more.
- Time snacks so they don't interfere with meals.
- Don't use food as a bribe or reward.
- Learn to recognize when your child is asking for food but really wants your attention.
- Resist serving meals and snacks while children are watching television, listening to stories, or absorbed in play. This can lead to overeating from habit.
- Don't get upset when your child eats everything one day and almost nothing the next; appetites can vary.
- Plan menus with attention to likes and dislikes, but don't be a short-order cook.

Fever

Pyrexia

In General:

Fever – an increase in body temperature – is one of the body's defences against outside attacks, such as infections. Less commonly, fever may indicate the presence of an internal threat, such as an auto-immune disorder. Normal temperature is not a single number but a range: 36° to 38°C, or 97° to 100.4°F. It also varies according to time of day, age, general health, and physical activity. Mild illness may push the temperature up a notch, but most doctors do not consider that a child has fever unless it climbs above 38°C (100.4°F).

Most fevers are caused by illness that isn't dangerous, but fever in a child who is under 3 months (see p. 10) or who has a condition such as sickle cell anaemia or immune suppression should be promptly investigated. In a few young children, fever can cause a febrile seizure (see Convulsions, p. 50), which, while frightening for parents, does not result in serious problems. A doctor should always examine a child after the first febrile seizure, however, to make sure that the cause is not a more serious condition. Youngsters generally outgrow febrile seizures by about age 6.

Sponging with tepid water and giving paracetamol or ibuprofen to reduce the temperature may make the child more comfortable and prevent dehydration from excessive sweating, but doesn't alter the course of an illness. A temperature of 40.5°C (105°F) or higher, however, is potentially serious. If your child has a high fever, call your doctor and take steps to reduce the temperature.

☎

Consult your doctor if your child has a fever along with any of the following:

- Age 3 months or under. (See p. 10.)
- Ill appearance, unusual drowsiness, or severe headache, regardless of age.
- Persistently ill appearance after the temperature has been brought down.
- Delirium, hallucinations.
- Refusal to drink.
- Underlying disorder or treatment affecting the immune system.
- Travel outside the country during the previous 8 weeks.

Warning

Never give aspirin to reduce fever in a child. The use of aspirin has been linked to an increased risk of Reye syndrome – a rare but serious disease affecting the brain and liver – following viral infections. Paracetamol or ibuprofen will help to reduce fever and make your child more comfortable. Don't exceed the recommended dose by giving a cold medication that also contains paracetamol. Do not give paracetamol or any other medication to a baby under 3 months without your doctor's advice.

Questions to consider	**If answer is**	**Possible cause is**	**Action to take**
Does your child also have a cough, runny nose, breathing difficulties, sore throat, and/or muscle aches?	**YES**	Common cold; influenza; other respiratory infection.	Call your doctor, who may examine your child and will advise you how to make her comfortable.
Is there a rash? Does your child also have a sore throat and/or swollen glands?	**YES**	Chickenpox; other viral illness.	Your doctor will see your child to diagnose the infection and recommend treatment accordingly.

QUESTIONS TO CONSIDER	IF ANSWER IS	POSSIBLE CAUSE IS	ACTION TO TAKE
Is your child dizzy, with pain or ringing in his ear? Is there a discharge from the ear?	YES	Ear infection.	Consult your GP. An ear infection may need to be treated. (See Earache/Ear Infection, p. 68.)
Does your child have swollen glands and a sore throat?	YES	Tonsillitis; streptococcal or viral infection; mononucleosis (glandular fever).	Consult your GP, who will determine the cause of the fever and recommend treatment.
Does your child have pain or burning on urination? Does she have abdominal pain?	YES	Urinary tract infection.	Your GP will examine the child and, if necessary, prescribe antibiotic treatment. If possible, take a urine specimen.
Does your child have nausea and/or vomiting, with diarrhoea and cramps?	YES	Infectious gastroenteritis (viral or bacterial).	Give your child clear drinks but no food for a few hours. If symptoms don't improve in 12 hours, call your doctor.
Is your under-5 irritable, lethargic, and feverish? Does she have a stomachache? Swollen glands in the neck? A rash, with reddened lips and tongue? Conjunctivitis? Are her hands and feet swollen?	YES	Kawasaki disease, with fever and inflammation affecting the blood vessels (also called mucocutaneous lymph node syndrome).	Call your doctor. The cause of this unusual disease is unknown, but your doctor will refer your child to a paediatric specialist straightaway.
Does your child also have vague symptoms such as fatigue and joint pains? Is there a rash?	YES	Lyme disease.	Your GP will examine the child and, if Lyme disease is suspected, order blood tests. Antibiotic treatment may be necessary.
Has your child been feverish for 5 days or longer?	YES	Condition requiring diagnosis and treatment.	Consult your GP for an examination.

Fever: a symptom not a sickness

Body temperature is controlled by a part of the brain called the hypothalamus, which balances signals from heat- and cold-sensitive receptors throughout the nervous system. Among the factors that influence temperature are infections; vaccines and medications; injury; inflammatory, auto-immune, and glandular disorders; and tumours. The temperature also rises with exercise or following prolonged exposure to heat.

In general, if a child with mild fever is older than 3 months, seems well, and has no other symptoms, treatment isn't required. But you should keep a close watch and be prepared to call your doctor in case new symptoms emerge.

Many doctors believe that fever may actually help to shorten the course of infections by activating the immune system. It's more important to find the cause of the fever and eradicate it than to get rid of the fever itself.

In General:

Fractures – breaks in the normal structure of the bone – are common injuries among children under 12. They can be very serious, with the bone broken in several places or pushing through the skin (so-called compound fracture). Less serious fractures, seen more often in children, involve a slight crack in the bone or a buckle (bulge) on the edge of the bone. Broken bones generally cause fewer problems in youngsters than in adults, because children's bones are more flexible and better able to absorb shock. They also heal faster than adults' bones.

Children's pliable bones often break in a greenstick fracture, in which the bone bends like green wood with a break only on one side, or in a buckle (torus) fracture, where the bone buckles on one side but is not separated.

Youngsters are vulnerable to one type of fracture that is not seen in mature bones. In children, fractures may damage the growth plates at the ends of the bones and cause the bones to grow improperly or not at all. That is why your child should have regular follow-up visits, especially for growth plate fractures, for at least a year after a fracture.

Most childhood fractures need only to be kept free of movement long enough for the bone to grow back together. A moulded cast of plaster or fibreglass is the usual treatment; surgical repair is seldom necessary. A little knot of bone, called a callus, forms over the fracture as a normal part of the healing process. Occasionally, it can be felt beneath the skin. It requires no treatment and will eventually get smaller and disappear.

☎

Call your GP or the orthopaedic surgeon treating your child's fracture if you note any of the following:

- Redness, swelling, and inflammation in the affected limb.
- Temperature over 38°C (100.4°F).
- Toes (for a leg cast) or fingers (for an arm cast) turning blue or pale, becoming painful or numb, or swelling.
- Increased pain in the fractured limb.
- Inability to wiggle the toes or fingers of the affected limb.
- The cast breaking or loosening, or the plaster getting wet or soggy.

Warning

Don't try to move a child who has broken her leg or suffered some other serious fracture (see Fractures, p. 217). Call 999 and make your child as comfortable as possible while you are waiting.

Questions to consider	If answer is	Possible cause is	Action to take
Did your child have a severe blow to the head or face? Is her nose swollen, crooked, and painful?	**YES**	Fracture of facial bones; broken nose.	Place a cold compress over the nose or other painful area to reduce pain and swelling. Call your doctor at once for further instructions.
Is your child having difficulty breathing following a fall or other accident? Does she have chest pain?	**YES**	Broken rib.	Take your child to the nearest hospital emergency department.
Is your toddler limping or refusing to walk? Is he guarding a painful limb?	**YES**	Fracture; sprain.	Call your doctor without delay for an examination, x-rays, and treatment, if necessary.

QUESTIONS TO CONSIDER	IF ANSWER IS	POSSIBLE CAUSE IS	ACTION TO TAKE
Is your active teenager limping? Does he have tenderness, but no bruising, over the shins?	**YES**	Shin splints or other stress injury.	Call your GP, who will examine the child and prescribe appropriate treatment. Rest may be advisable.
Does your child have swelling and pain at the site following injury to any bony part of the body, including fingers or toes?	**YES**	Fracture.	Call your GP, who will examine the child, order x-rays if advisable, and recommend any necessary treatment.
Has your child injured his head? Is there blood or clear fluid leaking from his nose or ears?	**YES**	Skull fracture.	Call 999 at once, or take your child to the nearest hospital emergency department.

Preventing childhood fractures

Many broken bones in youngsters could be prevented if parents always paid attention to the following simple safety measures:

- Never leave a baby unattended on a changing table or bed.
- When driving, always place children in well secured car seats in the rear seat.
- Don't start the car until all seat belts are fastened.
- Make sure your children wear any necessary protective gear when playing sports.
- Never allow your child to rollerskate, ride a bicycle, or go in-line skating or skateboarding without a helmet.

Types of fracture

*In a **displaced** or **compound fracture**, the broken ends of the bone must be realigned; a segment of bone may penetrate through the soft tissue and skin. In a **greenstick fracture**, the break is on only one side of the bone. A **simple fracture** breaks through but does not displace the bone sections.*

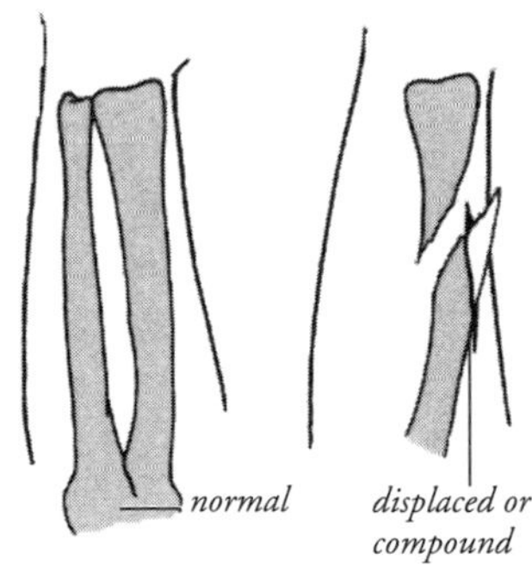

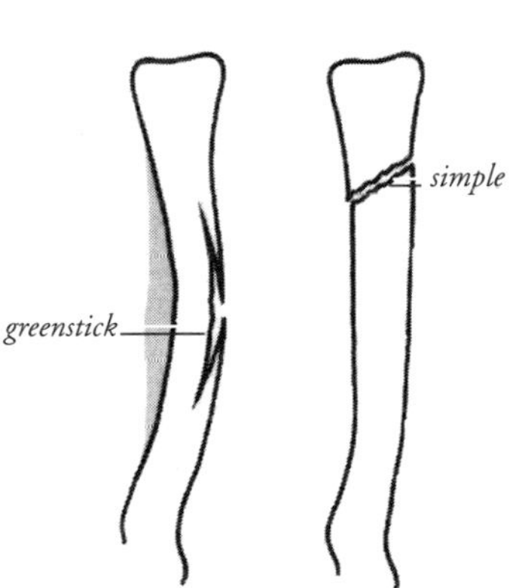

In General:

On average, normal pre-schoolers get six to eight colds and other upper respiratory infections a year, as well as at least two bouts of diarrhoea and vomiting. This phase gradually passes. Infection rates drop dramatically after children reach age 3 and their immune systems mature. It's not unusual, however, for a school-age child to have several colds, a skin infection (for example, impetigo) or conjunctivitis, and two or three viral stomach infections over the course of a year.

Children are more likely to develop an infection if they have breaks in the skin that let germs enter. Acute illnesses temporarily interfere with the immune system, and youngsters with chronic diseases such as cystic fibrosis or asthma have high rates of infections of the airways. Those undergoing treatments that temporarily suppress immunity, such as chemotherapy for tumours, need protection against infections until they can rebuild their defences.

A very small number of children often get sick because they have little resistance to infections. Some have an illness that temporarily affects their immune defences. Others have recurrent infections as a result of a rare inherited problem. Because their immune systems lack one or more components, these children fail to develop immunity to particular groups of germs. Treatment with a missing component, when it can be identified, may help to fight off infections.

Consult your GP if your child has any of the following:

- Recurrent fever with temperatures over 39°C (102°F).
- Frequently recurring boils or other symptoms of skin infection.
- Frequent sore throats, with or without a runny nose and cough.
- Three or more ear infections in a year.

Warning

If your GP prescribes a liquid antibiotic, use a calibrated measuring spoon or syringe to make sure your child gets the right dose. It's important to continue the medication for the time prescribed, even if symptoms seem to have cleared up after a day or two. Stopping an antibiotic before all the germs are eradicated can encourage the development of strains that are resistant to treatment with that medication.

Questions to consider	If answer is	Possible cause is	Action to take
Does your child constantly have a runny nose, coughing, hoarseness, and sneezing? Is his throat always sore? Does he sleep poorly? Does he often get headaches?	**YES**	Upper respiratory infections; hay fever (allergic rhinitis); sinusitis. (Also see Allergic Reactions, p. 26; Runny/Stuffy Nose, p. 126.)	Consult your doctor, who will examine the child and may perform diagnostic tests. Your doctor will recommend a plan to treat the symptoms and help prevent future bouts.
Does your child cough constantly? Does she wheeze, especially at night? Does she have trouble sleeping? Is she growing slowly?	**YES**	Asthma (also see Breathing Difficulty/ Breathlessness, p. 44); cystic fibrosis.	Consult your doctor, who will evaluate the child, perform diagnostic tests, and recommend treatment according to the results.

QUESTIONS TO CONSIDER	IF ANSWER IS	POSSIBLE CAUSE IS	ACTION TO TAKE
Has your child had more than three ear infections in the past year?	**YES**	Chronic middle-ear infection. (Also see p. 68.)	Check with your doctor, who may recommend preventive treatment or a consultation with an ear-nose-throat specialist.
Has your child had several attacks of boils, or infections around the fingernails?	**YES**	Recurrent skin infection; increased susceptibility to certain bacteria.	Consult your doctor, who will evaluate the child and prescribe treatment. If attacks are recurrent and severe, your doctor may order diagnostic tests.
Does your child often cough up thick mucus? Are his stools pale and foul smelling? Is he lethargic? Growing poorly?	**YES**	Cystic fibrosis or other condition requiring diagnosis and treatment.	Consult your doctor, who will examine the child and perform diagnostic tests.
Is your child pale and tired? Does she have fevers that come and go? Does she have fevers and sweats at night? Are her glands swollen?	**YES**	Blood disorder or other condition requiring diagnosis and treatment.	Consult your doctor for an examination and diagnostic tests.
Has your infant had thrush several times? Are his bowel movements pale and foul smelling? Is he irritable? Is he growing slowly?	**YES**	Malabsorption disorder or immune disorder requiring diagnosis.	Call your doctor promptly for an evaluation and diagnostic tests.
Has your child had numerous infections, such as pneumonia, blood infection, or meningitis? Is he growing poorly?	**YES**	Immune disorder requiring evaluation and treatment.	Consult your doctor, who will review the child's history, evaluate his condition, and possibly order tests to evaluate his immune system.

Inborn immune defects

True immune defects are rare. Most are passed from mothers to sons and are more common, therefore, in boys, although girls also are affected. In one type of immune defect, the lymphatic system (see p. 147) fails to produce enough protective antibodies. As a result, the body lacks resistance, especially to bacteria. In the second type, the body doesn't have enough lymphocytes (the white cells that engulf and kill invading germs) or the lymphocytes fail to do their job. The result is that the body cannot fight fungi, viruses, and the germs that cause tuberculosis. Some people have both defects at once.

With certain immune problems, the child develops the proper levels of protective cells or antibodies by adolescence and loses his susceptibility to infections. When antibodies are lacking, injection of donor antibodies can boost resistance. In special situations, long-term antibiotic treatment can also help protect against infections. In extremely rare cases, severe immune defects make children vulnerable to infections by germs that do not normally cause disease. Some of these children can be helped with bone marrow transplants and other treatments. The most severely affected are the 'bubble children', who have to live in germ-free domes, isolated from all outside contact.

In General:

Heredity, nutrition, and general health determine how tall a child will grow. Most children who are either tall or short do not have a growth disorder; they are simply growing the way they were genetically programmed. Parents often are surprised to learn that their baby's size at birth does not predict his likely adult height. At every physical examination, however, starting with the first one after birth, your doctor or health visitor will measure your baby's length (height) and weight, as well as the size of his head during the first year, to make sure he's growing at an appropriate rate. Nutrition is important to growth, and if a child takes in far too few calories, development and growth may be slowed. Picky eaters, however, usually have a normal growth rate even when they seem to eat very little.

It doesn't matter if your child is larger or smaller than others of the same age, as long as he's keeping to a steady rate of growth. Your health visitor will share your child's progress by showing his growth curves to you at each visit. Sometimes youngsters who are small for their age throughout childhood have a delayed growth spurt and end up taller than many of their friends.

Consult your doctor if your child:

- Either loses or fails to gain weight.
- Seems to be gaining too much weight.

Warning

Studies have shown that youngsters who are sedentary – spending too much time in front of the television or otherwise inactive – have poorer bone development than those who get plenty of physical activity. Children grow best when they exercise regularly.

QUESTIONS TO CONSIDER	IF ANSWER IS	POSSIBLE CAUSE IS	ACTION TO TAKE
Is your infant or toddler either losing or failing to gain weight? Is his growth rate slow?	**YES**	Failure to thrive; various causes.	Consult your doctor, who will measure and examine the child and review with you his diet, medical history, and other factors that may affect growth and weight gain. Your doctor will suggest an appropriate treatment plan.
Is your child healthy, but somewhat shorter than most others his age? Is he growing at a normal rate?	**YES**	Normal short stature.	Discuss your concerns with your doctor at your child's next regular checkup. Compare your child's growth with the ranges of height and build in both parents' families. Make sure your child gets a variety of food and plenty of exercise. Don't worry about his height.
Is your child exceptionally small for his age? Is he growing at a slow rate?	**YES**	Growth hormone deficiency; acquired hypothyroidism (underactive thyroid gland).	Consult your doctor, who will examine the child and may refer him for consultation with an endocrinologist.
Is your child exceptionally tall for her age? Is she normally proportioned and healthy?	**YES**	Tall stature.	Make sure your child eats a good diet and exercises well. Foster her self-confidence so that she maintains good posture. Discuss any concerns with your doctor.

QUESTIONS TO CONSIDER	IF ANSWER IS	POSSIBLE CAUSE IS	ACTION TO TAKE
Has your child been growing poorly or not at all since a bout of fairly severe illness?	**YES**	Slowing of growth due to illness.	Make sure your child has a selection of healthy foods and regular exercise. Consult your doctor if your child's appetite and growth rate do not return a few weeks after recovery or starting treatment.
Does your child have a chronic condition, such as inflammatory bowel disease or a thyroid or kidney disorder? Or was a chromosomal abnormality detected at birth?	**YES**	Systemic condition affecting growth.	Consult your doctor to make sure that your child is eating the right types of food and getting enough calories. Provide opportunities for regular exercise. Your doctor will also determine whether treatment is needed for the underlying condition.
Is your child exceptionally tall and slender? Does he have unusually long, thin arms, legs, fingers, and toes? Is he loose-jointed? Is his muscular development slow, although his mental development is fine?	**YES**	Marfan's syndrome, an inborn disease causing skeletal and possibly heart abnormalities.	Consult your doctor, who will examine the child and judge whether consultation with a specialist is needed.
Has your pre-schooler or school-age child abruptly started growing unusually fast? Do his head, hands, and jaw look disproportionately large? Have his features become coarser looking?	**YES**	Excessive levels of growth hormone due to an underlying condition.	Consult your doctor, who will examine the child and determine whether a consultation with a specialist is advisable.

Coping with growth disorders

When growth is excessive, the cause is usually a pituitary tumour releasing surges of growth hormone that particularly stimulates the growth of the long (arm and leg) bones and jaw. The condition can be treated with surgery, medications, or irradiation.

At the opposite end of the scale, inadequate levels of growth hormone cause a child to be unusually small. If a true growth hormone deficiency is diagnosed, hormone treatment during the growing years can help the child reach an acceptable adult height. This treatment is reserved for children with proven glandular (hormonal) problems. Paediatricians do not advise treating a healthy, short child with growth hormone just to make him taller.

Children may be abnormally small because they were exposed to an infection, drugs, or alcohol while in the womb; have chromosomal disorders; or were extremely premature. In almost all cases, these problems are detected before birth or just afterwards, and appropriate treatment is begun.

Occasionally, children adopted from overseas may have malnutrition resulting in decreased growth and delayed development. They need special help and more calories than normal to catch up to a level appropriate for their age. Adoption agencies can put you in touch with support groups for parents in similar situations, and your doctor will help you with advice and recommendations.

Hair Loss

Alopoecia

In General:

Within weeks or months of birth, a baby's first, fine hair is replaced by thicker hair, usually in a different colour. The practice of shaving a baby's head, traditional in some cultures, does not make the hair grow thicker or faster. Older children may lose their hair because of inflammation or infection, overstyling, medical treatment, or illness. Children's hair can be damaged by exposure to chemicals such as dyes and permanents or chlorine in swimming pools.

Your children's pattern of hair growth is part of their genetic package. If the hair is thin and dull, you can't make it grow full and lustrous. You can, however, help your youngster find a becoming style and shampoo the hair frequently to keep it in good condition.

Consult your doctor if your child has inexplicable hair loss along with:

- Fatigue.
- A red rash across the bridge of the nose.
- Fever or other symptoms of illness.
- Patches of inexplicable hair loss, including lashes and eyebrows.

Warning

Use a soft brush of natural or nylon bristles; hard bristles can break the hair and irritate the scalp.

Questions to consider	If answer is	Possible cause is	Action to take
Is your baby only a few weeks or months old? Is his hair falling out?	**YES**	Normal loss of baby hair (telogen effluvium).	Baby hair is gradually replaced by mature hair. Wash your baby's scalp frequently and use a soft hairbrush daily. If there's no sign of hair by 12 months, talk to your doctor.
Does your baby have a bald spot at the back or side of her scalp?	**YES**	Loss of baby hair caused by rubbing or lying in one position.	New hair will cover the spot as your baby becomes mobile. Changing your baby's position frequently can help. If several bald patches appear or the scalp is irritated, consult your doctor.
Does your baby have greasy, crusty patches on the scalp?	**YES**	Cradle cap (seborrheic dermatitis).	Wash the scalp frequently with a mild shampoo and gently towel-dry. Rub with baby oil or petroleum jelly before washing to help lift the crusts. If crusts are extensive, your GP may prescribe a cream.
Is your toddler or school-age child losing hair in round, scaly patches? Is his scalp itchy?	**YES**	Ringworm (tinea capitis).	Consult your GP, who will examine the child and prescribe antifungal medication if appropriate.
Is the loss especially noticeable around your child's hairline? Does she wear plaits or a ponytail? Does she use hot rollers or hair straightener, or have a permanent wave?	**YES**	Damage due to overstyling (traction) or chemicals.	Change your child's hairstyle to prevent damage from tight pulling. Avoid using chemical treatments such as dyes, straighteners, and perms. Use a mild shampoo and don't use a hair dryer.

QUESTIONS TO CONSIDER	IF ANSWER IS	POSSIBLE CAUSE IS	ACTION TO TAKE
Has your child lost a lot of hair following an illness with fever?	**YES**	Interruption of the hair growth cycle (telogen effluvium).	The hair usually grows back within 6 months, but bring the hair loss to your doctor's attention. (See Coping with hair loss, below.)
Does your pre-schooler or school-age child have dandruff? Do any members of the family have psoriasis or seborrheic dermatitis?	**YES**	Psoriasis; seborrheic dermatitis.	Consult your doctor, who will examine the child and refer you to a skin specialist (dermatologist) if necessary.
Does your child pull or twist her hair? Does she twist her hair while she sucks her thumb?	**YES**	Hair pulling (trichotillomania), sometimes related to stress.	Ask your doctor how to deal with this problem. Try to identify and remove sources of stress.
Has your child been diagnosed with an auto-immune disorder? Does he have Down's syndrome?	**YES**	Hair loss due to a chronic disorder.	Ask your doctor's advice for helping your child deal with the emotional stress of hair loss.
Is your physically maturing teenager losing his or her hair? Are family members on either side bald?	**YES**	Hereditary male-pattern baldness.	There is no proven treatment for baldness; medication is only partly effective. Help your child accept his or her hair loss and find attractive cosmetic solutions.
Is your older child or teenager losing clumps of hair?	**YES**	Alopoecia areata, related in rare cases to an auto-immune condition or stress.	Consult your doctor. In most cases, the hair eventually grows back. There is no proven, universal cure, although corticosteroid lotion is sometimes used.
Is your child being treated with irradiation or chemotherapy for a serious illness?	**YES**	Effects of treatment (toxic alopoecia; anagen effluvium).	The hair will grow back within 2 to 3 months of stopping the treatment. In the meantime, provide head coverings such as a scarf or cap. A particularly sensitive child might prefer a wig.

Coping with hair loss

Occasionally, a child suddenly loses hair in patches. The cause of this condition, called alopoecia areata, is unknown although other family members also have it in about a quarter of the cases. An auto-immune disorder is rarely present, and most youngsters with alopoecia areata are otherwise healthy. No predictable, safe, and effective treatment has been developed, but in most cases, the hair grows back within 6 to 12 months. Your doctor may refer you to a dermatologist. Treatment may involve topical corticosteroids or other medications. The condition may recur.

Headache

Cephalalgia

In General:

The three recurring pain symptoms that doctors most often see are stomachache, earache, and headache. Usually, headaches occur as a result of viral illness. In more than 90 percent of cases, the doctor can identify the cause of the headache with a physical examination and a review of the child's medical history. Extensive tests are seldom needed, and only in rare cases does headache signal a serious condition. Most headaches disappear with rest, food if the child is hungry, and the end of a viral illness. Paracetamol or ibuprofen can relieve pain.

Warning

If your child has frequent headaches, wakes up with a headache, has a sudden severe headache, or has vomiting as well, bring it to the attention of your doctor. Most recurrent headaches are benign; however, your doctor may want to rule out an underlying disorder.

Call your doctor if your child has a headache and any of the following symptoms:

- Unusual drowsiness.
- Reluctance to bend the neck forward.
- Repeated awakening with a headache but without other signs of illness.
- Irritability.
- Refusal to drink.
- Temperature higher than 39°C (102°F).
- Vomiting but no diarrhoea.
- Muscular weakness or loss of coordination.

Questions to consider	**If answer is**	**Possible cause is**	**Action to take**
Did your toddler have a bump or fall, but not lose consciousness?	**YES**	Mild trauma (serious injury is very rare with typical toddler falls and collisions).	Comfort your toddler and encourage him to nap; try a dose of paracetamol or ibuprofen. If sleep doesn't relieve the pain and upset, and the headache lasts for several hours or gets worse, call your doctor.
Is your child feverish and unwell? Does she have a sore throat, runny nose, or other symptoms?	**YES**	Common cold; streptococcal throat infection; other respiratory infection.	Headache often adds to the general sense of being unwell during infectious illness,. Consult your GP, who will perform diagnostic tests and prescribe treatment.
Does your child also have pain in the face and jaw? Is his nose runny? Is he tired and irritable?	**YES**	Sinusitis; dental problem.	Call your GP, who will examine the child and, if appropriate, prescribe treatment for sinusitis (see p. 127). She will advise you to call your child's dentist if a tooth is causing the pain. (See Dental Problems, p. 56.)
Does your child complain of a dull, nonthrobbing headache that feels like a tight band around his head?	**YES**	Tension headache possibly linked to emotional stress.	Give paracetamol for occasional headaches, but if they occur frequently consult your doctor. Try to uncover and remove sources of emotional stress.

Cephalalgia

QUESTIONS TO CONSIDER	IF ANSWER IS	POSSIBLE CAUSE IS	ACTION TO TAKE
Does your child complain of head pain when she has ice cream, chilled drinks, or other cold foods?	**YES**	Cold-foods headache (sensitive nerve); tooth sensitivity.	Some people get head pain when cold food touches the soft palate. The condition is harmless and wears off without treatment. If it's bothersome, avoid cold foods.
Does your child get headaches when reading or doing close work? Does she blink or squint a lot? Does she have neck and shoulder pain when working at a desk?	**YES**	Eyestrain; furniture needing adjustment; poorly placed computer screen.	Have your child's vision checked by an optometrist (optician). Adjustments to your child's regular work-station may also be required.
Does your child have a temperature over 39°C (102°F)? Is he sleepy and irritable? Is his neck stiff and sore? Does light hurt his eyes?	**YES**	Meningitis or another infection requiring urgent treatment.	Call your doctor at once. Bacterial meningitis is much less common since the introduction of the Hib vaccine, but your doctor will want to examine your child.
Is your child having severe and increasingly frequent headaches? Are they worse when she lies down, or on waking? Is she clumsy or walking oddly? Is she vomiting? Does the headache awaken her?	**YES**	Tumour.	Call your doctor without delay. Tests and referral to a paediatric neurologist or neurosurgeon may be needed to identify the cause of the headache.

Migraine headaches in children

Your child may have migraine if she gets recurrent headaches with symptom-free intervals and has at least three of the following features: throbbing head pain, usually on one side; nausea and/or vomiting; abdominal pain; a visual or sensory aura (such as blurring or flashes of light, or numbness of the hands and feet); relief of headache following sleep; and a family history of migraine.

Most migraine attacks in children are not severe and can be easily managed. More than half of childhood migraine sufferers stop having attacks at about age 10.

Attacks may be triggered by hormonal changes, food sensitivity (true food allergy is rare, see p. 27), stress, and other factors. If your child has symptoms suggesting migraine, your GP will recommend a treatment plan. Keeping a migraine diary can help a child identify and thus avoid migraine triggers. At the first sign of an attack, your child should rest in a quiet, darkened room. Paracetamol or ibuprofen is usually effective in relieving headache. In most cases, children with migraine have fewer, less severe headaches once they have been examined by a doctor and reassured that they do not have a serious condition.

In General:

A pronounced loss of hearing, or deafness, raises a barrier to communication that interferes with every aspect of a child's development. There are two main types of hearing loss. In the first, called conduction deafness, structural problems in the outer or middle ear block the transmission of sound. Common causes of conduction deafness are infections, injury, and wax buildup. Many children with this type of deafness can be helped by treatment for infection, or surgery or other measures to remove a blockage. The second type, sensori-neural hearing loss, may be inborn or caused by illness. Most people with sensori-neural deafness benefit to some degree from hearing aids.

In about half the cases of childhood sensori-neural deafness the cause is genetic, although deafness that runs in the family may not show up until later in life. Children are sometimes born deaf; in some cases because their mothers had a viral infection (German measles or rubella, for example) or took certain medications (such as the antibiotic streptomycin) during pregnancy.

Babies are usually tested for their response to sound at birth, and your health visitor will evaluate your youngster's hearing at regular checkups. Paediatricians recommend specialized testing for premature infants, those with a family history of deafness, and others at high risk for hearing impairment. Sensitive instruments can be used to measure hearing in babies under 3 months of age, often while the baby is sleeping. When needed, a hearing aid can be fitted before a baby reaches 6 months.

Wherever possible, hearing-impaired children should be educated with those who hear and speak normally. The best results are achieved with an approach that includes a combination of hearing aids, speech training, lip-reading, and sign language.

The cochlear implant, an electronic replacement for the inner ear, is a new treatment for severe hearing loss. This treatment remains controversial. The device is implanted surgically to carry the auditory signal. It can help many who are too deaf to use hearing aids but still retain some function in the auditory nerve. As with other treatments for deafness, the younger the child who receives an implant, the better the results are likely to be. For now, cochlear implants are performed only in children aged 2 years and older, but are under study in younger children.

Consult your GP if your child:

- Responds to your speech only when he can see your face.
- Is not speaking or making sounds appropriate to his age level.
- Doesn't seem to hear certain sounds.
- Cannot understand what's said on television or radio unless the volume is very high.

Warning

Always call your doctor if your child complains of ear pain. Left untreated, infections of the ears can cause permanent hearing loss.

Questions to consider	If answer is	Possible cause is	Action to take
Does your baby turn her head when you call? Does she respond when you clap, even when she's not looking at you?	**NO**	Hearing impairment.	Call your doctor without delay. After testing the child's hearing, the doctor may recommend consultation with a specialist, if necessary.

QUESTIONS TO CONSIDER	IF ANSWER IS	POSSIBLE CAUSE IS	ACTION TO TAKE
Does your baby of 6 or 7 months babble and imitate the tone of your voice? Does he respond to the sounds around him?	**NO**	Partial or complete hearing loss.	Consult your GP. She will test your baby's hearing and provide referral to a specialist, if needed.
Has your child been less responsive since having an ear infection?	**YES**	Fluid buildup following middle ear infection (otitis media with effusion).	Consult your GP, who will examine the child and provide appropriate treatment. If the problem persists, your GP may refer your child to an ENT specialist.
Has your child gradually become hard of hearing?	**YES**	Blockage of ear by foreign body or wax buildup.	Consult your GP, who will examine the ear, using a lighted instrument called an otoscope, and remove the blockage. Don't try to remove wax or other material yourself; you may force it farther in and injure the ear.
Has your child had an injury to the ear?	**YES**	Trauma; perforated ear drum.	Consult your GP, who will examine the ear and treat the child appropriately.
Has your child been hard of hearing since taking a recent plane journey or a roller-coaster ride?	**YES**	Injury due to change in ear/air pressure (barotrauma).	Hearing loss due to pressure change usually clears up by itself. If there's no improvement in 2 or 3 days, call your GP.
Does your child get severely dizzy and lose his balance? Does he have attacks of nausea and vomiting? Does he complain of ringing in the ears (tinnitus)?	**YES**	Neurological disorder.	Consult your GP, who will examine the child to determine whether he needs treatment.

Preventing injury from headphones

Children and teenagers often prefer to listen to music through headphones linked to a radio, stereo, or portable tape player. Kept at a volume similar to normal speech, headphones may do no harm. But if youngsters turn up the volume to block out external noise, they subject their ears to an assault that can cause permanent hearing loss. If others in the room can hear sound while the child is wearing headphones, the volume is at an unsafe level and should be turned down. Some experts believe there is no safe way to use headphones. They contend that one of the best ways to protect the hearing is not to use headphones at all.

Never allow your child to wear a portable headset while walking, skating, or cycling. Not only does it block out warning noises, but the risk is all the greater because the youngster concentrates on the music and is not alert to traffic and other potentially dangerous situations.

Heartbeat Irregularities

Cardiac arrhythmias, dysrhythmias

In General:

The heart is divided into four chambers: the left and right atria at the top, and the left and right ventricles on the bottom. These chambers are separated by valves that keep the blood moving through the heart in the proper direction, and the muscular walls of the chambers contract in rhythm to keep the heart efficiently pumping blood. The muscle contractions are triggered by electrical impulses from a group of cells in the right atrium, called the sinus, or sinoatrial, node. Each electrical impulse that powers a heartbeat arises in the sinus node, flows through the left and right atrial walls, and is relayed through a second group of pacemaker cells – the atrioventricular node – to the ventricles. An error at any stage of the conduction system may result in a disturbance of the heartbeat pattern known as the sinus rhythm.

At birth, a baby's heart beats as often as 120 to 140 times a minute, increasing to more than 170 with crying and slowing to between 70 and 90 during sleep. The very rapid newborn rate gradually slows, but the normal childhood range of heartbeats remains quite wide: from 70 to 100 per minute and averaging between 75 and 80. The rate speeds up during exercise and slows at rest. Adolescents in advanced athletic training may have a resting heart rate of only 40 to 50 beats a minute.

Minor variations in children's heart rate and rhythm, called arrhythmias or dysrhythmias, occur for many reasons. Occasional palpitations (strongly felt heartbeats) or flutterings are common and usually harmless. In most cases, a slight irregularity in the basic sinus rhythm is of no consequence; certain irregularities and patterns, however, may indicate a disorder and must be investigated. A change in rhythm is dangerous only when it is so pronounced and prolonged that it interferes with the heart's ability to pump blood efficiently. In the rare cases where treatment is necessary, the heartbeat can be regulated by medication or the use of an electric pacemaker for a time. Some cases may be treated surgically.

Call your doctor immediately if your child has a change in heart rhythm together with any of the following:

- Breathing difficulty.
- Chest pain.
- Dizziness, light-headedness, or pallor.
- Confusion.
- Loss of consciousness.

Warning

If the heartbeat is unusually slow or remains fast over a prolonged period, the change may be significant and should be brought to your doctor's attention.

Questions to consider	If answer is	Possible cause is	Action to take
Does your child's heartbeat seem irregular? Does it speed up when she breathes in, and slow down when she breathes out? Does her heart often 'skip a beat'? Is she otherwise well and active?	**YES**	Sinus arrhythmia, a normal variation in heart rate. The irregularity may be more noticeable after an illness with fever or during treatment with certain medications.	If the irregularity is worrying you, bring it to your doctor's attention. A simple examination will show whether further testing, such as an electrocardiogram (ECG or EKG), is needed.

Cardiac arrhythmias, dysrhythmias

QUESTIONS TO CONSIDER	IF ANSWER IS	POSSIBLE CAUSE IS	ACTION TO TAKE
Does your new baby's pulse seem unusually slow (less than 70 beats a minute)?	**YES**	Dysrhythmia; bradycardia, an abnormally slow heartbeat.	Consult your doctor, who will examine the baby's heart and determine whether further consultation is required.
Has your child's heartbeat felt uneven since he had an illness with fever?	**YES**	Uneven beats are common during recovery from illness with fever.	In most cases, the condition gradually resolves without treatment. If it persists or gets worse, discuss your concerns with your doctor.
Does your child complain that she can feel her heart beating faster while at rest? Does she drink several fizzy drinks, especially colas, most days?	**YES**	Excessive caffeine consumption, leading to fast and irregular heartbeats; dysrhythmia.	Caffeine can cause the heart to race or miss a beat. In children, this may be due to consumption of cola, coffee, and tea. Cut out chocolate, and replace colas and other caffeine-containing drinks with juices, milk, and water. If there's no change in a day or two, consult your doctor.
Has your child noticed a thumping or racing sensation in the chest while taking medication, such as an antihistamine for allergies, or a cold medication?	**YES**	Side effect of the medication.	Call your doctor, who will either withdraw the medication or prescribe a substitute medication.
Has your child previously been diagnosed and treated for a heart condition?	**YES**	Inborn or acquired heart condition.	Inborn heart disorders are usually associated with disturbances in heart rhythm. If irregularities newly appear or become more noticeable, bring them to your doctor's attention.
Is your child a baby over 3 months or a toddler? Is he having night terrors? Is he unusually tired and taking many naps? Is he irritable? Has he ever fainted? Does the mother have a history of auto-immune disease, such as lupus?	**YES**	Atrioventricular block, an abnormality in the heart's electrical system.	Consult your doctor, who will examine the child and refer him for an evaluation by a paediatric heart specialist, if necessary. This condition can usually be well controlled with use of medication and/or a pacemaker.
Can your child feel extra heartbeats? Or is her heart skipping beats? Does she have any other symptoms? Has she had a strep throat in the past several weeks? Is she anxious and generally unwell?	**YES**	Ectopic beats, which may be associated with various conditions, including thyroid disorders or rheumatic fever, a complication of strep throat.	Consult your doctor, who will examine the child to determine whether further tests and treatment are necessary.

Continued on next page

Heartbeat Irregularities

Cardiac arrhythmias, dysrhythmias

Questions to consider	**If answer is**	**Possible cause is**	**Action to take**
Is your child suddenly pale and tired? Is he sweating while at rest? Has he had several fainting episodes? Have other young members of the family ever had repeated fainting or a history of heart trouble?	**YES**	Arrhythmia leading to inefficient heart pumping; anaemia; prolonged QT syndrome (see below).	Consult your doctor, who will examine the child, order tests if appropriate, and possibly refer your child to a specialist.

Prolonged QT syndrome

A rare inherited condition may cause a child or adolescent to faint and have severe heartbeat irregularities during exercise or an emotionally stressful experience. This disorder is known as the prolonged QT syndrome because of the characteristic pattern – an abnormal lengthening of the QT interval – seen when an electrocardiogram is performed during carefully monitored exercise. Occasionally, the condition is not inborn but occurs with another form of heart disease. When inherited, it may also be associated with deafness. If one member of your family is diagnosed as having prolonged QT syndrome, the others should also be tested. The disorder can be controlled by medication.

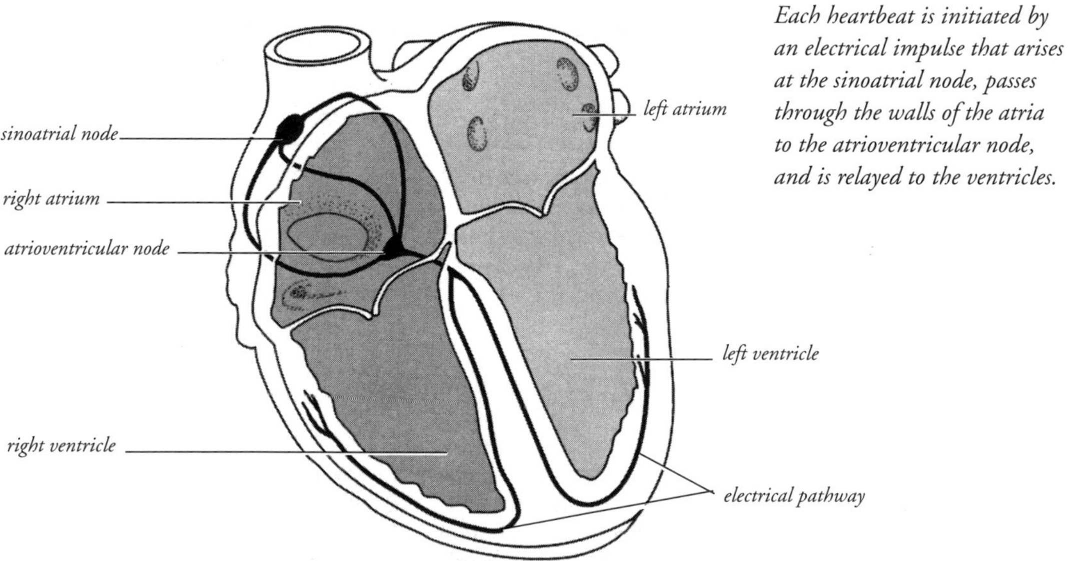

Each heartbeat is initiated by an electrical impulse that arises at the sinoatrial node, passes through the walls of the atria to the atrioventricular node, and is relayed to the ventricles.

Attention deficit hyperactivity disorder

Consult your doctor promptly if your child fits the following general picture:

- Gets overexcited and loses control.
- Is falling behind in schoolwork.
- Fights with others or has trouble keeping friends.
- Doesn't complete tasks.

IN GENERAL:

All children get bored and fidgety once in a while. Many tend to be impulsive, and, at times, find it hard to give a task their full concentration. What's different about youngsters with hyperactivity and attention deficits (termed attention deficit hyperactivity disorder or ADHD) is that their symptoms are much more intense than in other boys and girls the same age. They rarely sit still. They are impulsive and distracted almost all the time and in any situation, causing disruption and disturbing people everywhere they go. Their behaviour causes social difficulties. Teachers can't manage them, other children reject them, family outings are a trial, and family tensions may reach an unbearable pitch. Children with ADHD may also have behaviour problems (see p. 34), and have a hard time paying attention. They are easily distracted and find it difficult to see a task through to the end. Often, these youngsters struggle with criticism, failure, and disappointment as their self-esteem is whittled away.

Warning

Medication does not cure ADHD, but it helps control hyperactivity and lets the child make use of his other faculties.

About 4 out of every 100 children have ADHD; boys are affected six times more often than girls. Researchers believe there may be numerous causes. Recent studies indicate that the brains of youngsters with ADHD may function differently from those of other children. In many families, there is a history of similar attention difficulties in a close relative, suggesting that the condition may be at least partly genetic. Whatever the causes may be, ADHD is not due to poor parenting. However, there are ways parents and children can develop special techniques for coping with ADHD. If your child has ADHD, you may feel overwhelmed by the strain of dealing with his boundless energy 24 hours a day. Don't hesitate to talk it over with your doctor. Ask for her help, too, in linking up with a support group where you can hear how others cope.

QUESTIONS TO CONSIDER	IF ANSWER IS	POSSIBLE CAUSE IS	ACTION TO TAKE
Is your child overly fearful? Does she laugh or cry uncontrollably? Has she experienced frightening events? Does she have friends and do reasonably well at school?	**YES**	Overanxious disorder; anxious child.	Consult your doctor, who may recommend a plan to help the child deal with her fears and control her behaviour.
Does your school-age child still have temper tantrums? Does he get overexcited and overtired? At other times, does he stick to tasks and get along with other family members and friends?	**YES**	Temper tantrums. (Also see p. 148.)	Keep to a schedule for sleep, play, and meals so your child doesn't get overtired or hungry. Talk with him to work out a plan for coping with frustrations without losing his temper. But don't reason with him as with an adult. If these measures don't help, discuss your concerns with your doctor.

Continued on next page

Hyperactivity/Attention Deficit Disorder

Attention deficit hyperactivity disorder (ADHD)

Questions to consider	If answer is	Possible cause is	Action to take
Is your school-age child having difficulties at every level: home, school, and social activities? Is he always on the move? Does he sleep very little? Is his behaviour causing difficulties?	**YES**	Hyperactivity; attention deficit disorder; learning problems; family stress; temperamental mismatch; inappropriate expectations.	Consult your GP, who may recommend further evaluation and treatment.
Is your child impulsive and easily distracted? Does he have a short attention span?	**YES**	Attention deficit disorder (without hyperactivity).	Discuss your concerns with your doctor, who may advise further evaluation.

Recognizing warning signs of ADHD

Doctors look for hyperactivity, impulsiveness, and inattention in diagnosing ADHD, but many children with attention deficits are not hyperactive. They just 'space out', and their behaviour can be equally difficult to deal with. Diagnosing ADHD is important because similar symptoms may accompany other conditions such as depression (see p. 176) or other stress, or learning problems (see p. 106). In these cases, the approach to treatment will be different.

There is no simple test for diagnosing ADHD. It can be difficult to diagnose because different standards of behaviour apply at different ages. A pre-schooler, for example, shouldn't be expected to show the same level of concentration as a child at junior school. Your doctor doesn't rely on her observations during a single consultation, when the child may be on his best behaviour or even a bit fearful. Instead, she sifts out a pattern of behaviour from repeated observations, school reports, and the comments of parents, teachers, and other care-givers. Generally, for a firm diagnosis, all the main symptoms have to be present most of the time. Problems are picked up in many children aged 10 to 13, when they are unable to keep up with the increased need to pay attention. These children may be bright, but they're hampered by their inability to concentrate.

ADHD can be diagnosed only by a physician or psychologist. Teachers cannot make a diagnosis, although they can identify problems that should be evaluated by your GP or specialist. Attention deficits and learning problems are often present together and each can make the other worse. If your child has several of the following symptoms and they are interfering with his progress at school or his relationships with other children, consult your doctor.

- Inability to keep his mind on a task.
- Distractibility.
- Impulsiveness.
- Low frustration level; impatience.
- Constant fidgeting with hands and feet.
- Restlessness; uncontrollable energy.
- Tendency to interrupt others constantly.
- Overexcitability.
- Schoolwork below class level.
- Lack of organization.
- Disobedience.
- Mood swings; irritability.
- Difficulty carrying out instructions.
- Trouble in making and keeping friends.

QUESTIONS TO CONSIDER	IF ANSWER IS	POSSIBLE CAUSE IS	ACTION TO TAKE
Does your child daydream at school? Is he a loner? Is he hard to deal with because he doesn't get things done? Is he being picked on?	**YES**	Attention deficit disorder; learning disorder; lack of social skills; emotional problems; inappropriate expectations.	Consult your doctor, who may advise evaluation and recommend a plan for treatment.
Is your child always disobedient and hard to control? Is he defiant when you correct him?	**YES**	Testing behaviour; temperamental problems; school problems; family stress; unreasonable expectations.	When both of you are calm, review problem areas with your child. Agree on a plan of action involving cooperation in specific areas. Set up a scoring system. If a 2-month trial is unsuccessful, ask your doctor to evaluate the situation.
Is your child always on the move? Is he impulsive, reckless, and unable to concentrate? Was he slow in reaching developmental milestones?	**YES**	Neurological or physical condition requiring medical evaluation.	Consult your doctor, who will examine the child and may refer you for consultation with a specialist.

Coping with ADHD

There isn't a 'quick fix' for ADHD, although some children outgrow the symptoms in adolescence and, with treatment, others learn to control symptoms and channel their energy productively. Successful treatment depends on cooperation by the parents, the GP and/or specialists, teachers, and – most of all – the child himself. Doctors often prescribe medication, which can help the youngster block out distractions and concentrate on tasks. Treatment usually involves educational measures, including tutoring, and psychological counselling. Behavioural management and training in social skills may help a youngster with attention problems make friends for the first time. Your therapist will guide you to programmes for parent training and support. Some families benefit from family therapy. The aim of treatment is to give the child a sense of being in control and make him more productive, so he can take credit for his progress. Maintaining and improving his self-esteem are crucial.

All children function best in a structured environment. ADHD youngsters have more trouble than most with organization and rules, and need a consistent schedule. Give your child extra attention to help him focus on tasks such as getting dressed or doing homework. Social events and outings may be easier if you let the youngster know beforehand how you expect him to behave. But don't expect any child, hyperactive or not, to sit still throughout events that are far beyond his capacity to understand or enjoy.

Controversial treatments such as additive-free diets, sugar restriction, and mega-dose vitamins haven't held up when tested scientifically. Talk to your doctor before trying any treatments.

Indigestion

Gastroesophageal reflux

Consult your doctor if your infant has:

- Persistent vomiting.
- Poor weight gain.

In General:

An attack of indigestion brings general discomfort, a feeling of overfullness, wind relieved by belching, and heartburn, a burning feeling caused when acid stomach contents flow back into the oesophagus and irritate its lining. This backward flow, or gastroesophageal reflux, also causes the sour taste that sometimes occurs after a heavy or fatty meal. A certain amount of reflux is normal; only when it is repeated and persistent is it likely to cause a problem. Babies frequently have reflux but it generally wears off after infancy and doesn't recur until much later in childhood.

Despite claims for over-the-counter remedies, indigestion is caused not by too much acid, but by acid in the wrong place. The trigger is sometimes too much food. A sphincter at the end of the oesophagus relaxes to let food pass, then closes tight to keep it in the stomach. Various triggers, however, can make the sphincter open at the wrong time. Pressure due to an overfull stomach, obesity, or lying down after eating may force it open. A meal heavy in fats slows down stomach emptying and contributes to overloading. Foods that can make the sphincter muscle relax include tomato-based products, chocolate, caffeine, and peppermint. Certain medications, such as some used to treat asthma, may also have this effect.

Provided your child is growing at a normal rate, it is very unlikely that a serious gastrointestinal problem is present.

Warning

Don't treat your child's indigestion with over-the-counter antacids and acid-suppressant remedies or homemade concoctions of bicarbonate of soda. Regular use of antacids and certain pain medications can injure the stomach lining. Use these and all medications only on the advice of your doctor.

Questions to consider	If answer is	Possible cause is	Action to take
Is your baby between 2 and 6 weeks old? Does he vomit every feeding? Is the vomiting projectile or forceful? Is he failing to gain or even losing weight?	**YES**	Pyloric stenosis. (See Feeding Problems in Infants, p. 9.)	Contact your GP straightaway.
Is your baby aged 6 weeks or older vomiting each feeding (though not forceful projectile vomiting)?	**YES**	Chalasia, spitting up due to relaxation of the sphincter between the oesophagus and stomach; gastroesophageal reflux (GER).	Consult your GP, who will examine the baby and possibly recommend thickening the formula with cereal or another dietary change. Some vomiting or spitting up is normal; most children outgrow the problem by about 1 year. (See p. 16.)
Is your child vomiting after every meal, and has he been diagnosed with a serious developmental delay?	**YES**	Gastroesophageal reflux due to developmental disorder.	Consult your doctor; your child may need further evaluation, or medical or surgical therapy.

QUESTIONS TO CONSIDER	IF ANSWER IS	POSSIBLE CAUSE IS	ACTION TO TAKE
Does your infant or toddler often gag and regurgitate food? Does she chew on food hours after eating? Is she sometimes difficult?	**YES**	Rumination (repetitive gagging, regurgitation, and swallowing of food).	Your child requires an examination to rule out serious, treatable conditions. After observing how you feed and handle your baby, your doctor may have constructive suggestions for alleviating the problem.
Is your child complaining of a stomachache and an occasional sour, burning taste in the throat?	**YES**	Gastritis (inflammation of the stomach); peptic ulcer possibly linked to *Helicobacter pylori* infection.	Consult your GP. If the diagnosis of peptic ulcer is confirmed, your child may benefit from a course of medications, possibly including an antibiotic.
Does your child have burning in the chest, hoarseness, chronic cough, or wheezing? Has he had pneumonia? Is he gaining weight only slowly?	**YES**	Respiratory effects of gastroesophageal reflux.	Your doctor will examine the child and may review his diet with you. The child may benefit from medical treatment as well as cutting down on fatty foods, tomato-based products, and colas.
Is your child taking a theophylline medication for asthma?	**YES**	Side effect of theophylline.	Consult your doctor, who may modify the prescription to decrease the side effects.
Does your child have a burning pain in his chest? Does he rush his food or sometimes eat too much? Does he have wind or bloating?	**YES**	Swallowed air (aerophagia); overeating; oesophagitis; eating too fast.	Pace meals so that the whole family eats in a more relaxed fashion. Your GP will examine the child to determine whether his condition requires treatment.
Does your school-age child or teenager have frequent wind, bloating, cramps, and diarrhoea after meals? Is he growing slowly?	**YES**	Malabsorption disorder such as lactose intolerance; coeliac disease; Crohn disease; colitis; irritable bowel syndrome; ulcerative colitis.	Consult your GP, who will examine the child and may provide a referral to a specialist, if necessary. Dietary changes may be advised.

Coping with gastroesophageal reflux

Time the evening meal so your child has an hour or two of quiet relaxation but nothing more to eat or drink before bedtime. She should sit up in a straight chair, reading, doing homework, or involved in some other calm activity to give the digestive process time to work. Lying down soon after eating encourages the reflux of stomach contents into the oesophagus. She may sleep more comfortably if you raise the head of her bed with a wedge, available from chemists by prescription. Sleeping with the upper part of the body elevated uses gravity to discourage reflux.

If your child is troubled by indigestion or other symptoms related to gastroesophageal reflux (GER), your doctor may also prescribe a medication to improve the motility of her digestive tract.

Irritability

Call your GP if your child is unusually irritable and has:

- A fever over 38°C (100.4°F).
- Pain, including a sore throat or stiff neck.
- Unusual drowsiness.
- A headache.
- Vomiting without diarrhoea.

Warning

Don't ignore irritability and hope it will go away by itself. If the cause is physical, the condition should be addressed. And if stress is making your child testy, the cause should be identified and, if possible, eliminated.

In General:

Each child is born with a temperament – a personality and disposition – that emphasizes certain characteristics over others. Parents are often astonished to find that their newborn already seems adventurous or hesitant, impatient or accepting, outgoing or shy. Although children's basic natures are inborn, their temperament and outlook are influenced by their experiences, interactions with parents and others, and sense of self-worth.

Like grown-ups, most children feel irritable and short-tempered at times. If the child can't tell you why, it may be because he either cannot pinpoint the trouble or can't yet express himself in words. In general, an acute physical cause for irritability leads a child to act very differently from his everyday behaviour. If a child often seems irritable, there may be an underlying condition or stressful factors in the family or school environment. It is important to recognize the difference between a passing mood and the fretful crying that shows a young child needs your attention to deal with fever, pain, cold, heat, hunger, or other physical reasons for irritability. An occasional irritable mood may not be significant, but a child who is usually irritable may need medical attention. Many babies from about 2 weeks up to 6 months have daily bouts of irritable crying and colic (see p. 6). Although upsetting to the parents while it lasts, this irritability isn't a symptom of illness and usually disappears on its own by the time the baby is 6 months or before. A child between the ages of 18 months and 3 years may often be increasingly irritable as she works up to one of the tantrums (see p. 148) that punctuate this age, which is known for good reason as the 'terrible twos.' This phase passes as the child becomes more independent. Finally, it's not unusual for a teenager to be irritable during the mood swings (see p. 190) associated with hormonal changes during adolescence.

Questions to consider	If answer is	Possible cause is	Action to take
Is your baby over 3 months old? Is his temperature over 38°C (100.4°F)? Is he fretful?	YES	A viral or bacterial infection.	Contact your GP, who may want to examine the baby and will prescribe any necessary treatment.
Does your infant or older child have sniffles and a runny nose? Is she coughing?	YES	Common cold; other upper respiratory tract infection.	If symptoms last more than 2 days call your GP for advice. (See Cough, p. 52; Breathing Difficulty/Breathlessness, p. 44; Runny/Stuffy Nose, p. 126.)
Is your toddler limping or guarding a limb? Is there swelling, redness, or warmth?	YES	Fracture, infection, or injury in the leg or hip.	Consult your GP for an examination and x-rays, if necessary. (See Fracture/Broken Bones, p. 78.)

QUESTIONS TO CONSIDER	IF ANSWER IS	POSSIBLE CAUSE IS	ACTION TO TAKE
Does your child wake up irritable every morning? Does he often breathe through his mouth because of a stuffed-up nose? Is he always tired?	**YES**	Allergy; interrupted sleep due to enlarged tonsils or adenoids and upper airway blockage; sleep apnoea.	Consult your GP, who will examine the child for signs of chronic allergy (see p. 26), tonsil or adenoid enlargement, and upper airway blockage (see p. 126), and prescribe any necessary treatment.
Are your child's stools hard pellets? Has she failed to move her bowels for several days? Does she complain of a stomachache?	**YES**	Constipation.	Make sure your family's diet includes plenty of fresh vegetables and fruits and other sources of fibre; encourage your child to drink several glasses of water or diluted juices each day. (See Constipation, p. 48.)
Is your school-age child constantly irritable and fatigued? Does he go to bed late? Does he have any symptoms of illness? Is he involved in many after-school activities?	**YES**	Not enough sleep; disorder requiring treatment.	Your youngster's schedule may include more than he can manage. Where possible, provide for more rest and make sure he's getting enough exercise. If these measures don't help, or if the child has other symptoms, consult your GP for an evaluation.
Is your school-age youngster irritable, anxious, or easily distracted?	**YES**	Emotional stress due to academic or social problems at school; tension in the family.	If the family is under stress, explain the situation without overburdening the child; try to keep the daily impact to a minimum. Questioning may give you an idea of what's bothering your child at school. Speak with teachers to identify problems.
Is your child just grumpy, without any symptoms of illness?	**YES**	Copying the behaviour of others; frustration.	Examine the behaviour of other family members; discuss coping techniques with your doctor. Let the child make his own choices when there is room for reasonable compromise.

Coping with irritability

Although your child has her own unique disposition, she also copies the examples she sees. If she usually gets an irritable, impatient response to her questions, sooner or later she may mimic this behaviour and treat others the same way. If your child often seems grouchy and irritable, but has no health problem that could be causing discomfort, take a look at the examples she's getting at home and at school. Avoid placing your child in double-bind situations, let her express her opinions, and don't ask if she wants to do something when you really mean you want her to do it.

Itching

Pruritus

In General:

When a child gets an itchy rash, he may recently have been exposed to an irritant or may have a viral infection. Itching without a rash occurs for many reasons, especially in children with dry skin or eczema (atopic dermatitis), and when central heating and winter air dry out the skin. Fungal and yeast infections can be itchy although – apart from ringworm or nappy rash due to yeasts – they are not often seen before adolescence.

Some children scratch from habit, which irritates the skin and prompts further scratching. Those with allergies are especially vulnerable to the itch-scratch-itch cycle. Eventually, the skin gets cracked and sore and may become infected.

Itchy skin without a rash is linked to a few systemic conditions, but these are rare in children. Girls may be embarrassed by itching due to vulvovaginitis (see p. 156), and teenage boys are prey to the itchy fungal infections known as dhobi itch and athlete's foot. Your GP may recommend over-the-counter products to treat these latter two conditions, and you should encourage your youngsters to dry themselves thoroughly after showering or bathing.

☎

Consult your GP if:

- Your child has itching together with swelling of the lips or face.
- A patch of eczema is showing signs of infection, such as swelling, warmth, and pus.
- Your child's nervous habit of scratching is causing skin problems or social difficulties.

Warning

If your child has itchy skin, use mild soap for laundry and avoid detergents that contain dyes and perfumes. Rinse clothes thoroughly, and put them through a second plain water cycle, if necessary, to remove soap residue.

Questions to consider	If answer is	Possible cause is	Action to take
Does your baby have patches of red, rough skin? Do other family members have allergies?	YES	Eczema (atopic dermatitis).	Your GP will examine the child and recommend treatment. Don't dress your baby in wool.
Does your child have red, flaky patches or a moist rash? Do the affected areas come into contact with allergens such as dyes in clothing or nickel in jewellery? Have you switched brands of soap or detergent?	YES	Allergic contact dermatitis.	Use cold compresses to soothe the irritation. Try to identify and avoid the source of irritation. If the rash is severe, consult your GP, who will examine the child and recommend treatment.
Has your child developed a blistering rash after being outdoors? Are the marks of the rash in lines?	YES	Poison ivy, oak, or sumac; nettles or other stinging plants.	Wash the area with soap and water and rinse for 10 minutes. Wash the clothes. Apply cool compresses. If the rash is severe, call your doctor for advice.
Does your child have an itchy rash in an exposed area? Or are there bumps with red spots in the centres?	YES	Bites of insects, such as jiggers, mosquitoes, or fleas.	Apply cool compresses. (Also see Bites and Stings, p. 36.) If the rash persists or bites show signs of infection, consult your doctor.

Questions to consider	If answer is	Possible cause is	Action to take
Is your child constantly scratching? Can you see either nits (egg cases) in her hair or reddish tracks in her skin?	**YES**	Skin parasites such as head lice (on the scalp) or scabies (on the body).	Call your GP, who will recommend treatment and measures to eradicate the parasites from your home. Notify your child's school or childcare centre.
Does your child have itchy ring-shaped patches on the skin and/or bald patches on the scalp?	**YES**	Ringworm.	Consult your GP, who will prescribe treatment and advise how to stop the infection from spreading.
Has your child broken out in an itchy rash after a cough, fever, and upper respiratory symptoms?	**YES**	Rash due to virus such as chickenpox (varicella).	Consult your GP, who will examine the child and prescribe any necessary treatment.
Has your child developed a rash while taking a medication, such as an antibiotic?	**YES**	Medication side effect.	Consult your GP, who will examine the child and prescribe another antibiotic, if necessary, and treat the skin condition.
Does your child have itching around the anus? Is it more intense at night?	**YES**	Pinworms. (See Rectal Pain/Itching p. 124.)	Your GP will examine the child and prescribe appropriate treatment. Ask your GP how to prevent the spread of infection.
Does your adolescent son complain of itching around his genital area?	**YES**	Dhobi itch (fungal infection); dermatitis in the skin folds (intertrigo).	Your GP will recommend appropriate treatment. Encourage your son to soap thoroughly during showers and baths and dry thoroughly before dressing.

Dealing with eczema

Eczema is another term for atopic dermatitis: reddened, itchy skin sometimes covered with blister-like bumps that weep and crust over. In long-term eczema, the skin thickens, becoming scaly and deeply scored.

Eczema typically occurs in children whose families have a tendency to develop eczema and allergies, even though the child's irritation may not be caused by allergy. It may appear at any age. In babies between 2 and 6 months, atopic dermatitis appears as itching, redness, and bumps on the face and scalp, perhaps spreading to the arms and trunk. In about half the cases, the rash disappears by 2 or 3 years. Many children outgrow it by about age 6, others by puberty. In others it may recur from time to time.

If you suspect certain foods are causing the rash, serve alternatives. Your GP will advise you in this regard. Apply moisturizers while the skin is damp. Use a pH-neutral soap that is perfume-free. Limiting baths to one to three a week may help in some cases. Your GP may recommend an antihistamine. It's best to give antihistamines to youngsters at night to avoid problems of drowsiness at school, although non-sedating antihistamines are now available. A topical steroid may be needed when a child has severe eczema.

Jaundice

Icterus

IN GENERAL:

Jaundice, a yellow-green discoloration seen in the skin and usually the whites of the eyes, is caused by excessive blood levels of bilirubin. This pigment, formed when red blood cells break down at the end of their natural cycle or are damaged, is normally processed through the liver and then excreted in the stools. Jaundice is often seen in newborn babies because their immature livers cannot keep up with the amount of bilirubin that is being produced (see Treating jaundice in a newborn baby, opposite). Many breast-fed babies develop prolonged jaundice. This is not a cause for alarm, but your doctor will examine the baby to rule out unusual and serious causes of jaundice.

In older children and adults, jaundice indicates that an infection or other disorder is interfering with the function of the liver. A child of any age with jaundice must be seen by a doctor, who will identify the cause and recommend appropriate treatment.

Consult your GP immediately if:

- Your child develops a yellow colour in the skin and the whites of the eyes.

Warning

If your child is diagnosed with viral hepatitis (a common cause of jaundice), ask your doctor how to prevent the spread of infection. Remind family members to wash hands thoroughly after using the toilet and before every meal. Do not share drinking glasses and eating utensils.

QUESTIONS TO CONSIDER	IF ANSWER IS	POSSIBLE CAUSE IS	ACTION TO TAKE
Is your baby more than 1 day but less than a week old?	**YES**	Physiologic jaundice.	Consult your doctor or midwife, who will examine the baby and prescribe any necessary treatment (usually, none is required).
Has a yellowish colour appeared in your baby aged 2 to 7 days or older? Are you breast-feeding?	**YES**	Breast-feeding jaundice; other condition requiring investigation and treatment.	Call your doctor, who will examine the baby and determine the cause of the jaundice. Some babies remain mildly jaundiced for a prolonged period; this is not harmful.
Is your baby over 2 weeks and still jaundiced? Are his stools unusually pale?	**YES**	Biliary atresia (blockage of the bile ducts); other obstruction to bile flow.	Call your doctor at once. Further testing will be necessary to identify the cause and determine treatment.
Is your child taking a prescribed medication, such as an antibiotic or an anticonvulsant medication?	**YES**	Medication side effect.	Call your doctor, who will examine the child and prescribe an alternative treatment, if necessary.

Icterus

Questions to consider	If answer is	Possible cause is	Action to take
Is your toddler or older child looking yellowish? Are her stools pale and her urine dark? Has she lost her appetite? Is she nauseated or vomiting and generally unwell? Does she have a stomachache?	**YES**	Hepatitis (probably viral).	Call your GP, who will examine the child and treat her as necessary. Ask your doctor when the child may return to her childcare centre or school.
Has your child's skin turned yellow, although the whites of his eyes still look white?	**YES**	Carotenaemia, possibly due to frequent consumption of yellow, orange, and red (carotene-containing) vegetables.	Consult your GP, who will examine the child to rule out a serious disorder. This condition usually appears in children who are eating large amounts of carrots or tomatoes, and is harmless.

Treating jaundice in a newborn baby

Many healthy babies develop a yellowish tinge in the skin and the whites of their eyes during the first few days of life. This condition, called physiologic jaundice, shows that the blood has an excess of bilirubin, a chemical that is released during the normal breakdown of old red blood cells. Everyone's blood contains bilirubin, but newborns often have higher levels because babies have extra red blood cells at birth. Bilirubin is processed and cleared away through the liver. The livers of newborn babies, however, are not yet working at full capacity. Most babies with mild jaundice regain their healthy pink colour without special treatment.

Bilirubin is generally harmless in a healthy baby. If allowed to build up to an unusually high level, however, bilirubin may cause brain injury in a newborn. If the blood level of bilirubin is exceptionally high or your baby is susceptible because of prematurity or illness, your doctor may prescribe phototherapy. In this treatment, exposure to special lights called bili lights for 1 to 2 days helps eliminate bilirubin until the baby's liver is more mature. These lights do not produce ultraviolet light. Even with this treatment, the bilirubin may remain elevated for several days or weeks. Natural daylight through a window is also helpful, but never put your baby outside in direct sunlight. Your doctor may treat your baby with phototherapy at home, or may recommend that he spend a few days in the hospital, where he can be continually monitored by medical personnel. Sometimes doctors prefer to treat mildly jaundiced babies with more frequent feedings of breast milk or formula to help pass the bilirubin out in the stools.

Joint Pain/Swelling

Arthralgia, Arthritis

In General:

Pains resulting from a minor injury to the arm or leg are usually short-lived. But children may also have persistent pain in the joints as a result of infection, allergy, or arthritis. If your child has joint pain that lasts longer than a day or two, and seems reluctant to move the affected limb, bring it to your doctor's attention. (Also see Fracture/Broken Bones, p. 78, and Knee Pain, p. 188.)

Call your GP if your child has joint pain along with:

- Fever.
- A rash.
- Warmth, swelling, or tenderness.
- Difficulty using an arm or leg.

Warning

Don't ignore complaints of joint pain, especially if your child is an active sports player or dancer, or takes part in other regular athletic activities. Joint pain in children is not normal and should be evaluated by your doctor.

Questions to consider	If answer is	Possible cause is	Action to take
Does your child have joint pain following an injury caused by a fall or a sudden movement? Can she move her limb?	**YES**	Bruise; muscle or ligament strain.	Apply an ice pack to the sore joint; use a cold compress but no ice if your child is under 2 years. If the pain is no better after 24 hours, consult your GP.
Is your child suddenly limping? Does he have pain in one hip? Is he between 2 and 10 years of age? Has he recently had a mild respiratory illness?	**YES**	Inflammation of the hip joint (called toxic or transient synovitis), probably caused by a viral infection.	Consult your GP. If viral synovitis is confirmed, the doctor may recommend rest and paracetamol or ibuprofen. This acute hip pain usually clears up with no aftereffects.
Is your toddler or pre-schooler holding her arm close to her side? Is the elbow very tender? Does she resist if you gently try to straighten her arm? Was the child recently pulled or swung by the arms?	**YES**	Pulled elbow, also called nursemaid's elbow, caused when soft tissue becomes trapped in the joint.	Call your doctor straightaway for an examination. Fold a scarf or soft towel to make an arm sling, but don't try to treat the injury or give food, drink, or pain medication until your doctor says it's all right. Your doctor may manipulate the elbow to release the trapped tissue and discuss how to avoid such injuries.
Does your child have severe pain and some swelling in the joint at the tip of a finger? Is he an active ball player?	**YES**	Ball finger.	Apply an ice pack to this minor injury which occurs when a ball bends a fingertip back. If the finger is still painful and swollen after a couple of days, consult your GP.
Does your child have soreness and stiffness in the hands, wrists, knees, and ankles? Did she recently have symptoms suggesting a viral infection?	**YES**	Postviral joint pain.	Joint pains following a viral infection usually go away within 1 to 2 weeks. If your child has a fever or isn't better after a week, call your doctor.

Questions to consider	If answer is	Possible cause is	Action to take
Does your child have pain, redness, and warmth in one or more joints? Is her temperature higher than 38°C (100.4°F)? Is she having trouble moving her limbs? Did she recently have an infection or a tick bite?	**YES**	Inflammation and/or infection; septic arthritis; juvenile rheumatoid arthritis; Lyme disease (see Preventing Lyme disease, below); rheumatic fever; lupus.	Your doctor will examine the child and order laboratory tests to clarify the diagnosis. Long-term treatment may be required. Your doctor may also refer you to a specialist in joint disorders.
Does your son limp because of pain in the hip, thigh, or knee? Is he generally free of symptoms other than leg pain? Is he between about 4 and 9 years of age?	**YES**	Perthes disease (usually in boys; rare in girls) or other condition requiring diagnosis and treatment.	Consult your doctor, who will examine your son and determine whether he needs further tests and treatment.
Does your child also have a purple rash on the legs, feet, and/or buttocks? Does he have pain in the abdomen?	**YES**	Henoch-Schönlein purpura, an autoimmune condition.	Consult your doctor, who will examine the child, order appropriate diagnostic tests, and prescribe necessary treatment.
Does your teenager (ages 10 to 13) have hip and knee pain? Is he having trouble walking? Is he overweight?	**YES**	Displacement of the head of the thigh bone (slipped capital femoral epiphysis).	Consult your doctor, who will examine the youngster and determine whether treatment is required.

Preventing Lyme disease

Lyme disease is an infection caused by bacteria transmitted in the bites of deer ticks. These creatures, about the size of a poppy seed, live in grassy, wooded, and marshy regions, especially in Scotland. They can be found year-round but are most plentiful in spring, summer, and autumn.

The most distinctive symptom is a circular rash, which usually appears 3 to 10 days after the tick bite. The rash doesn't always follow a bite, however, and for some people Lyme disease is signalled only by influenza-like symptoms such as headache, fever, fatigue, swollen glands, and aches in the muscles and joints. Antibiotic treatment is usually effective if given within a month of the bite. Left untreated, Lyme disease may cause severe symptoms, including visual disturbance, facial paralysis, and joint pain and arthritis.The infection is harder to treat in the later stages.

Dress your children protectively when they venture into wooded areas. They should wear long-sleeved shirts and tuck their trouser legs into their socks. A hat can help keep ticks away from favoured spots along the hairline and behind the ears.

By removing a tick as soon as you see it, you lower the chance of your child getting Lyme disease, because a tick needs to be attached to the skin for about 24 hours in order to transmit the infection.

IN GENERAL:

A child who is having trouble at school may have a learning problem. This doesn't mean the youngster is less intelligent than others; it's just harder for him to learn. Failure in school may make the affected youngsters and their families increasingly disappointed and frustrated. Occasionally, a learning problem is at the root of an apparent behaviour problem (p. 34), temper tantrums (p. 148), or attention deficit/hyperactivity disorder (p. 93). The behaviour generally improves once the learning problem is recognized and dealt with.

In rare cases, learning difficulties follow a head injury or brain infection. Often, no definite cause can be found, but learning problems tend to run in families.

Some youngsters have problems with basic skills such as reading, writing, spelling, and numbers. Others have trouble with language skills, including listening, understanding, remembering, and speech. A third group have difficulty with balance, writing, and coordination – skills that require the child to integrate messages from the motor (muscle) and sensory systems. Poor social skills often hamper youngsters with learning problems. They misunderstand and respond inappropriately to friends, teachers, and parents. Social and emotional problems, like learning problems, need to be dealt with as soon as possible. Problems may be obvious before a child enters nursery or kindergarten or show up only when he can't keep up in the later grades.

Your child's teachers can refer you to other resources available in your local district. They will also work out classroom strategies and suggest steps you can take at home. Psychological counselling may be advised. If your doctor diagnoses serious attention problems, she will refer your child for further expert assessment and treatment.

Consult your doctor as well as your child's teachers if your child:

- Has trouble reading words or numbers.
- Is not achieving class level.
- Has tantrums or behaviour problems.
- Seems depressed.
- Tries to avoid going to school.

Warning

Despite claims and publicity, treatments such as megavitamins, patterning exercises, eye exercises, and additive-free diets haven't been found to benefit children with learning disorders. Seek the advice of your doctor before starting any treatment.

QUESTIONS TO CONSIDER	IF ANSWER IS	POSSIBLE CAUSE IS	ACTION TO TAKE
Is your child's speech hard to follow? Does she have trouble finding words or organizing her thoughts? Does she often misunderstand you? Does she have trouble with recall?	**YES**	Slow development; language/speech disability; attention and/or memory problems.	Consult your doctor, who will evaluate the child and advise whether treatment is necessary.
Does your school-age child speak well but have trouble writing? Does he put off assignments or fail to complete written projects? Does he get others to write for him?	**YES**	Writing difficulty (dysgraphia); fine motor problems.	Ask your child's teacher for an evaluation by an educational psychologist. Request a meeting to discuss the specific problem and possible solutions. The school's special needs department, if any, may provide help with organization and writing mechanics, or outside tutoring may be recommended.

QUESTIONS TO CONSIDER	**IF ANSWER IS**	**POSSIBLE CAUSE IS**	**ACTION TO TAKE**
Does your child find it hard to understand what she reads, though she can follow what is read to her? Does she have trouble remembering printed information?	**YES**	Visual learning difficulty; dyslexia; poor vocabulary; difficulty with concepts; attention problems.	Ask your child's teacher to ask an educational psychologist to evaluate the problem. Find out if the school special needs department can provide appropriate help or whether further tutoring is advisable.
Does your child have problems memorizing? Is it hard for her to retell a story in the right sequence? Does she have trouble with maths?	**YES**	Memory/thinking difficulty; attention problems; few memory strategies.	If these problems are causing difficulties at school, ask for an evaluation and possibly referral to the special needs department. Get advice on improving your youngster's memory, organizational skills, and concentration.
Is your child's behaviour causing concern? Is he aggressive toward other students or teachers? Is he defiant at home? Is he failing to keep up?	**YES**	Learning problem; behaviour problem (see p. 34); hyperactivity (ADHD) (see p. 93); depression (see p. 176).	Ask your child's teachers to identify areas of concern and get their recommendations for management. Consult your doctor, who can advise as to whether psychological counselling is needed.

Gifted children need help, too

Children who have high abilities in reading, language, mathematical reasoning, science, performing or fine arts, or sports are often considered gifted. These youngsters usually have lots of interests, read more – and more difficult – books than others the same age, and are often able to work on their own at an early age. Their outstanding talents give them a great potential for achieving personal satisfaction as well as for making a contribution to society.

Just as children with learning problems need help, gifted children also deserve special programmes to develop their talents. Without such programmes, some gifted children do not meet their potential in the classroom. Failing to get emotional rewards from their achievements in school, they lose faith in themselves and feel increasingly unsuccessful and isolated from their peers. They may become bored and disruptive.

Providing programmes for gifted children is not always easy. Without special training, teachers may find it difficult to deal with the advanced thinking of a gifted student. School budgets often do not allow for employing teachers who are trained to work with gifted youngsters. Most gifted youngsters benefit from an approach that combines independent study, advanced special classes, and use of outside resources, where appropriate. A student with outstanding ability in one field, such as music or performing arts, may be considered for application to a specialized school.

Limb/Leg Pain

In General:

Temporary pain in children's arms or legs is usually the result of minor falls, collisions, or muscle strains. Your doctor's attention is usually not warranted, and a cold compress and pain medication (paracetamol or ibuprofen) is the only treatment that's normally necessary. On the other hand, pain due to an obvious, more serious injury, such as a fracture, requires medical care at once. And even when there's no sign of injury, your child should be seen by a doctor if limb or leg pain lasts more than a day or two, or grows more intense.

Consult your doctor if limb pain is severe or is accompanied by:

- Limping.
- A lump in a bruised muscle that doesn't go away within a week or two.
- Difficulty in moving the affected limb.
- Swelling or pain that continues to increase after 24 hours.

Warning

Don't ignore limb pains and muscle aches. Your doctor may identify a physical cause that can be treated. Stress, too, can cause nonspecific symptoms such as pain.

Questions to consider	If answer is	Possible cause is	Action to take
Did the pain come on suddenly with movement? Is there any swelling or stiffening at the site of the pain?	**YES**	Muscle strain or sprain.	Apply cold compresses to relieve soreness and swelling and have your child elevate and rest the affected area. If pain persists, consult your doctor, who may want to examine the child.
Does your child complain of cramping pain in the muscles of the thigh, the calf, or the arch of the foot? Does the pain usually come on at night after an active day?	**YES**	Muscle spasms from overuse.	Gently but firmly rub the area to relieve discomfort.
Does your school-age (age 5 to 10) child have pain in the legs almost every night? Is he otherwise well and without symptoms?	**YES**	'Growing pains' (nonspecific pains of unknown cause).	If the pains are worrying your child, discuss your concerns with your doctor. She may want to examine the child to rule out serious causes of pain and will discuss ways to deal with stress at school and home.
In addition to aches in the limbs, does your child have a temperature over 38.3°C (101°F)? Does he also have symptoms such as a runny nose, sore throat, and watery eyes?	**YES**	Viral infection.	Make the child comfortable; give cold drinks to soothe the sore throat, and paracetamol to reduce fever and ease discomfort. If symptoms persist or get worse over the next 48 hours, or the temperature rises above 38.3°C (101°F), call your doctor.

Questions to consider	If answer is	Possible cause is	Action to take
Is your adolescent limping since taking part in a vigorous exercise or sports program? Are one or both of his shins painful? Can you feel a slight swelling over the tender area?	**YES**	Shin splints.	Apply a cold compress to reduce pain and swelling; rest the limb until the pain is gone. Have your child resume exercise gradually and prevent further problems by conditioning. Begin and end exercise sessions with warm-ups and stretching. Paracetamol or ibuprofen may be given for pain relief.
Does your child have pain and swelling in any joints? Does he also have fever and/or a rash?	**YES**	Infection requiring diagnosis and treatment; juvenile rheumatoid arthritis; juvenile polyarthritis; Lyme disease.	Consult your GP. (Also see Joint Pain/Swelling, p. 104.)
Does your child have severe pain in one area? Is the surrounding skin swollen, warm, and tender?	**YES**	Infection of bone (osteomyelitis), skin, or joint.	Consult your GP, who will examine the child and perform diagnostic tests, including x-rays. If a bone infection is present, your GP will advise consultation with a specialist.
Is your child complaining of frequent, severe leg pain? Is she unusually pale and tired? Does she have swollen glands? Does she have an unusual number of bruises?	**YES**	In rare cases, a tumour, blood disorder, or other condition requiring diagnosis and treatment.	Consult your GP, who will examine the child, perform appropriate diagnostic tests, and recommend any necessary treatment.

Avoiding overuse injuries

Exercise that is too much for your child's state of development or physical condition may result in overuse injuries such as sprains, strains, stress fractures, shin splints, and tendinitis. Pain in legs and limbs often results from such injuries to bones, soft tissues, and the growth cartilage that is found only in children. Youngsters are especially vulnerable to overuse injuries, as bone length grows at a faster rate than muscle mass, placing uneven stresses on the musculoskeletal system.

Unless carefully managed, overuse injuries may cause adverse long-term effects. To avoid overuse injuries, encourage your child to stick to the following guidelines:

- Begin and end every sports or exercise session with warm-up exercises, such as walking, slow jogging, or riding a bicycle, followed by gentle stretching exercises.
- Gradually work up to new levels in the frequency, duration, and intensity of exercise.
- Don't overtrain.
- Follow your coach's instructions when learning an activity.
- Check your shoe size at least every 3 months and buy athletic shoes at a shop where the salespeople are trained in fitting sports shoes for youngsters.

Masturbation

In General:

As babies discover the different parts of their bodies, they learn to associate particularly pleasurable feelings with touching their genitals. This is not sexual activity; it's just a comforting sensation. Parents should neither discourage nor call needless attention to a youngster's normal curiosity. There'll be time to teach about privacy and modesty later on.

Masturbation – stimulation of the genitals – is normal and, up to about age 6, common among both boys and girls. From that age until puberty, self-stimulation may decline as children develop a greater social awareness and sense of modesty. Nevertheless, masturbation remains a normal activity and usually continues in private. As hormones and sexual tensions surge during puberty, healthy adolescents may accept self-stimulation as an expression of their emerging sexuality.

Some parents find it difficult to accept the notion of masturbation, possibly because it implies an acknowledgment that children are sexual beings. Those who cling to now-dispelled myths may react with embarrassment and outrage. Most parents who are aware of their child's masturbatory activity can accept it as part of normal development. They may even recognize it as an opportunity for teaching youngsters about sexuality and the differences between public and private behaviour.

Consult your doctor if your child:

- Engages in compulsive masturbation every day, whether in private or in public.
- Persists in public masturbation even after you have told him that such activity is acceptable only in private.
- Masturbates and shows symptoms of emotional disturbance, such as bed-wetting or faecal soiling, aggressiveness, destructive behaviour, or social withdrawal.
- Exhibits sexual activity or talk inappropriate for his age.

Warning

At times, excessive masturbation or a public display may be a sign that your child is under emotional strain, is overly preoccupied with sex, or is not receiving the emotional comfort she or he needs. It may also indicate that a child is being sexually abused. If you have any concerns, discuss them with your doctor.

Questions to consider	If answer is	Possible cause is	Action to take
Does your baby boy frequently have penile erections when you remove his nappy or when he's asleep?	YES	Normal response to pleasurable sensation; full bladder.	This is quite normal in a healthy little boy. Babies revel in the playful feeling when their nappies are off.
Does your baby or toddler reach for her genitals when you change her nappy?	YES	Normal exploration and familiarization with her body.	Young children find it comforting to feel their bodies. This activity will gradually grow less frequent as increasing independence enables your child to explore the world outside her body.

Questions to consider	If answer is	Possible cause is	Action to take
Does your toddler or pre-schooler cover or rub his crotch, or expose his genitals, when he needs to urinate?	**YES**	Confusion about physical sensations and urges.	Some children are confused by the sensations they feel when their bladders are full or they need to defecate. Teach your youngster to tell you when he feels the urge so you can help him get to the potty or lavatory in time.
Does your pre-schooler or school-age child often rub her genitals when others are around?	**YES**	Emotional tension.	Try to eliminate the source of tension and reassure your child. Ask your doctor to examine the child to rule out any physical cause. When your child stimulates herself in public, suggest that she might be more comfortable on her own but can rejoin the family when she feels ready.

Signs of inappropriate stimulation

Inappropriate sexual behaviour, including public masturbation and sexual posturing, may be a sign that your child has been exposed to stimulation far beyond his emotional capacity. It may even be a tip-off that your child is being sexually abused. Youngsters who are enlisted into sexual activity frequently become preoccupied with sexual matters. Their unusual behaviour may be a cry for help, which is especially urgent when a sexual predator has sworn the child to secrecy. Cable television and the Internet are also sources of explicit sexual material, much of it frankly pornographic. Although you may not allow such material in your own home, your child may have access to it at the homes of friends and schoolmates.

If you suspect sexual abuse, or have concerns about the influence of other children or adults with whom your youngster has been spending time, consult your doctor. He or she will examine your child for signs of abuse and may be able to elicit information that your youngster is shy of discussing with those closer to him. If abuse has occurred, your doctor will suggest a course of action to lessen the impact of abuse and may recommend counselling for the child and your whole family.

Mouth Pain

Stomatalgia

In General:

Pain in the mouth is most often caused by infections, allergies, canker sores, or injury. Pain arising from the throat is often confused with mouth pain.

Warning

If a child's mouth is sore he may be reluctant to drink. Encourage your child to drink enough to keep his tissues properly hydrated.

Consult your GP if your child:

- Is refusing to drink because of mouth pain.
- Complains of mouth pain along with swelling of the lips or breathing difficulty.
- Has a mouth ulcer that lasts longer than 1 week.
- Has swellings on the gums, roof of the mouth, or lips.

Questions to consider	If answer is	Possible cause is	Action to take
Has your breast-fed baby developed small, ulcerated patches on the roof of her mouth?	**YES**	Pterygoid ulcers.	These minor, superficial ulcers are not painful; they are caused by nipple pressure during breast-feeding and disappear after weaning. If they look inflamed, or the baby is refusing to feed, consult your doctor.
Is your baby drooling a lot and keeping his fist in his mouth most of the time? Is he between about 4 and 8 months old?	**YES**	Normal behaviour that occurs with teething.	Give the baby a smooth teething ring or a dummy, if he finds it comforting. (See Dental Problems, p. 56.)
Is your baby hungry but unwilling to feed? Does she have whitish patches on her tongue and inside her cheeks? Has she been taking an antibiotic?	**YES**	Oral thrush (yeast infection).	Consult your GP, who will examine the child to determine the cause of her discomfort and prescribe appropriate treatment. Yeast infections are fairly common in newborn babies; in older children they may occur when antibiotic therapy upsets the normal flora of the mouth.
Is your older child complaining of pain on swallowing due to a sore throat?	**YES**	Viral or streptococcal infection of the throat.	Consult your GP, who will examine your child and then prescribe appropriate treatment if needed.
Does your child have painful ulcers on the inside of his lower lips, his cheeks, or his tongue?	**YES**	Canker sores (aphthous ulcers).	If these ulcers do not disappear in a week or if they recur repeatedly, consult your GP. The exact cause is unknown.

Questions to consider	If answer is	Possible cause is	Action to take
Does your child have painful, yellowish spots in her mouth? Are the glands in her neck swollen? Does she have a fever? Is there a red, crusted blister (fever blister, cold sore) on your child's lip? Are the gums reddened, swollen, or painful? Are there blisters on the tongue?	**YES**	Mouth infection caused by virus such as herpes or Coxsackie.	Consult your GP, who will evaluate the child's general health and recommend methods to reduce discomfort, including a soothing mouthwash or a pain medication to apply to the sore area. Cold liquids may be comforting.
Does your child have dry, reddened lips? Are they scaling and cracked in the corners of her mouth?	**YES**	Chapped lips (cheilitis), possibly caused by sensitivity to foods and worsened by alternate wetting and drying.	Apply a bland lip salve or petroleum jelly, especially during cold weather. Don't apply lanolin-based salves, which may cause further problems with sensitivity.
Does your child have a sore on the end or side of her tongue, or one sore spot on the inside of her cheek?	**YES**	Sore caused by chipped tooth; self-injury caused by biting (nervous habit).	If the sore is caused by a rough spot on a tooth or filling, consult your child's dentist, who will examine the teeth and file off any sharp points. On sympathetic questioning, most children usually admit to causing self-injury and try to avoid it in the future.
Does your child have sore patches on his tongue or inside his mouth? Is he taking a prescription drug such as an anticonvulsant or an antibiotic?	**YES**	Medication side effect.	Consult your GP, who will examine the child and adjust his medication if necessary.

Geographic tongue

The normal tongue is a healthy pink, its upper surface covered with papillae – hairlike projections of tissue – encircled by taste buds. Occasionally, parents are alarmed to see that their child's tongue is covered with bright red patches with white borders forming a maplike pattern. The painless patches tend to fade and reappear in new sites on the tongue. This condition, known as geographic tongue or benign migratory glossitis, is irritating but not serious. It doesn't require treatment. The exact cause is unknown, although the tendency seems to run in families.

Muscle Pain

Myalgia

Consult your doctor if muscle pain is accompanied by:

- Inability to move the affected area.
- A persistent swelling or lump.

Warning

Use ice – never heat – to treat new muscle injuries. Heat increases the blood flow to the injured area, in turn increasing haemorrhage and making inflammation worse.

In General:

Minor injuries incurred during sports and play are the most frequent cause of muscle pains in children. Many parents are familiar with 'growing pains' caused by normal wear and tear (see Limb/Leg Pain, p. 108), and children often have temporary aches and pains when they increase their athletic activity, begin a new sport that requires unaccustomed movements, or play an old sport at a higher level.

Some viral illnesses, especially influenza, can cause achy muscles but are usually accompanied by fever, fatigue, and a feeling of being generally unwell. Emotional tension and anxiety may also take the form of muscle pain in the neck and shoulders, particularly in adolescent girls. A child who has tight, painful muscles due to stress must learn to unwind. Exercise is among the best ways because it promotes the release of endorphins, the body's natural painkillers and mood elevators. Youngsters who are physically active may have a few bumps and scrapes, but they are much less likely to have nagging stress-related pain than their more sedentary friends.

Even children with chronic diseases can keep fit and have fun with physical activity. A child with a disability should be encouraged to become as active as possible without taking unnecessary risks. Your doctor can advise you about suitable sports.

Questions to consider	If answer is	Possible cause is	Action to take
Is your child complaining of sharp, cramping pain in the calf or thigh? Does the muscle feel hard and tense? Has she either spent an unusually active day or been confined in one position (such as in a car) for a long period?	**YES**	Muscle cramp due to fatigue or reduced circulation.	Rub the area to increase the circulation. If the pain doesn't improve after an hour, or your child has frequent muscle cramps, consult your doctor.
Did the pain begin suddenly during sports or strenuous activity? Is the area slightly swollen?	**YES**	Muscle strain.	Have your child rest and apply the RICE treatment (see box opposite). If the pain and swelling get worse, call your GP. Encourage your child to begin and end activity sessions with warm-up exercises and stretching to help prevent strains.
Did severe pain follow an injury, such as twisting an ankle or falling on a wrist? Is the area rapidly swelling?	**YES**	Sprain (torn ligament); fracture.	Consult your GP.

Myalgia

QUESTIONS TO CONSIDER	IF ANSWER IS	POSSIBLE CAUSE IS	ACTION TO TAKE
In addition to aching muscles, does your child have symptoms such as a fever, runny nose, sore throat, or cough?	**YES**	Influenza or other viral infection.	If your child's temperature is 38.3°C (101°F) or higher, call your GP. Otherwise, encourage the child to rest and give paracetamol or ibuprofen to relieve muscle aches and reduce fever. Make sure drinks are available to replace lost fluids.
Is your child complaining of pain and stiffness in the shoulders, upper arms, and neck? Is she otherwise healthy? Could she be under unusual stress because of events at home or school?	**YES**	Emotional tension; functional pain.	Try to identify sources of stress and deal with them. Encourage your child to exercise regularly. If pain and tensions persist, discuss your concerns with your GP.
Does your child have a persistent lump in a muscle?	**YES**	Tumour (rare).	Consult your GP, who will examine the child and perform diagnostic tests.

RICE treatment for muscle injuries

If your child strains a muscle or injures a limb, apply the following RICE treatment to minimize swelling. Don't use any other treatment, including pain relievers, until a doctor has examined the child and diagnosed the injury. If your child is injured while playing a sport, keep her from putting weight on the injured limb as you help her off the playing field.

1. Rest: stop the activity and rest the injured part.
2. Ice: place an ice bag (a packet of frozen vegetables from the freezer will do) wrapped in a towel over the injured area. If the child is under age 2, use a cloth wrung out in cold water; excessive cold can damage delicate tissues in young children. Don't apply ice directly to the skin and do not leave the wrapped ice bag on the skin for longer than 20 minutes or apply it more often than every 2 hours; excessive exposure to cold can damage tissues.
3. Compression: remove clothing from the injured spot. An elastic bandage may be helpful to prevent swelling and promote healing; however, it is very important to make sure the bandage is not too tight, as an overly tight bandage can cut off circulation.
4. Elevation: raise the injured arm or leg higher than the level of the child's heart, and keep it elevated until the pain and swelling begin to go down.

Place an ice bag over the injured area. Protect the child's skin with a towel.

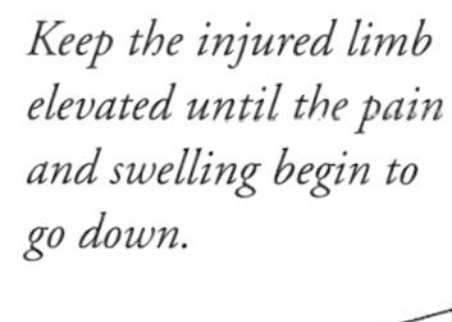

Keep the injured limb elevated until the pain and swelling begin to go down.

Nosebleeds

Epistaxis

In General:

Even slight damage to the delicate mucous membrane lining the nose may rupture tiny blood vessels and cause bleeding. Babies rarely have nosebleeds, but toddlers and school-age children often do. Fortunately, by the teenage years, most youngsters outgrow this common, sometimes alarming, but almost never serious event. A tendency to nosebleeds often runs in the family. Many children have nosebleeds for no apparent reason.

A nosebleed usually comes on suddenly, with blood flowing freely from one nostril. A child who has nosebleeds at night may swallow the blood in her sleep and vomit it up or pass it in the stools. Most nosebleeds stop by themselves within a few minutes, but for persistent bleeding, see Stopping a nosebleed, opposite.

Nosebleeds are unlikely to indicate serious disease, although bleeding can result from injury. Children may cause bleeding by picking their noses; toddlers often injure the nasal membranes by forcing objects into their nostrils. Youngsters are especially likely to have nosebleeds during colds and in the winter months when the mucous membranes become dry, cracked, and crusted, or when a chronic condition such as allergic rhinitis harms the membrane.

A child with a chronic disease that causes forceful coughing, such as cystic fibrosis, may have frequent nosebleeds. And parents of those with inborn disorders affecting the blood's ability to form clots, such as haemophilia or von Willebrand disease, should be watchful about harmful habits such as nose-picking.

☎

Call your GP immediately if:

- Your child is pale, sweaty, or not responding to you.
- You believe your child has lost a lot of blood.
- Your child is bleeding from the mouth, or vomiting blood or brown material that looks like coffee grounds.
- Your child's nose is bleeding after a blow or injury to any part of the head.

Warning

Don't use medicated nose drops or nasal sprays to treat conditions affecting the nose and respiratory passages. Although sold over the counter for the relief of congestion, these medications actually increase congestion after a few days' use. The rebound effect can be even more uncomfortable and hard to treat than the original problem.

Questions to consider	If answer is	Possible cause is	Action to take
Does your child have a runny nose due to a cold or hay fever (allergic rhinitis)? Does he have allergies?	YES	Swelling and irritation of nasal tissue.	To stop bleeding, pinch the soft part of the nose. Use of a cold air humidifier in your child's bedroom at night may help relieve stuffiness and keep the membranes moist. Do not add medications or aromatic preparations to the humidifier. If your child has not been evaluated for allergies, consult your doctor.
Do you live in a very dry climate? Or is your house overheated? Is the winter air very dry?	YES	Drying of nasal mucous membranes.	Try a cold air humidifier in the child's room at night. Saline nose drops may help to keep tissues moist. If bleeding is severe or recurrent, consult your doctor.

Epistaxis

Questions to consider	If answer is	Possible cause is	Action to take
Has the child had a fall or a bump on the nose? Or does he pick his nose? Or has he blown his nose very hard?	**YES**	Injury (trauma) to nose.	Follow the steps in Stopping a nosebleed, below. If the bleeding doesn't stop after two 10-minute attempts, or if the child had a severe blow to the head, call your GP at once.
Does your child have frequent, fairly severe nosebleeds for no apparent reason?	**YES**	Abnormal formation of blood vessels in the nose; polyps or other growths in the nose; bleeding disorder. (See Bleeding and Bruising, p. 38.)	Consult your GP, who will examine the child and provide a referral, if advisable, to an ear-nose-throat specialist.
Is your child taking medication, whether a doctor's prescription or an over-the-counter product such as medicated nose drops or nasal spray?	**YES**	Side effect of the medication.	Stop any over-the-counter medication. Consult your GP, who will prescribe an alternative treatment, if necessary.
Has your child previously been diagnosed with a blood-clotting disorder?	**YES**	Abnormal blood clotting; bleeding following self-injury such as nose-picking or scab-picking.	Explain how self-injury is causing nosebleeds and make a deal with your child to stop it; a contract providing an award for doing so may be helpful. Seek your GP's advice about alternative approaches.
Does your child have a chronic illness that causes forceful coughing? Or does she need medications or extra oxygen for a chronic disorder?	**YES**	Pressure injury due to forceful coughing; effect of medications on nasal mucous membrane.	Consult your GP, who will recommend measures to keep the nasal tissues moist and prevent nosebleeds.

Stopping a nosebleed

- Stay calm; the nosebleed is probably not serious, and you should try not to upset your child.
- Keep your child sitting or standing, and leaning slightly forward. Don't let her lie down or lean back as this will allow blood to flow down her throat and may make her vomit.
- Don't try to stuff tissues or other material into the nose to stop the bleeding.
- Firmly pinch the soft part of your child's nose – using a cold compress if you have one, otherwise your fingers – and keep the pressure on for a full 10 minutes. Do not look to see if the nose is bleeding during this time; you may start the flow again.
- If the bleeding hasn't stopped after 10 minutes, repeat the pressure. If bleeding persists after your second try, call your doctor or take the child to the nearest hospital emergency department.
- Although most nosebleeds are benign and self-limited, a child with severe or recurrent bleeding, or bleeding from both nostrils, should be evaluated by an ear-nose-throat specialist.

Paleness

Pallor

IN GENERAL:

If your child looks unusually pale, your doctor will examine the nailbeds, lips, the creases of the palms, and inside the lower eyelids. As long as these areas are rosy pink and there's no weakness or unusual fatigue, your child is probably quite healthy. A naturally fair child may look even paler during the winter months, when there are few opportunities to play outdoors. And the impression of pallor is sometimes heightened when a child has dark blotches under the eyes as a result of allergies (allergic shiners) or tiredness.

Warning

A child with mild anaemia usually has pale-to-normal skin colour and few symptoms. When anaemia is advanced, the child is pale, irritable, and lacking in energy. The symptoms may develop so gradually, however, that parents have difficulty recognizing them.

☎

Consult your doctor if your child looks unusually pale and also:

- Has bruising in places that don't usually get injured.
- Has swellings in the neck or abdomen.
- Feels weak and extremely tired all the time.
- Has prolonged bleeding, including nosebleeds lasting more than 10 minutes or menstrual periods longer than 7 days.

QUESTIONS TO CONSIDER	IF ANSWER IS	POSSIBLE CAUSE IS	ACTION TO TAKE
Is your child pale but active and healthy? Is he eating and sleeping well?	**YES**	Normal fair complexion.	Your child is naturally fair. Pay special attention to sun protection when he plays outdoors.
Is your child between 8 months and 2 years? Does she seem pale, fretful, and lethargic?	**YES**	Anaemia of infancy; iron-deficiency anaemia.	Your doctor will examine the child and may order laboratory tests. If your child is anaemic, your doctor will review her diet and, if necessary, prescribe extra iron.
Does your child have dark blotches under his lower eyelids? Has he had several late nights or unusual activity? Is he otherwise healthy?	**YES**	Tiredness; allergies.	If your child is overtired, make sure he gets enough rest to make up for daytime activities. If he also has a stuffy nose or other symptoms of allergies (see p. 26), ask your doctor's advice.
Has your child recently had a viral infection? Or has she been taking a prescribed medication, such as an antibiotic?	**YES**	Temporary, normal decrease in red blood cell production following acute illness.	Your doctor will examine the child, order blood tests, and – if the diagnosis is confirmed – explain a treatment plan.
Has your child been diagnosed with an auto-immune disease or other chronic illness? Does she have digestive problems?	**YES**	Auto-immune haemolytic anaemia; anaemia secondary to a chronic illness.	Consult your doctor, who may order blood tests and, if necessary, prescribe treatment, including iron supplements.

QUESTIONS TO CONSIDER	IF ANSWER IS	POSSIBLE CAUSE IS	ACTION TO TAKE
Does your child have unexplained bruising? Is he sometimes feverish?	**YES**	Leukaemia; tumour.	Your doctor will examine the child and order necessary diagnostic tests.
Is your baby about 6 months old? Are his hands or abdomen swollen? Does he seem fretful and in pain? Does he have ancestors from Africa or the Mediterranean?	**YES**	Sickle cell anaemia.	Call your doctor, who will examine the child, perform blood tests, and, if appropriate, prescribe treatment.
Is your baby between 6 and 12 months? Is he fretful? Is he losing or failing to gain weight? Does your family have ancestors from a Mediterranean country?	**YES**	Thalassaemia (an inherited blood condition that mainly affects people from the Mediterranean).	Call your doctor, who will examine the baby, order blood tests, and prescribe any necessary treatment.
Does your toddler or preschooler often eat non-food items such as paint chips? Does she seem less advanced than others of her age? Does she often have stomachaches and vomiting?	**YES**	Lead poisoning.	Consult your doctor promptly for treatment as well as advice on getting rid of lead in your home and environment.

Managing anaemia

Iron deficiency is the most common nutritional anaemia, although it is rarely a cause of severe problems. It is often seen in children under 3 years who drink a lot of milk, as well as in adolescent girls who need a good supply of iron to make up for losses in menstrual blood. There are two kinds of iron in our diet. Haeme iron is found in animal products, especially red meat, shellfish, and fish. Non-haeme iron occurs in a variety of plant foods such as legumes (peas and beans), fortified breads and cereals, and dried apricots. On average we absorb only about 10 percent of the iron we eat. Our absorption of non-haeme iron can also be decreased up to 50 percent by other foods we eat, including the tannins in tea, compounds called phytates in grain products, and oxalic acid, which occurs in leafy greens such as spinach and chard as well as in rhubarb. On the other hand, we absorb more iron from plant foods if we eat foods containing vitamin C at the same meal. Good sources of vitamin C include citrus fruits and juices, strawberries, cantaloupe, watermelon, sweet potatoes, sweet peppers, broccoli, and many other fruits and vegetables.

Different kinds of anaemia may also be caused by several diseases, occur as a reaction to medication, or follow a viral infection. If your doctor suspects that your child may be anaemic, he will order a blood test to determine the amount of haemoglobin – the oxygen-carrying pigment that gives blood its red colour – in her blood. Another test, called a haematocrit, shows how much of the blood is made up of red blood cells, and an evaluation of red cell size can indicate what type of anaemia is present. If the tests confirm the diagnosis, your doctor will prescribe a treatment plan for the anaemia and treat any underlying disorder.

In General:

As a developing baby approaches the time for birth, his spine begins to straighten out from its original C-curve in preparation for the dramatic changes in posture and movement that will be highlights of the next few years. After the birth, the neck (cervical spine) curves forward in readiness to support the head. At the same time, the chest (thoracic spine) curves backward and there is a corresponding inward curve of the lower spine. This graceful curvature protects the spine from undue stress. Changes in posture can alter the natural curve and place stress on the vertebrae, the interlocking bones of the spine.

To find the balance needed for walking, the toddler curves his lower back inwards, at the same time pushing his belly and buttocks out in the typical, pot-bellied, 2-year-old stance. As the body matures, the posture becomes more erect until, at maturity in the late teens, the spine is properly curved and the young adult is standing tall. At regular check-ups, your doctor evaluates your child's spine, shoulders, and hips, along with his gait and stance, for symmetry and balance, and makes careful note of any abnormal curves. If your doctor detects any abnormalities, she will determine the cause and provide any necessary treatment.

Consult your doctor if your child has a change in posture together with:

- Persistent or increasing back pain.
- Fever, weight loss, and feeling generally unwell.
- Weakness in the legs.
- Persistent vomiting.
- Evidence of a curved spine, such as one shoulder or hip consistently higher than the other.

Warning

Conditions that interfere with good posture should always be brought to the attention of your doctor. While some require treatment, others eventually correct themselves. When your doctor recognizes that a disorder will clear up without treatment, she will advise you that the best course is careful observation with no intervention. In the meantime, both parents and child must be patient.

Questions to consider	If answer is	Possible cause is	Action to take
Does your youngster usually slouch, keeping his shoulders rounded and his chest sunken? Is he otherwise healthy, with no complaints of pain?	**YES**	Postural kyphosis (round back), caused by habitual poor posture.	Encourage your child to correct his faulty posture in order to avoid problems later on. If kyphosis persists, consult your GP, who will examine the youngster to rule out serious problems.
Does your child keep her shoulders hunched? Does she have back pain? Is she unable to straighten up?	**YES**	Idiopathic kyphosis; Scheuermann disease.	Consult your GP, who will examine the child and provide a referral to a specialist. Treatment usually involves exercises and braces; surgery is rarely required for this relatively common condition.
Is your youngster holding his head to one side, with his chin up? Is his neck painful, with limited motion? Has he recently had an upper respiratory infection?	**YES**	Wryneck (torticollis), possibly linked to a viral illness.	Consult your GP, who will examine the child and recommend any necessary treatment.

QUESTIONS TO CONSIDER	IF ANSWER IS	POSSIBLE CAUSE IS	ACTION TO TAKE
Does your child seem to be holding one shoulder higher than the other? Are the hips uneven? Does the spine appear curved when your child bends over?	**YES**	Curvature of the spine (scoliosis); asymmetry; unequal leg length.	Consult your GP, who may refer your child to a paediatric orthopaedic specialist (Also see Back Pain, p. 30.)
Is your child walking with difficulty? Does he have pain or stiffness in the lower back and hips? Are his joints painful?	**YES**	Inflammatory disorder such as juvenile rheumatoid arthritis or other condition requiring diagnosis and treatment.	Call your doctor, who will examine the child and determine whether referral to a specialist is advisable.
Does your toddler seem to be slow in walking? Do his legs seem weak? Is he unusually clumsy? Is his belly particularly prominent, while his spine curves backward?	**YES**	Neuromuscular condition, metabolic disorder, or bone disease requiring investigation and treatment.	Consult your doctor, who will evaluate the child and determine the appropriate management.

Good posture now may prevent back problems later

Habits of poor posture adopted by children become exaggerated in self-conscious adolescents: slouching, slumping, head down, and shoulders rounded. Boys may slouch because they don't want to stand out from the crowd, and girls stoop because they are afraid of appearing taller than their friends, especially boys. Poor posture starts around the time of breast development in many girls; some are embarrassed because their breasts are growing, others because they're not.

Encourage your child to practise good posture. Whether sitting, standing, or exercising, the body should be straight but relaxed, with head level, shoulders down and back, and abdomen and buttocks tucked in.

Wryneck, or torticollis, causes a child to hold his head in an abnormal position. He may lean his head towards one shoulder and, when lying on his stomach, always turn the same side of his face towards the mattress. If not treated, wryneck may lead to permanent deformity and restricted head movement.

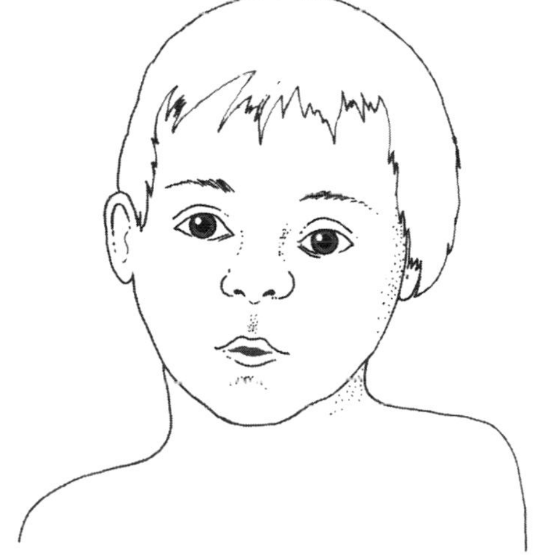

Rectal Pain/Itching

Proctalgia, Proctodynia/Pruritus Ani

In General:

Frequent causes of rectal discomfort in children include ringworms and constipation. Pain associated with bowel movements may lead to constipation and an anal fissure, a painful tear in the mucous membranes lining the anus, which often leads, in turn, to further constipation because of stool holding and pain. To many children, the itching caused by ringworms, which is usually most intense at night, is just as distressing as the pain associated with constipation or anal fissure. Scratching the itch further irritates the skin and increases the risk of infection. Streptococcal infection can cause dermatitis with redness and intense discomfort around the anus.

Serious causes of rectal pain are uncommon in children, as are haemorrhoids. Common and uncomfortable but usually less serious in adults, haemorrhoids may be a symptom of more serious disease in children.

Any bruising near the anus should alert parents to the possibility that their son or daughter has been sexually abused, especially if the child is reluctant to give a reason for the bruising and discomfort.

Consult your doctor if your child has:

- Rectal pain and bleeding.
- Severe constipation and rectal discomfort.
- Haemorrhoids.
- Itching that is more intense at night.
- A sore, red rash around the anus.
- Bruising near the anus.

Warning

An anal fissure will not heal unless measures are taken to soften hard stools that can tear the anus. This may require help from your doctor to retrain the youngster so that she stops withholding stool and learns to respond to the urge to defecate.

Questions to consider	If answer is	Possible cause is	Action to take
Does your child fidget and scratch her anus? Is the itching worse at night? Are there white, threadlike worms less than 1cm (½ in) long moving in her stools?	**YES**	Ringworms. (See Itching, p. 100; Managing ringworms, opposite.)	Consult your GP, who will examine the child to confirm the diagnosis and prescribe appropriate treatment. Ask whether other family members should also be treated to prevent the spread of infection.
Does your child have pain when he moves his bowels and for several minutes afterward? Is there fresh blood on the toilet paper, on the stool, or in the toilet bowl?	**YES**	Anal fissure.	Consult your doctor, who can diagnose an anal fissure by examining the anus. Most anal fissures occur during passage of hard stools (see Constipation, p. 48). Treatment may involve stool softeners to break the cycle of hardened stools, laceration, and stool withholding.
Does your infant or preschooler have a sore, red rash around the anus?	**YES**	Perianal dermatitis caused by streptococcal infection.	Call your doctor, who will examine the child and, if necessary, prescribe an antibiotic. Clean the child's anus with plain water after bowel movements and apply zinc oxide ointment or a similar barrier cream to protect the skin.

QUESTIONS TO CONSIDER	IF ANSWER IS	POSSIBLE CAUSE IS	ACTION TO TAKE
Is your child having painless bleeding from the anus? Does she seem healthy and active otherwise?	**YES**	Inflammatory polyps; Meckel diverticulum, a saclike pouch in the small intestine (ileum).	Consult your GP, who will examine the child to determine whether the bleeding is due to polyps and should be referred to a specialist.
Has your child's rectum protruded through the anus and stayed outside after a bowel movement? Was he straining on the toilet? Or has he previously been diagnosed with a chronic condition such as cystic fibrosis?	**YES**	Rectal prolapse.	If your child is not in pain, cover your finger with toilet tissue and push the rectum back into its proper position. (Pieces of toilet tissue that stick will pass out with a bowel movement.) If your child finds it hard not to strain, suggest that he keep his feet on a low footstool while seated on the toilet. Consult your doctor if you can't replace the rectum or if it is tender or bleeding.
Is your toddler or pre-schooler walking oddly and showing signs of rectal pain? Does she resist suggestions that she use the potty or lavatory? Can she tell you if she may have something inside?	**YES**	Foreign body in rectum (your child's natural curiosity).	Call your doctor to examine the child and identify the foreign object. A small object can sometimes be left to pass on its own; if it is large, sharp, or otherwise dangerous, your GP will refer you immediately to hospital.
Does your child have pain and a sore, red swelling or 'pimple' near the anus?	**YES**	Perianal abscess and/or fistula; Crohn disease.	Consult your GP, who will examine the child to determine whether treatment is necessary.

Managing ringworms

Ringworms are found everywhere, at every age and economic level. Especially common in children, they are easily transmitted from one child to another in childcare centres and schools. The infection is annoying but harmless, although ringworms may carry faecal bacteria to the female genital tract and cause vulvovaginitis (see p. 156).

Children ingest ringworm eggs carried under fingernails, on clothing or bedding, or in house dust. The eggs hatch in the stomach and the larvae migrate to the intestine where they mature into white worms about 1cm (about ½in) long. At night, female worms deposit eggs near the child's anus. The child scratches the itching this causes and traps more eggs under the fingernails – only to ingest them again or shed them where they will find their way to new hosts.

If your child has itching, is unusually fidgety, or has trouble getting to sleep, press surgical tape to the skin around the anus in the morning. Show this to your doctor; adhering eggs and worms will confirm the diagnosis.

Ringworms can be eradicated with a short course of medication. Because re-infestation is common, the treatment may need to be repeated at intervals. Wash bedding and clothing in hot water to get rid of eggs and stop ringworms from spreading.

In General:

Head banging and rocking are quite common among normal children and are also seen in those with developmental problems. In normal children, repetitive head banging and rocking, while alarming to parents, are harmless and gradually stop over a period of months. If they continue longer, the child should be evaluated by a doctor.

Some experts theorize that the actions begin as normal behaviour and are part of the child's efforts to master movement as she gradually gains control of her body. Thus, a child who starts head rocking as early as 4 or 5 months may be rocking her whole body at 6 to 10 months as she develops more skills.

Nobody knows why children bang their heads and rock, but it's interesting that these rhythmic habits – body rocking, head banging, and head rolling – all stimulate the vestibular system of the inner ear, which controls balance. They are not usually associated with developmental delay, although children who have certain types of disabilities often repeat movements, as do autistic children and others with oversensitive nervous systems.

Children usually outgrow rocking, rolling, and head banging between 18 months and 2 years of age, but repetitive actions are sometimes still seen in older children and adolescents.

Consult your doctor if your child is frequently nodding or shaking her head and:

- Doesn't interact with her parents.
- Has developmental delays.

Warning

Children are rarely, if ever, harmed by this behaviour, but if you are concerned that your child may injure himself, or the behaviour is not diminishing over months, consult your doctor.

Questions to consider	If answer is	Possible cause is	Action to take
Does your baby of about 6 months rock vigorously in his cot for up to 15 minutes at a time, or even longer? Does this activity often occur when he's left alone to fall asleep or listen to music? Is there any particular event or stimulus that either triggers or stops the behaviour?	**YES**	Body rocking as part of a baby's normal development.	Body rocking is harmless and seems to comfort the child. It will gradually stop as your child becomes more mobile, and is usually gone by the age of 2 or 3, although some form of body movement may last through adolescence.
Does your child bang his head hard and often – as many as 60 to 80 times a minute – against solid objects such as his cot? Does the head banging follow a head-rolling or body-rocking phase? Does your child also suck his thumb or rub a blanket as he bangs his head?	**YES**	Head banging.	This inexplicable behaviour seems to comfort the child but distresses the parents, who fear that their baby will hurt himself. In fact, it doesn't seem to worry babies (more often boys) who often look relaxed and happy while they bang their heads. It usually starts at about 6 months and stops by the time a child is 2 years old.

QUESTIONS TO CONSIDER	IF ANSWER IS	POSSIBLE CAUSE IS	ACTION TO TAKE
Has your baby rubbed a bald spot with her constant head rolling or shaking? Is she otherwise active and happy? Do her eyes move normally?	**YES**	Head rolling or rubbing.	This harmless habit may also appear in a child who can sit up. It may start as early as 6 months and usually disappears before the child reaches 2 years.
Does your developmentally disabled child bang her head or perform other rhythmic actions? Are you concerned that she may injure herself?	**YES**	Developmental disorder or autistic behaviour.	Consult a paediatrician, who may prescribe a short-term medication to calm the child and recommend a helmet to protect her head.

Coping with head banging

Your baby will eventually outgrow head banging and body rocking. In the meantime, however, the movement and noise that seem to give him pleasure may cause a great deal of wear and tear on your family's nerves. You can't restrain the baby or make him stop the activity, but you can take a few simple steps to keep the noise at the lowest possible level.

Pull the cot away from the wall and place it on a thick rug. Fit rubber or plastic carpet protectors on the legs of the cot to lessen noise and make it harder for your baby to move the cot as he rocks. Use a padded cot bumper that goes all the way around the cot. Secure it with at least 6 ties to keep it from falling away at the sides. Trim the ties to no more than 15cm (6in) long and double-knot them. Some paediatricians suggest using a metronome or playing music with a strong beat to regulate the head banging.

Place a mobile over the cot to divert your baby with different shapes and bright colours. A mobile with a built-in music box that plays a repetitive tune can be soothing for a baby trying to fall asleep. Your baby may have fun with a gym across the top of the cot or an activity centre attached to the side. Watch your baby's reaction to mobiles and gyms, however; some babies find them frightening and cry until they are removed. In any case, mobiles, gyms, and cot bumpers must be removed at 5 months, which is when many babies are making serious attempts to sit, get up on all fours, or pull themselves to a standing position. Even very young babies love to get ready for naps by spending several minutes looking at a picture book, or hearing their parents singing songs or nursery rhymes. Music playing softly in the room may put your baby in the mood for sleep.

Runny/Stuffy Nose

Rhinorrhea/Nasal Congestion

In General:

A runny or stuffy nose usually clears up in a few days without any need for medication or medical care. The most common cause is an upper respiratory viral infection such as a common cold (rhinovirus) or, in winter, flu (influenza). When a runny nose is accompanied or followed by other symptoms, your child may have a more serious problem. In such cases, you should consult your doctor.

Warning

Do not treat your child's stuffy nose with nonprescription nasal sprays unless your doctor gives the go-ahead. These medications may provide temporary relief, but there is sometimes a rebound effect that can worsen the problem.

☎

Consult your GP if the runny or stuffy nose is accompanied by:

- Unusual sleepiness or lethargy.
- Difficulty breathing.
- A fever over 38°C (100.4°F) in a child under 3 months and 38.3°C (101°F) in one over 3 months.
- Neck pain or stiffness.
- An earache or sore throat.
- Swollen glands.
- Eye redness or swelling.
- A rash.

Questions to consider	If answer is	Possible cause is	Action to take
Is the major symptom a clear, watery discharge? And is your child as active as usual with little or no fever?	**YES**	Common cold.	You may want to keep your child at home for a day or two, but no special action or medication is needed; a cold will run its course in 4 to 7 days.
Does your child also have an earache? Is she fussy and irritable?	**YES**	An ear infection.	Ask your GP to examine the child and confirm the diagnosis. An antibiotic might be needed. (See Earache/Ear Infection, p. 68.)
Does the child also have a sore throat? Are the throat symptoms severe?	**YES**	Most likely a cold, but other infections should be ruled out.	See your GP, who will examine the child and treat if necessary. (See Sore Throat, p. 136.)
Is your child feverish and unusually sleepy or lethargic?	**YES**	Complications of an upper respiratory infection.	Consult your GP, who will examine your child and recommend treatment.
Are the neck and glands swollen and tender?	**YES**	An infection, which may be viral or bacterial.	See your GP, who will want to examine the child and may recommend treatment.
Has your child's nose been runny for more than a week, or does this symptom recur periodically? Is the nose itchy? Are the eyes red, itchy, or watery?	**YES**	Hay fever (allergic rhinitis) or another allergic response.	Consult your GP, who may want to arrange tests for specific allergies. (See Allergic Reactions, p. 26.)

QUESTIONS TO CONSIDER	IF ANSWER IS	PROBABLE CAUSE IS	ACTION TO TAKE
Has the discharge lasted more than 10 days? Is it thicker or changed in other ways? Is there a headache?	**YES**	Sinus infection.	See your GP to confirm the diagnosis. He will prescribe appropriate treatment (see Treating sinusitis, below).
Is the discharge foul-smelling and coming from only one nostril?	**YES**	Foreign object in the nostril.	Consult your GP, who will examine the child and, if necessary, arrange to have the object removed.
Does the child have trouble breathing? Does he snore? Wake up frequently?	**YES**	Enlarged tonsils and adenoids.	Ask your GP to examine the child and, if necessary, perform diagnostic tests.
Has the child had a recent fall or facial injury?	**YES**	Nose injury (such as deviated septum) or other structural problem.	Consult your GP for tests and x-rays, if necessary.

Treating sinusitis

The sinuses are air spaces in the bones above and adjacent to the nose. Each of the eight sinuses is lined with mucous membranes that drain into the nose.

An acute sinus infection is usually set off by a cold, influenza, or hay fever. If the sinus membranes become inflamed, swollen, and possibly infected, your child may complain of a headache, stuffy nose, and perhaps tenderness around the eyes or other parts of the face. The nasal discharge is likely to become unusually thick and tinged with green or yellow. There also may be a fever and your child will probably act sicker than he does when he has an ordinary cold.

Treatment depends upon the underlying cause. Antibiotics may be prescribed to clear up a bacterial sinus infection. Taking a steamy shower, placing a misting humidifier in your child's bedroom, or using a saline nasal spray may help to drain the blocked sinuses. Ask your GP for advice on the best approach for treating your child.

The size and shape of sinuses vary from one person to another, but this illustration shows a typical conformation. The frontal sinuses, which develop at about age 8, are situated in the forehead and are a frequent cause of sinus headaches. The maxillary (upper jaw) sinuses, located to the side of the nostril, are the largest. The sphenoid sinuses are more towards the centre of the head; the ethmoid sinuses are made up of many air pockets on each side of the nose.

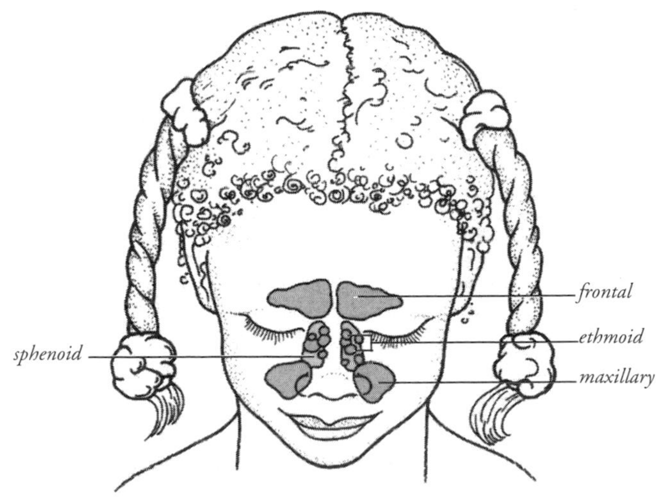

Sexual Maturation

Puberty

IN GENERAL:

The secondary sexual characteristics emerge under hormonal control at puberty. In girls, the first physical sign of sexual maturation is breast development, which begins somewhere between 9 and 13 years of age. Boys generally commence puberty a year or so later than girls, as the testes and penis begin to grow between ages 10 and 14. Even before the earliest physical signs appear, parents usually notice that youngsters need more food to keep up with their rapidly accelerating growth rate. With the adolescent growth spurt that follows about 2 years after the early signs, the height increases by about 25 percent while the weight may almost double.

Girls begin to menstruate on average at about 12 to 13 years of age. Studies in ballet dancers, athletes, and girls with eating disorders (see p. 178) show that those who have an abnormally low percentage of body fat tend to have their first menstrual period (menarche) later than average. Ovulation may be established only after a girl has experienced irregular or unusually heavy periods for several months.

In boys, ejaculation first occurs somewhere between 11 and 15 years, although the range of 8 to 17 years is considered normal. Growth of the larynx (Adam's apple) and deepening of the voice coincide with the first appearance of facial hair, and the increase in height is matched by a corresponding increase in muscle mass.

In girls, growth gradually stops within a year or so after menarche. In boys, full height is usually reached by age 17 or 18, although young men may continue to grow until 21 years and many keep on filling out their lanky frames with muscle bulk into their early twenties.

Consult your GP if you notice:

- Signs of sexual development in your daughter under age 8 or your son under age 9.

Warning

The timing of sexual maturation varies widely and is influenced by a host of factors, including genetic background, nutrition, and body mass. If, however, there's no sign of sexual development in a girl of 13 or a boy of 14, see your GP.

QUESTIONS TO CONSIDER	IF ANSWER IS	POSSIBLE CAUSE IS	ACTION TO TAKE
Does your pre-adolescent daughter have a painful swelling underneath each nipple?	YES	Normal development.	This is a normal phase of breast development; the tenderness will decrease in time.
Is your 13-year-old daughter showing no signs of physical maturation, such as breast development, body hair, or increased growth?	YES	Delayed puberty.	Discuss your concerns with your GP. Your daughter may be following a family pattern, but your doctor will evaluate her status and determine whether referral is required.
Has your son shown no signs of development yet? Has he reached his 14th birthday?	YES	Delayed puberty.	Your GP should examine the youngster to determine whether a problem exists and referral is necessary.

QUESTIONS TO CONSIDER	IF ANSWER IS	POSSIBLE CAUSE IS	ACTION TO TAKE
Has your young school-age child (under age 8) started to show unusual signs such as enlargement of one or both breasts or growth of body hair?	YES	Precocious puberty; premature menarche. (See Breast Swelling, p. 43).	Consult your GP, who will determine whether the child should be tested and be seen by a specialist.
Is your teenage son developing at a normal rate, but worried that his breasts are growing?	YES	Breast enlargement (gynaecomastia).	This breast swelling is normal and temporary; it usually disappears without treatment. If your son is embarrassed by his appearance, ask your GP to reassure him that he's normal.
Is one of your daughter's breasts larger than the other? Is her development otherwise normal?	YES	Normal asymmetrical development of the breasts.	Reassure your daughter that many women have somewhat asymmetrical breasts. The difference may grow less obvious, but if it remains very marked after she has attained her full growth, treatment is possible.

Hormonal control of puberty

In both boys and girls, puberty begins when a part of the brain called the hypothalamus secretes gonadotropin-releasing factor (GRF). This prompts the nearby pituitary gland to release follicle-stimulating hormone (FSH) and luteinizing hormone (LH).

In girls FSH and LH act on the ovaries, stimulating them to produce progesterone and oestrogen, female hormones that are instrumental in regulating the menstrual cycle and monthly release of egg cells (ova). Also under hormonal control are the secondary sexual characteristics including breast development, pubic and armpit hair, and the increased fat stores that give a girl a womanly figure.

In boys, the pituitary hormones act on the testes to produce testosterone, which stimulates the growth of the genitals and the production of sperm. Secondary sex characteristics under testosterone control include the growth of facial and bodily hair, enlargement of the larynx with deepening of the voice, and an increase in muscle mass.

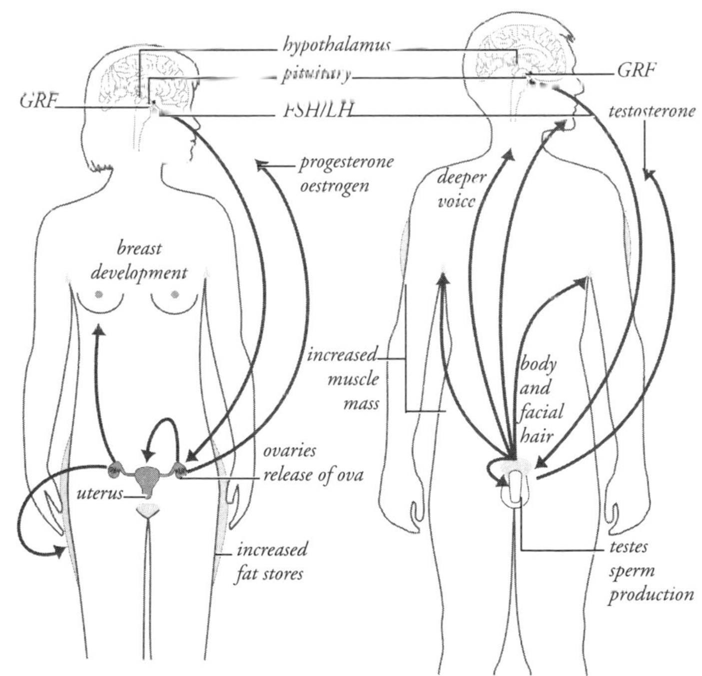

In General:

Despite its rigid, rocklike appearance, bone is in a state of constant change, renewing its cells and remodelling itself according to the nutrients available and the load it is required to bear. This process of renewal and remodelling continues throughout life.

Between birth and age 4, your child's skeleton doubles in size from an average length of 50cm (20in) to about 100cm (40in). Bone growth continues at a steady but somewhat slower rate until puberty, when a gain of 10cm (4in) in a single year is not unusual. The rate of growth is influenced by growth hormones and sex hormones. Malnutrition, lack of vitamin D, and chronic illness slow bone growth and may interfere with the correct formation of the bones. Long-term treatment with certain medications (for example, prednisone and other steroid drugs) can also impair bone development.

Glandular disorders, such as thyroid problems, sometimes interfere with skeletal development, causing short stature and disproportionately short limbs that can resemble dwarfism in severe cases. Pituitary disorders and a few other very rare conditions may cause a child to grow abnormally tall, with disproportionately large hands and feet, bony deformities, and developmental problems.

Consult your GP if:

- Your toddler walks with a limp.
- Your child's spine appears crooked or his limbs are asymmetrical.
- Your child seems to be growing slowly, his head appears unusually large, and his arms and legs look bowed.
- Your child seems to be growing abnormally fast and her hands and feet look disproportionately large.

Warning

At birth, many babies have what appear to be leg or foot deformities that reflect the effects of a confining position in the womb. In most cases, the bones straighten out without treatment during the first year of life.

Osseous (bony) or skeletal dysplasia (abnormal formation) is a term applied to unusually short stature with abnormal proportions. More than 300 such disorders are known. Each affects the skeleton in different ways and may also involve other organs. In many cases, skeletal dysplasia is detectable at or before birth, although some conditions become apparent only later. When the head, limbs, and trunk are out of proportion and certain bones are misshapen, the dysplasia is termed dwarfing. If the body is extremely small but the proportions are normal, the medical term is nanism and the individual is, in nonmedical terms, a midget, not a dwarf. (Also see Growth Problems, p. 82.) Excessively tall stature together with specific skeletal deformities is known as gigantism.

All skeletal dysplasias appear to have a genetic basis, except for rare conditions that affect a baby when the expectant mother takes certain medications (such as a blood thinner) or has a severe lack of certain vitamins (especially vitamin K). In a few extremely rare inherited conditions, children are stillborn because severe bone dysplasia is just one of many congenital abnormalities that are present.

Your GP or health visitor checks proportions by holding your baby's arms straight at her sides. He or she may recommend further evaluation if the infant's hands do not reach to the middle of the pelvis or – in a child over 1 year – do not extend past the upper thigh. Where a child's spine and limbs are out of proportion, however, the arms may extend well below the middle of the thigh. The family history is an important part of the examination because most forms of skeletal dysplasia are genetic. Similar malformations or extremely short stature in other family members may point to the diagnosis. Children who have skeletal dysplasia but no other severe disabilities usually have normal health, intelligence, and life expectancy.

Questions to consider	If answer is	Possible cause is	Action to take
Does your newborn baby's head look misshapen? Has it become flattened on one side in the weeks since his birth?	**YES**	Normal moulding of skull.	A baby's skull is subject to great pressure during birth; this causes no harm and the head will gradually resume a normal shape. If flattening has occurred since birth, it is simply the result of pressure and will disappear as the baby is able to change his position.
Has your toddler recently started to walk unaided? Is she limping?	**YES**	Disorder of the hip or other condition requiring treatment.	Consult your GP. Although usually diagnosed at birth, this condition may not be apparent until a child starts to walk. Your doctor will refer the child to a specialist.
Is one of your child's shoulders higher than the other? Do her hips look uneven? Is her spine curved?	**YES**	Curvature of the spine (scoliosis).	Consult your GP who will determine whether your child should be seen by an orthopaedic specialist. Treatment may be required. (See Back Pain, p. 30.)
Does your infant always hold his head toward one shoulder? When he lies on his stomach, does he always keep the same side of his head on the mattress?	**YES**	Wryneck (torticollis).	Consult your GP who will examine the baby and may recommend special exercises. (Also see Posture Defects, p. 120.)
Is your pre-adolescent or teenager worried because one side of his ribcage looks much smaller than the other?	**YES**	Thoracic (ribcage) asymmetry.	This common phenomenon is normal. It is always present from birth but may not be noticeable until ages 9 to 13, or when growth speeds up at puberty. The condition has no medical significance and no treatment is needed.

Funnel chest and pigeon breast

Minor abnormalities of development in the chest are usually no cause for worry, though they give unwarranted concern to self-conscious adolescents. Youngsters may go through a stage of being reluctant to change in the locker room or strip for swimming.

A frequently seen abnormality is 'funnel chest' (pectus excavatum or hollowed chest), where the breastbone (sternum) is sunken and the chest cavity correspondingly narrowed. Funnel chest is usually just an isolated congenital abnormality and may, in fact, run in the family. Occasionally it may indicate the presence of an unusual connective tissue disorder such as Marfan's syndrome (see p. 83) or the now-rare nutritional disorder rickets. Youngsters with chronic obstructive disease of the airways may develop a funnel chest deformity, which becomes less noticeable or even disappears when the underlying condition is successfully treated. Funnel chest is rarely a cause for concern and surgery to correct it is seldom necessary.

An unusually prominent sternum causes the shape known as pigeon breast (pectus carinatum, meaning keel-shaped chest). In an otherwise healthy and well-formed youngster, this is of no consequence.

In General:

Children's skin problems are often caused by allergic reactions (see p. 26) or infections, but many of the skin disorders that plague adults are also seen in children. Skin disorders can usually be identified by a simple inspection backed up by detailed questioning and a physical examination. In some cases, however, diagnostic tests may be necessary, especially if the problem is confused by injury, infection, or attempts at treatment.

Treatment of skin problems is based on the general rule that inflamed, oozing lesions normally need to be dried out, whereas chronic, dry conditions should be moisturized. A condition should be diagnosed before treatment is started. If the skin problem is an allergic reaction, it will recur unless the child avoids contact with the offending substance or it is eliminated from the diet.

Soaps containing perfumes and deodorants may be too harsh for those with sensitive skin. Many doctors recommend nonsoap cleansing lotions for babies, and neutral, full-fat soaps for toddlers and older children. Laundry soap or detergent residue on clothing and bedding can also irritate sensitive skin. Use a laundry product that's free of dyes and perfumes, and double rinse to eliminate irritating chemicals. Soaps and lotions containing lanolin may be irritating to those with atopic dermatitis. Children who cannot tolerate woollen clothing next to the skin are likely to be hypersensitive to lanolin-based products. If you're in doubt about any product, use plain warm water to wash your child. When a moisturizer is needed, it should be applied to damp skin immediately after a bath or shower.

Some synthetic fabrics and the dyes and other chemicals used in manufacturing also can be irritating to sensitive skins. Washing new clothes before wearing may help. If not, wear undyed cotton clothing next to the skin.

Consult your GP if your child has:

- Ring-shaped, red or scaly patches on the body or scalp.
- Spreading blisters that turn crusty and scaly.
- A rash while taking a prescribed medication.
- Many small, itchy, red lumps and track marks in the skin.

Warning

Doctors warn against the use of all-purpose over-the-counter skin medications, which may contain substances that can sensitize the child's skin and worsen the irritation. Use these and all medications only on your GP's advice.

Questions to consider	**If answer is**	**Possible cause is**	**Action to take**
Has your baby developed a raised, spotty rash a day or two after getting over a fever? Did he have only mild, vague symptoms while his temperature was elevated?	YES	Roseola infantum, an infection usually caused by herpes virus 6.	Consult your GP; if roseola seems the likely diagnosis, treatment may be advised to lower the fever.
Have bright red, warm, raised patches suddenly appeared on your child's cheeks? Does he also have mild symptoms such as slight fever? Is the rash spreading?	YES	Fifth disease (erythema infectiosum), a viral infection.	Call your GP, who may examine the child to make sure the rash is due to fifth disease. This mild parvovirus infection usually clears up within 10 days, but the rash may recur.

Questions to consider	If answer is	Possible cause is	Action to take
Has your child developed several blister-like spots surrounded by red halos on her face and body? Is she feverish and irritable?	**YES**	Chickenpox (varicella).	Consult your GP if you are unsure of the diagnosis. Paracetamol may relieve discomfort. Calamine lotion helps the itching, and your GP may also prescribe a medication. If any spots get very red, warm, and tender, they may be infected, in which case antibiotic treatment may be required.
Does your child have itchy red patches with small blisters and scaling or crusting? Was the skin exposed to a possible allergen, such as soap, jewellery, or new clothing?	**YES**	Contact dermatitis.	If you can trace the patches to a particular irritant, remove it and see if the rash improves (see Allergic Reactions, p. 26). If you can't, or if patches don't disappear, consult your GP, who may prescribe treatment.
Does your child have a cold sore or fever blister near her mouth?	**YES**	Herpes virus infection. (See Mouth Pain, p. 112.)	Consult your GP, who may recommend measures to make the child comfortable until the sore heals.
Have hardened, red patches developed in areas that itch or started as eczema?	**YES**	Lichen simplex (neurodermatitis).	This roughening of the skin occurs when the child repeatedly scratches an irritation. It will gradually disappear without treatment.
Has your toddler or older child developed a dusting of brown spots on parts of the body exposed to sunlight?	**YES**	Freckles (ephelides).	Freckles are common and run in families. Darker in summer, paler in winter, they are not dangerous, but indicate sun damage. Protect your child's skin with a sunscreen, T-shirt, and hat.
Are occasional small, brown spots appearing on your child's face and body?	**YES**	Moles (nevi).	Most people get moles in childhood and adolescence. A mole does not require attention unless it's disfiguring or could become irritated (such as on the shaving area of a teenage boy's face). But if you see a change in the size, colour, or shape of a mole, consult your GP, who may refer you to a dermatologist.
Does your child have six or more noticeable spots about the colour of milky coffee (café au lait) on his body?	**YES**	Condition requiring diagnosis and treatment (such as neurofibromatosis).	Consult your GP, who will examine the child and refer you, if necessary, to another specialist.
Does your child have spreading red blisters that are forming crusty scabs?	**YES**	Impetigo (streptococcal or staphylo coccal infection).	Call your GP; if the child has impetigo, antibiotic treatment will be required. Impetigo is highly infectious.

Continued on next page

Questions to consider	If answer is	Possible cause is	Action to take
Does your child have one or more painful, red, warm lumps under the skin? Is a lighter area visible at the top of each swelling?	**YES**	Boils (infected hair follicles).	Apply hot compresses to relieve pain and swelling. Do not squeeze the boil. Cover it with an adhesive bandage if it is open or exposed. If it fails to heal or more boils appear, call your GP, who may prescribe an antibiotic and other treatments.
Does your child have several painless, rough-surfaced lumps on her hands or elbows?	**YES**	Warts.	Warts are caused by a virus and eventually disappear without treatment. If the warts make it difficult for your child to use her hand or are disfiguring, your GP may advise removal or topical treatments.
Does your child have a lump on the sole of his foot? Is there a small opening in the swelling? Is it slightly painful?	**YES**	Plantar (sole of the foot) wart, also called verruca; callus.	Consult your GP, who will prescribe treatment or advise on footcare to remove the callus. She may refer you to a chiropodist.
Has your 9- or 10-year old's facial skin begun to look oily and coarser? Is she developing whiteheads and pimples in oily areas?	**YES**	Acne.	Skin changes are normal as children near puberty. Make sure your child cleans her face each night and morning. If she develops pustules or a rash, consult your GP, who may recommend more specific acne treatment.
Does your child have numerous small, itchy bumps? Can you see nits (egg cases) on her hair? Or are there red or greyish lines near the itchy bumps?	**YES**	Infestation with parasites such as lice or scabies.	Consult your GP, who will examine the child and recommend treatment, as well as measures to eradicate the parasites. Notify your child's school or childcare facility. Ask your GP if your child should stay home to avoid spreading the infestation.
Does your child have red, scaly, spreading rings with paler centres on his body? Is there patchy hair loss on his scalp?	**YES**	Ringworm (tinea corporis on body; tinea capitis on scalp).	Consult your GP, who will prescribe appropriate treatment.
Does your youngster complain of itching between his toes or on the soles of his feet? Is the skin scaling or peeling in these areas? Are his fingernails or toenails yellowish?	**YES**	Athlete's foot (tinea pedis).	Consult your GP, who will prescribe an antifungal cream or ointment. If the infection is severe, oral medication may be needed. If weather permits, your child should wear open sandals to help clear up the infection.

Questions to consider	If answer is	Possible cause is	Action to take
Does your school-age child or teenager have a rash with oval, coppery patches of scaly skin? Is the rash on his trunk? Did it start with a single, 'herald' patch?	**YES**	Pityriasis rosea.	Consult your GP to make sure of the correct diagnosis. If pityriasis rosea is confirmed, the rash will disappear on its own in 4 to 8 weeks. Your GP may recommend a cream to ease itching. Baths and showers should be tepid; heat may make the itching worse.
Has your school-age child developed thick, whitish, scaly patches on his face and body? Are they particularly noticeable on his elbows and knees? Does he also have dandruff?	**YES**	Psoriasis (attacks are often linked to stress, such as exam-time at school).	Consult your GP, who will examine the child. If the lesions appear to be psoriasis, referral to a dermatologist might be advised.
Does your child have a hard knot of skin over a recently healed skin injury? Has a skin tag begun to form on an area that was intentionally pierced, such as an earlobe?	**YES**	Keloid.	Consult your GP. These skin overgrowths are not harmful but they can grow to unsightly proportions. They are more common in dark-skinned people, especially those of African descent.

Pigmentation disorders

Apart from the common pigmented birthmarks, freckles, and moles, disorders of skin pigmentation are more often due to a lack, rather than an excess, of pigment. Albinism, an inborn lack of pigment in the skin, eyes, and hair, varies in intensity from a piebald pattern, with a few or many de-pigmented patches, to total albinism, with complete absence of pigment. Albinos are extremely vulnerable to the sun's effects; they should not venture outdoors unless well protected with clothing, sunglasses, and sunblock.

Vitiligo turns the skin white in patches that often appear in a symmetrical pattern. Patches frequently occur around the mouth and eyes, and over prominent bones. Vitiligo may be linked to auto-immune disorders (such as diabetes mellitus or thyroid disease) or have no apparent cause. In some cases, pigment gradually returns, although the skin may remain lighter. Patches burn easily and should be protected with high-power sunblock.

Patches of darker pigmentation frequently appear on the skin following inflammation. These are best left alone as they generally fade with time.

Sore Throat

Pharyngitis

In General:

Parents who have been through a winter or two with young children won't be surprised to learn that a sore throat is one of the most common complaints in school-age children. Often, it's the first symptom of a common cold. But while sore throats and colds are more common in the winter, sore throats due to viruses also occur during the summer months, especially among toddlers and pre-schoolers.

Antibiotics can help bacterial sore throats. However, most sore throats are caused by viruses, and for these antibiotics don't work. Treatment involves making the child more comfortable by reducing his temperature and giving cool drinks and soft foods that are easy to swallow. Viral throat infections usually clear up by themselves in 3 to 5 days, but bacterial sore throats may very occasionally lead to complications if left untreated.

Some children wake up almost every morning with throats that are sore and dry from breathing through the mouth. One reason may be a blocked nose due to allergies, large adenoids, or other conditions. The discomfort usually disappears once a child has had a drink to remoisten the back of the throat. If you choose to bring your child to your GP for these recurring sore throats and an allergic cause is diagnosed, your doctor will recommend treatment of the allergies. This should improve the problem of recurrent sore throat. A cool-mist humidifier in the bedroom may also be helpful. Occasionally, you may notice white spots on your child's tonsils when she doesn't have a sore throat. The spots are food particles in the tonsil pits. If the child is otherwise well, no attention is required.

Call your GP if your child has a sore throat along with:

- A temperature of 39°C (102°F) or higher.
- Ear pain.
- A rapid onset of new symptoms such as nausea; swollen glands; rash; severe headache; breathing difficulty; or red, tender joints.
- Dark urine up to 3 or 4 weeks after the sore throat.
- A rash.
- Pus (light-coloured flecks) on the tonsils.

Warning

If your GP prescribes an antibiotic, do make sure your child takes all the medication for the full time prescribed, even though the sore throat may feel better after a day or two. Stopping the medication before all the germs are eradicated may allow the sore throat to return.

Questions to consider	If answer is	Possible cause is	Action to take
Has your child developed a sore throat over the space of a few days? Does he also show symptoms such as a runny nose or cough?	YES	Common cold or other viral infection of the upper respiratory tract.	Keep your child comfortable, with plenty of drinks to replace lost fluids (see Runny/Stuffy Nose, p. 126). Paracetamol may be given to reduce fever. In children over 5 years, sucking a sweet or throat lozenge may give some relief; for those age 8 or older, gargling with salt water (half-teaspoon of salt in 240ml (8oz) of warm water) may soothe the pain. Consult your GP if the cold isn't better within a week or other symptoms develop.

QUESTIONS TO CONSIDER	IF ANSWER IS	POSSIBLE CAUSE IS	ACTION TO TAKE
Is your child's throat red and inflamed? Can you see pale flecks on her tonsils? Does she have swollen glands in her neck or a stomachache? Is her temperature 38.3°C (101°F) or higher?	**YES**	Strep throat; infectious mononucleosis (glandular fever); or another throat infection.	Consult your GP, who will determine the diagnosis and advise on treatment, which may include an antibiotic. The child may go back to school or other activities 24 hours after the start of treatment, provided her temperature is 38°C (100.4°F) or lower.
Is your child complaining of a sore throat during the summer months? Can you see blisters on his throat?	**YES**	Infection by Coxsackie or another virus.	Call your GP, who will examine the child and advise appropriate treatment. (See Mouth Pain, p. 112.)
Is your baby refusing to drink or to take solid food? Is she irritable? Can you see white patches on her tongue and gums?	**YES**	Thrush.	Consult your GP, who will examine the baby. If she has this common yeast infection, treatment will be prescribed. (See Mouth Pain, p. 112.)
Is your child in a lot of pain, feverish, and drooling? Is she having difficulty breathing?	**YES**	Serious cause of throat pain such as epiglottitis, abscess, tonsillar infection, or foreign body.	Take your child to the nearest hospital A&E department or call 999. (See Breathing Difficulty/Breathlessness, p. 44.) This is an emergency.
Is your child having severe pain, especially on drinking or eating? Is he drooling? Do his gums and tongue hurt the most? Does he have a fever? Are his neck glands swollen?	**YES**	Herpes infection of the mouth (herpes gingivostomatitis).	Call your GP promptly for an examination and treatment recommendations.

Tonsils in or out?

Before antibiotics showed their value in curing throat infections and preventing complications, tonsils were removed almost routinely in children who had frequent sore throats. Now physicians recommend leaving the tonsils in place because they help fight infections.

Specialists still recommend removal of the tonsils and adenoids when the tonsils swell so much that they interfere with swallowing or breathing, or when a child has recurrent, severe abscesses around the tonsils. This procedure may also be advised when a child has had more than five strep throats in one year.

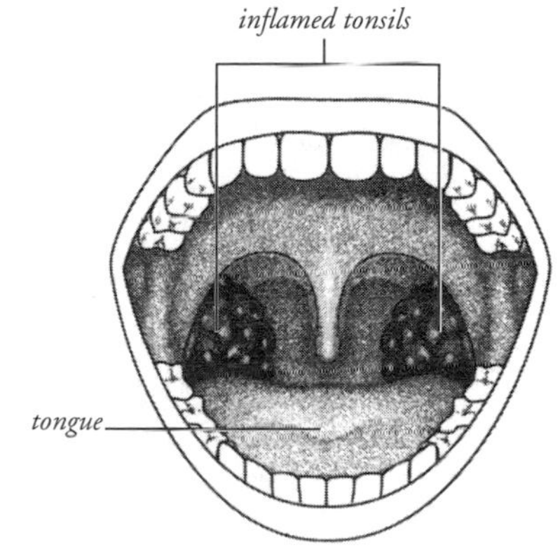

The tonsils are clumps of lymphoid tissue located in the rear of the throat.

IN GENERAL:

By their first birthday, many children can say several words clearly and can attempt the strongest syllable of many others. During the second year, most toddlers begin to talk intelligibly, and after the second birthday they bubble over with increasingly complex sentences, ideas, and questions. On average, girls speak a little earlier than boys, but many factors influence speech development, including genetics, birth order, and interactions with parents. For some children, a period of stammering occurs when the ability to speak can't keep up with the flow of thoughts. It's not usually a sign of future speech problems, and will pass provided the parents speak clearly and resist the urge to finish their child's sentences and overcorrect his mistakes.

In evaluating how well a child speaks, it's important to distinguish between speech and language. Speech is the production of understandable sounds, whereas language is the underlying mental function and includes both expressive (speaking) and receptive (understanding) speech. Common causes of speech problems are hearing loss (see p. 88), developmental delay (see p. 58), and lack of verbal stimulation. Early detection can help to prevent a speech problem from interfering with learning. If your doctor believes your child may have a speech or language problem, he will examine her and test her hearing and, if necessary, refer her for further evaluation and treatment. Many schools also monitor children's speech and recommend further assessment for those with potential problems.

Consult your doctor if, at about 2½ years:

- Your child's speech is very hard to understand.
- Your child doesn't use two-word sentences.
- Your child doesn't follow simple verbal instructions.

Warning

Some parents are so eager to have their baby speak that they intimidate the child. Don't pressure your child, but provide verbal stimulation with books, singing, and repetitive rhymes.

QUESTIONS TO CONSIDER	IF ANSWER IS	POSSIBLE CAUSE IS	ACTION TO TAKE
Is your child making no effort to speak at 2 years? Is she active and healthy? Does she understand you and communicate nonverbally?	YES	Slower rate of speech development.	Your child's speech may be slower than her motor skills. If she is surrounded by talkative siblings or others in childcare, she may not feel the need to speak. Read and speak with her one-on-one, giving her plenty of opportunities to reply.
Does your child respond to your voice only when he can see your face?	YES	Hearing problem.	Consult your GP who will examine the child and test his hearing. Consultation with a specialist may be advised.
Does your pre-schooler hesitate, stammer, repeat syllables, or confuse word order?	YES	Normal period of nonfluency.	Your child is learning to coordinate his thoughts with his motor skills. Speak clearly and read to your child. Don't overcorrect him or finish his sentences. This stage usually passes quickly.

Questions to consider	If answer is	Possible cause is	Action to take
Does your pre-schooler still use 'baby' sounds, such as d- for th- or w- for l-?	**YES**	Normal development.	Many children don't master consonants until age 5. Speak clearly without drawing attention to the problem sounds; read to your child.
Does your school-age child lisp or consistently mispronounce consonants?	**YES**	Lisp or other speech impediment.	If the impediment is marked, ask your GP to recommend referral to a speech and language therapist for an evaluation.
Is your school-age child stuttering or hesitating? Does he grimace when trying to get words out?	**YES**	Stammering or stuttering.	Consult your doctor, who may recommend an evaluation by a speech and language therapist.
Does your school-age child often repeat phrases or odd sounds? Does he sometimes repeat 'bad words' aloud? Does he also make unusual movements?	**YES**	Tourette's syndrome (a disorder marked by tics and involuntary utterances) or another neurological condition.	Consult your GP, who will examine the child and provide a referral to a paediatrician, if necessary.
Does your child avoid communicating? Is he between 2 and 5 years old? Does he seem to be in a world of his own? Has he lost skills he used to have?	**YES**	Communication disorder or autism.	Consult your GP, who will evaluate the child and recommend referral to appropriate specialists.
Are your child's motor functions also delayed?	**YES**	Developmental problem with many possible causes.	Consult your GP, who will evaluate the child's development and recommend referral to a specialist, if necessary.

Language milestones for the first 5 years

- By the end of the second year, your toddler should be able to speak in two- to three-word sentences. She should also be able to follow simple instructions and repeat words heard in conversation.
- By the end of the third year, your child will be able to follow an instruction with two or three steps, recognize and identify practically all common objects and pictures, and understand most of what is said to her. She should speak well enough to be understood by those outside the family.
- By the end of the fourth year, your child asks abstract (why?) questions, and understands concepts of same versus different. She has also mastered the basic rules of grammar as she hears it around her. Although your child should be speaking clearly by age 4, she may mispronounce as many as half of her basic sounds; this is not a cause for concern.
- By age 5, your child should be able to retell a story in her own words and use more than five words in a sentence.

In General:

The colour, consistency, and frequency of stools can vary widely in the same child, as well as among children of similar ages who are eating almost identical diets. Babies who are breast fed may pass stool as infrequently as once every 3 to 7 days or so. In contrast, healthy toddlers may have several movements every day. Once children are eating the same food as the rest of the family, however, they generally settle into a routine of one or two daily bowel movements. As long as the stools are soft and well formed – neither liquid diarrhoea (see p. 62) nor hard, dry pellets indicating constipation (see p. 48) – the child's bowels are functioning normally and he is simply following his own timetable.

The colour of stools is not important unless they are blood streaked or black and tarry, indicating possible gastro-intestinal bleeding, or are excessively pale, indicating a possible liver disorder.

☎

Call your GP if your child is passing:

- Tarry-looking stools.
- Blood in the stool.
- Very pale stools and has a yellow cast to the skin.
- Bulky, greasy stools that float and are foul smelling.

Warning

The stools of toddlers and older children may contain fragments of undigested food. This is usually due to incomplete chewing and does not indicate malabsorption (see Diarrhoea, p. 62). In contrast, stools that are bulky or greasy, or float in the toilet bowl are signs of possible malabsorption.

Questions to consider	If answer is	Possible cause is	Action to take
Are there streaks of fresh blood on the toilet paper or around the anus? Is there blood on the stool or in the toilet bowl? Does the child have rectal pain? Is she constipated but otherwise healthy?	**YES**	Anal fissure. (See Rectal Pain/Itching, p. 122.)	Consult your GP, who will examine the child and, if the diagnosis is confirmed, recommend measures to heal the fissure.
Has your child been passing watery stools since starting a prescription medication, such as an antibiotic?	**YES**	Medication side effect.	Call your GP, who will review the medication and prescribe an alternative, if appropriate.
Are your child's stools extremely dark in colour? Has she been taking iron supplement tablets, or eating large servings of dark-green, leafy vegetables, such as spinach? Is she otherwise healthy?	**YES**	Normal effects on the stool of diet and/or medication.	No action is necessary; the child is healthy.

Questions to consider	If answer is	Possible cause is	Action to take
Are your child's stools unusually pale? Is there a yellow tinge to his skin and the whites of his eyes?	**YES**	Viral hepatitis (see Jaundice, p. 102); congenital malformation (atresia).	Call your GP, who will examine the child and recommend appropriate assessment.
Has your child been passing stools that are pale, bulky, and unusually foul smelling?	**YES**	Malabsorption disorder.	Consult your GP for an evaluation and recommendations for management.
Is there red or maroon blood in the stool? Does the child feel ill? Is there fever?	**YES**	Inflammatory disorder of the digestive tract causing bleeding (haematochezia).	Call your GP straightaway; your child needs an examination and treatment.
Are your child's stools black and tarry looking? Or do they contain material resembling coffee grounds?	**YES**	Bleeding in the digestive tract causing blood in the stool (melaena).	Call your GP at once for an examination, diagnostic tests, and appropriate treatment.

Stool colour and consistency

Variations in the colour and consistency of children's stools are quite normal. It's true that in unusual conditions, bright red streaks or a tarry black colour may indicate the presence of blood and should be investigated at once. A change to a very liquid consistency with or without mucus signals diarrhoea, especially if the child is irritable or in pain. And very pale, foul-smelling stools that float in the toilet bowl may be a sign of a malabsorption disorder. In these cases, too, your child should be seen by your doctor. A child with whitish, clay-coloured stools and brownish urine may have a liver problem and requires prompt medical attention.

Day-to-day changes, however, just show what the child has been eating. A breast-fed baby passes soft, almost runny stools that resemble light mustard. They may contain seedlike particles. In formula-fed babies, normal stools are tan to yellow and somewhat firmer than in breast-fed infants, but should still be no firmer in consistency than peanut butter. If stools are hard or very dry, your baby may not be getting enough fluid, or may be losing too much fluid through perspiration, fever, or illness. Hard stools in a baby eating solid foods can be a sign that the diet contains foods that he's not yet ready to handle, except in small quantities. When a baby has had a large serving of cereal or another food that takes an effort to digest, the process may slow down and the stools, when they pass, will be greenish. Iron supplements can turn the stools black.

After a meal including beetroot, or food or drink containing red dye, a youngster's stools may be tinged an alarming red. Some children also pass pinkish urine. Stools of a brilliant blue, purple, or other rainbow hue probably show that your child taste-tested her crayons. Don't be alarmed; in all these cases, the colour will disappear as soon as the food or crayon has left your child's digestive tract. It's reassuring to know, too, that manufacturers of crayons as well as foods have to meet strict safety standards when using dyes in products meant for children.

Stool Incontinence

Encopresis

In General:

Doctors recognize two patterns of soiling. In the more common one, primary encopresis, the child has always soiled and has never been successfully toilet trained. Youngsters with secondary encopresis, by contrast, start soiling again after they have been trained for months or years. When a child over age 4 repeatedly passes stool in his underwear or other inappropriate places, there may be one or several causes. Perhaps the youngster has never developed good toilet habits, or unusual emotional stress could be causing him to lose control. In many cases, the cause is a physical disorder. About one child out of every 100 about the age of 7 has difficulties with stool soiling. The problem is several times more common in boys than in girls. Whatever the reason for soiling may be, children rarely soil themselves on purpose and they need help to achieve control. Unless he gets help, the child with soiling, or encopresis, may become socially isolated and develop emotional difficulties.

Encopresis sometimes begins when a child repeatedly ignores the urge to defaecate and holds the stool back. Gradually, the nerve sensations in the area grow weaker and the intestines become less able to contract. The stools themselves become larger, harder, and more painful to pass, which makes the child afraid to have a bowel movement. Eventually, hardened faeces block the passage, but liquid stool occasionally leaks around the solid mass and stains the underwear and bedsheets. The child may not be aware that he's passing liquid stools, but parents see the stains and wrongly believe their child has developed diarrhoea (also see Constipation, p. 48). A child with encopresis needs prompt help because the longer the problem goes on, the harder it may be to deal with.

Consult your GP if your child:

- Is over age 4 and has not yet learned to control his bowel movements.
- Has started soiling his pants after a period of apparent control.

Warning

Enemas and medications such as stool softeners are sometimes needed to empty impacted stools and help the child retrain his bowels. Use only the medications your doctor prescribes; taken without a doctor's supervision, over-the-counter products may make the problem worse and even harm your child's health.

Questions to consider	If answer is	Possible cause is	Action to take
Does your child regularly soil his clothing or have bowel movements in inappropriate places? Is he over age 4? Has he resisted efforts to start toilet training?	**YES**	Primary encopresis.	Consult your doctor, who will examine the child and recommend a plan for management.
Does your school-age child often have diarrhoea-like movements? Are there stains on his clothing or sheets?	**YES**	Faecal retention, impaction, and leakage. (See Diarrhoea, p. 62 and Constipation, p. 48.)	Consult your GP, who will examine the child and may prescribe treatment including medications and retraining.

QUESTIONS TO CONSIDER	IF ANSWER IS	POSSIBLE CAUSE IS	ACTION TO TAKE
Has your child been soiling occasionally since having a bout of diarrhoea or gastroenteritis?	**YES**	Upset of normal bowel habits.	Remind your child to take regular breaks to go to the toilet. Her normal schedule should return within a week. If it doesn't or the child has other symptoms, consult your GP.
Has your formerly toilet-trained child started soiling since beginning or changing school? Is she otherwise active and doing well?	**YES**	Behavioural response to difficult situation.	Your child may dislike the school toilets or the schedule may not mesh with her usual rhythms. Ask that school toilets be repaired or cleaned, if necessary. Encourage regular visits to the lavatory at home and allow extra time to ensure complete movements.
Has your child begun soiling after a period of control? Is he under unusual stress? Is he having learning or social difficulties at school?	**YES**	Stress.	If your family is going through a trying time, explain the situation but don't overburden your child. Talk to teachers to identify and deal with problems. Consult your doctor about how to help your child retrain his bowels and manage stress.
Is your child impatient or impulsive?	**YES**	Impulsiveness; lack of concentration.	Encourage your child to spend enough time in the lavatory; use a reward system if it helps. Seek your GP's advice if the problem doesn't improve.

Managing stool retention and soiling

Stool-holding is a fairly common phenomenon among young children. If this becomes a problem, your doctor can recommend a plan with the following goals: (1) to help the child set regular bowel habits; (2) to help the child recognize and respond to the urge to defaecate, and to hold stool only until the right time and place for a bowel movement; (3) to lessen the family's concerns; and (4) to provide a diet that will promote normal movements.

Doctors usually begin treatment with medication to help the child pass impacted faeces. This lets the bowel shrink to a normal size. In the next phase, the child takes daily doses of stool-softening medication to ease stool passage. Your doctor will review the child's diet to make sure it includes fibre in the form of vegetables, fruits, whole-grain cereals and breads, together with plenty of fluids. Air cooked popcorn without butter is a high-fibre snack that promotes regular bowel function.

If soiling is the problem, a reward system can encourage a youngster who really wants to succeed. You could try gold star stickers on a calendar for 'non-soiling' days, or a toy or book to mark a week without an accident. Relapses are not uncommon, and treatment may take months or years. Reassure your child that you know he's trying and in time he'll reach his goal.

IN GENERAL:

When a child has an isolated bump or swelling confined to a small area, the most likely cause is an infection or cyst. Trauma can also lead to swelling around an injured area and bruising can be felt as a lump under the skin. From time to time, some children develop the acute, lumpy swellings of angioedema because they are highly sensitive to a food, cold, or other stimulus. In this case, if the child has hives as well (see Allergic Reactions, p. 26), it's a further sign that the reaction is allergic in nature. This kind of reaction can also occur in response to a viral infection. (For Swollen Glands, see p. 146.)

Consult your doctor if your child develops:

- A painful lump.
- A red, warm, and tender lump.
- A persistent and growing lump that can't be explained.

Warning

If your child has a lump that can't be explained, bring it to your doctor's attention. Although tumours in children are rare, it's better to err on the side of caution than to ignore a possible warning sign.

QUESTIONS TO CONSIDER	IF ANSWER IS	POSSIBLE CAUSE IS	ACTION TO TAKE
Does your child have one or more painful, red, warm lumps under the skin anywhere on the body? Is a lighter area visible at the top of each swelling?	**YES**	Boils (infected hair follicles).	Apply hot compresses to relieve pain and swelling. Do not squeeze the boil to draw out the contents. Cover it with an adhesive bandage if it is open or exposed. If it fails to heal or more boils appear, your doctor will examine the child and may prescribe an antibiotic and additional treatment.
Does your child have several painless, rough-surfaced lumps on her hands or elbows?	**YES**	Warts.	Warts, which are caused by a virus, eventually disappear without treatment. If the warts make it difficult for your child to use her hands, are disfiguring, or seem to be spreading, consult your doctor, who may advise treatment.
Does your child have a soft, painless swelling in the groin? Does it disappear when lightly pressed?	**YES**	Inguinal hernia.	Consult your GP, who will examine the child and provide a referral to a surgeon for further treatment, if necessary. (Also see Abdominal Swelling, p. 24.)
Does your son have a soft, painless swelling on one side of his scrotum? Does one testicle appear a lot larger than the other? Does the swelling look smaller when he lies down?	**YES**	Hydrocele; hernia.	Consult your GP, who will examine the child to determine whether the child has a hydrocele, a minor inborn condition that allows fluid to accumulate in the scrotum. If your child has a hernia, your GP will provide referral to a surgeon for treatment.

Questions to consider	If answer is	Possible cause is	Action to take
Does your child have a lump on the sole of his foot? Is there a small opening in the swelling? Does it hurt a bit when he walks on it?	**YES**	Plantar (sole of the foot) wart, also called verruca.	Consult your GP, who will prescribe treatment if it is painful.
Does your child have swellings that look like bruises over the lower part of his legs, although he can't remember injuring himself? Has he recently had an upper respiratory infection? Is he taking any medication?	**YES**	Erythema nodosum, an inflammatory skin disorder.	Consult your GP, who will examine the child and perform diagnostic tests.
Is your child complaining of a painful swelling over a bone?	**YES**	Infection; tumour or other condition requiring diagnosis and treatment.	Call your GP for a consultation as soon as possible.

Lumps on the wrist

A child sometimes develops a fluid-filled cyst called a ganglion (plural, ganglia). A ganglion forms when synovial fluid – the lubricant that makes our joints work smoothly – leaks through a perforation in the capsule surrounding a joint and builds up in the tendon sheath. The joint most often involved is the wrist, and the ganglion is usually seen on the back of the hand or wrist.

Most ganglia are harmless and not painful; they gradually disappear without treatment. If, however, your child has a ganglion that is unusually large or painful, or that keeps the child from fully using the wrist, your doctor may recommend treatment. A ganglion that interferes with proper hand function can be treated with surgery to cut out the cyst and seal off the leakage of fluid.

Don't attempt to treat a ganglion yourself. In the past, ganglia were commonly called Bible bumps because they were treated by being hit with a Bible or other heavy book. This approach can do more harm than good because it may break the small bones in the hand.

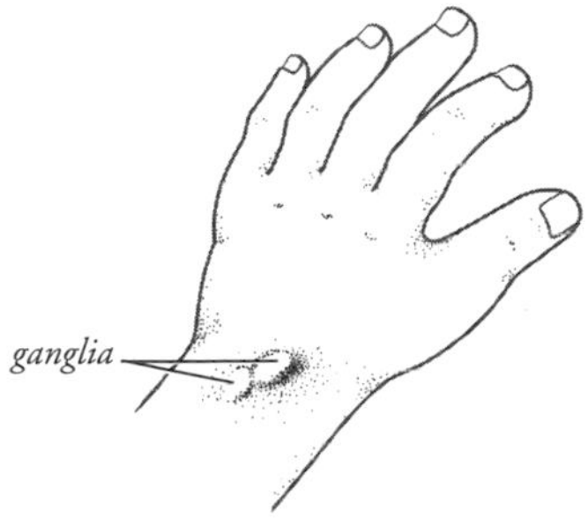

ganglia

A ganglion (plural, ganglia) is a firm, smooth lump, usually about the size of a pea, just under the skin surface. A ganglion most often develops on the back of the wrist, but may also occur on an ankle joint or a finger.

Swollen Glands

Lymphadenopathy

In General:

Children's lymph glands lie close to the surface of the neck, armpit, and groin. When they become swollen, it's usually because the child has developed an infection. In toddlers and older children, painless swollen glands in the neck caused by minor infections usually disappear once the illness is over and do not require treatment. If your child has swollen glands that are tender, persist longer than a few days or get larger, or aren't related to a recent infection, your GP should examine them. Don't feel your child's glands more than once or twice a day, however, as rubbing can make glands more tender and swollen.

Contact your GP if your child has:

- Swollen glands and is a baby of 12 months or younger.
- Swollen glands for 7 days or longer.
- Swollen glands together with a temperature over 38.3°C (101°F) for 5 days or longer.
- Swelling of glands throughout the body.
- Rapidly enlarging glands along with a colour change in the overlying skin.

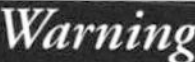

Warning

Swollen glands in babies under 1 year are not always easy to classify and should be brought to your doctor's attention.

Questions to consider	If answer is	Possible cause is	Action to take
Does your child have painless swellings at the front and sides of the neck? Has she recently had a temperature of at least 38°C (100.4°F) as well as a runny nose, sore throat, or other symptoms of a respiratory infection?	**YES**	Viral infection; infectious mononucleosis (glandular fever); tonsillitis.	If the child is feeling better, check the size of the swellings in a day or two to make sure they're going down. If the swelling is unchanged after 1 week, consult your doctor.
Is there a swelling just under your child's jawbone? Does she have pain in a tooth or elsewhere around the mouth?	**YES**	Infection in the tooth, the gum, or the cheek.	Consult your GP, who will examine the child and prescribe therapy, if needed. If the infection appears to be in the teeth or gums, your GP will refer you to your child's dentist.
Does your child have swollen glands only in the groin or armpit? Does he have a sore, a boil, or redness, pain, and warmth suggesting infection in the leg or arm on the same side of the body?	**YES**	Infection (probably bacterial).	Consult your GP, who will examine the child and provide necessary treatment, including an antibiotic, if required.
Has your child developed swollen glands while on medication for a chronic condition such as epilepsy?	**YES**	Side effect of medication.	Consult your GP, who may adjust the medication.

Questions to consider	**If answer is**	**Possible cause is**	**Action to take**
Has your child developed tender, swollen glands since being scratched or bitten by a cat? Does she also have a mild fever and headache? Is she generally not her usual self?	**YES**	Cat-scratch disease, an infection contracted through a scratch or bite from a (usually) healthy cat.	Consult your GP, who will examine the child and prescribe any treatment required. Warm compresses and paracetamol can help alleviate discomfort.
Does your child have swollen glands all over his body? Does he also have a temperature over 38°C (100.4°F) or other symptoms of illness?	**YES**	General illness, most often a viral or another infection requiring diagnosis and treatment.	Consult your GP, who will examine the child to determine whether diagnostic tests and treatment are required.
Does your adolescent have swollen glands just above the collarbone? Are there swollen glands elsewhere on his body?	**YES**	Condition such as chest infection or tumour requiring prompt diagnosis and treatment.	Call your doctor to arrange an examination as soon as possible.

The lymphatic system

The lymphatic system is the body's major line of defence against invasion by infecting bacteria and viruses. The system consists of the spleen (the largest organ in the lymphatic system) and groups of smaller lymph glands or nodes linked by separate vessels called lymphatics that carry lymph. The lymph glands, found in the neck, armpits, groin, and many other parts of the body, act as barriers against the spread of germs. Lymph is a watery fluid that contains large numbers of white blood cells called lymphocytes. Produced in the spleen, lymph glands, and bone marrow, lymphocytes recognize foreign cells and germs and take part in the body's immune reaction to these and other unwelcome substances. Lymphocytes produce antibodies to disarm or destroy infecting germs; the antibodies stay in the bloodstream for long periods and help the body to resist future invasion by the same agent. At times when the body is under attack by germs, the lymph glands swell noticeably as the lymphocytes increase and produce antibodies.

The main sites of the lymph nodes are shown below. Lymph circulates freely in the tissues of the body, and lymphatic vessels are present wherever there are blood vessels. Unlike the blood, lymph has no central pump, although valves in the large lymphatic vessels prevent backflow. The lymph nodes filter out germs and produce disease-fighting lymphocytes. The lymphatic system is also important in carrying fats, transporting nutrients and wastes, and preserving the fluid balance throughout the body.

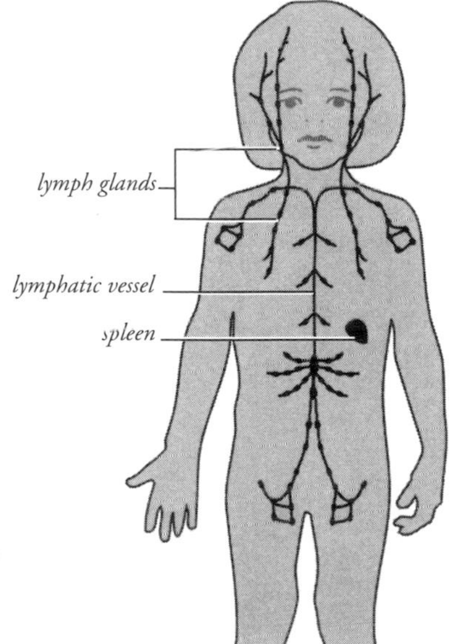

IN GENERAL:
At around 2 years, a toddler's confusion about her growing independence often leads to crying and full-blown tantrums. During these outbursts, the child may fling herself on the floor, kick and fight, and even hold her breath until she passes out (see Dealing with breath-holding, p. 41). Parents may be confused because the triggers for outbursts are often trivial: for example, being asked to wear a hat on going outdoors, or being offered a different kind of cereal. When your toddler has a tantrum, remind yourself that this is part of normal development and does not reflect badly on your ability as a parent.

While tantrums are normal between about 18 months and 4 years (the 'terrible twos'), frequent emotional storms in a child of elementary school age may be a cause for concern. Socially immature children may express their negative or hostile feelings by being destructive (see Behaviour Problems, p. 34). This kind of behaviour is a red flag for problems of adjustment later on. A youngster with such problems should be evaluated and treated by a specialist in behavioural and emotional disorders.

Yelling, losing your temper, or spanking your child won't help and may make the situation worse. When your child has a tantrum, it's best to ignore it if you can, or lead the youngster to her room for a 'time-out'. If a child still has tantrums after age 4, your doctor may recommend a consultation with a child psychiatrist or psychologist. A parent education group may be helpful for further support.

Consult your doctor if your child has tantrums involving any of the following:

- Breath-holding and fainting.
- Outbursts lasting and growing more intense after age 4 years.
- Injury to himself or others, or damage to property.
- Frequent nightmares, severe problems with behaviour and toilet-training, fearfulness, or overdependence.

Warning

Try to keep toddler tantrums within manageable limits by seeing that your child doesn't get overtired, overstimulated, or needlessly frustrated. Set reasonable guidelines for behaviour: children are more likely to have frequent tantrums if parents either are too strict or fail to set any limits at all.

QUESTIONS TO CONSIDER	IF ANSWER IS	POSSIBLE CAUSE IS	ACTION TO TAKE
Does your toddler or preschooler respond to almost every question with 'No!'? Is he refusing foods he used to like? Does he sometimes do the opposite of what you tell him? Does he often cry for no apparent reason?	YES	The 'terrible twos', a normal phase of development lasting from about 18 months (and even younger) to 4 years.	Help your child become increasingly independent by letting him have his own way when it won't make a difference to important plans. Don't punish these outbursts; they'll grow less frequent over time. Provide playthings so he can work out his frustrations; be ready to comfort and joke with him when he's back to his normal, happy self.
Is your child over age 4 having tantrums? Does she have daytime soiling? Does she find it hard to get along with other children?	YES	Behavioural disorder.	Consult your doctor, who will determine whether a consultation with a children's mental health specialist is advisable and may suggest that you take part in a parent support group.

QUESTIONS TO CONSIDER	IF ANSWER IS	POSSIBLE CAUSE IS	ACTION TO TAKE
Is your child having tantrums at school? Is he aggressive toward teachers or other children?	**YES**	Behavioural disorder; learning difficulty.	Consult your child's teachers to identify problems that are causing frustration. Consult your GP; vision and hearing should be tested in case hidden problems are causing learning difficulties. Teach your child to resolve conflicts with words, and review the behaviour he sees within the family. Your GP may advise consultation with a behavioural specialist.

Coping with tantrums

When your toddler starts to get worked up, try a diversionary tactic: 'Let's see what's in this storybook,' or 'Did you hear the doorbell?' If the storm clouds continue to gather, it may help to leave the room or just ignore the behaviour. It's best to let the tantrum run its course, then be ready to cuddle the child and resume interrupted activity as soon as she has cooled off. Don't put up with physical assaults, however; if the youngster lashes out, let her know that smacking and kicking are unacceptable from her, just as they would be from you. If a tantrum happens away from home, calmly carry your toddler to another room or outside so she can weather the storm away from onlookers.

While some tantrums are normal during the 'terrible twos' (from about 18 months to 4 years), there's no need to trigger extra outbursts by subjecting your toddler to unbearable indecision or making unrealistic demands. Give her reasonable freedom in making decisions, but keep choices simple. Let her choose within a structured framework: an apple or a banana, for example, but not the whole fruit bowl. Above all, choose your battles and make it clear that you cannot negotiate issues relating to health and safety, such as going to bed or riding buckled up in the car seat. Once a choice has been made, stick to it and be consistent but not rigid. Soften your discipline with a joke or whimsy and keep in mind that toddler tantrums are a phase that will pass.

After a show of temper in an older child, suggest alternative ways of behaving. Show that while you disapprove of the behaviour, you still love the child. Time-out in the child's room may help with cooling off. Be fair; watch your children to make sure that an apparently non-aggressive sibling isn't secretly teasing, cheating, or physically hurting another.

If your child is past the pre-school years and still having tantrums, tantrums are out of control, or you're afraid of losing your self-control when your child has an outburst, ask your doctor or health visitor's advice. Many community organizations, including churches, temples, and parent-teacher associations, sponsor parent-effectiveness training courses and support groups.

IN GENERAL:

In contrast to most seizures (see Convulsions, p. 50), the muscle spasms known as tics never involve a loss of consciousness. Unlike the involuntary movements of cerebral palsy and other conditions resulting from injury or oxygen deprivation at birth, tics are coordinated movements of the voluntary muscles. Transient tics are surprisingly common; it's estimated that 10 percent of the population has a tic that lasts a month or more but eventually disappears without treatment. Habit tics stem from a compulsion to repeat certain movements and are made consciously, at least initially. Common examples include sniffing, grimacing, blinking, neck stretching, and shoulder shrugging.

Rhythmic tremors, particularly of the chin or leg, that resemble spasms are normal in healthy newborn infants. This jitteriness, which is most noticeable when the baby is crying or being examined, disappears after the second week of life. Older children may have inherited tremors that sometimes can be severe enough to interfere with writing and other motor activities. Some medications also cause tremor. Spasms may involve jerking of the whole body, often during sleep. These benign movements often occur just as a child is falling asleep. A few rare disorders involving muscle spasms are inherited, and some are caused by metabolic diseases that prevent the body from processing a substance such as copper or iron. A child who develops rheumatic fever following a streptococcal throat infection may have Sydenham chorea, a tic disorder formerly known as St. Vitus' dance.

Consult your GP if your child:

- Is making sounds along with repetitive movements.
- Becomes anxious when prevented from carrying out apparently meaningless rituals.

Warning

Certain medications may trigger tics in susceptible children, especially those with attention deficit hyperactivity disorder. If your child is being treated with a stimulant medication, bring any unusual movements or sounds to your doctor's attention.

QUESTIONS TO CONSIDER	IF ANSWER IS	POSSIBLE CAUSE IS	ACTION TO TAKE
Do your child's limbs jerk once or twice as she's falling asleep?	**YES**	Nocturnal myoclonus.	These normal muscle jerks require no treatment. They may persist into adulthood.
Does your child have a recurrent twitch in the eyelid or another muscle?	**YES**	Fatigue; stress.	The twitching is annoying but harmless; it disappears as your child gets over his fatigue or stress, but may often recur.
Does your child make repetitive movements or sounds? Does he have a cough that disappears during sleep? Can he suppress the actions when asked? Are they stronger or more frequent when he's under stress?	**YES**	Transient tic of childhood or habit spasms.	Transient tics of childhood usually disappear without treatment within several weeks, but may last up to a year. If the movements become more marked or new ones develop, consult your GP for an examination.

QUESTIONS TO CONSIDER	IF ANSWER IS	POSSIBLE CAUSE IS	ACTION TO TAKE
Does your child make repetitive movements for up to 30 seconds at a time? Is she unable to suppress these actions? Is she awake and aware?	**YES**	Simple partial seizures (see Convulsions, p. 50); Tourette's syndrome; habit spasm.	Consult your GP, who will examine the child and may recommend treatment or consultation with another specialist.
Does your child repeat movements involving three or more muscle groups at once? Do other family members have movement disorders?	**YES**	Chronic motor tic disorder.	Check with your GP, who will examine the child to rule out any physical problems and may recommend treatment.
Has your child developed movements since starting medication for hyperactivity?	**YES**	Side effect of medication.	Call your doctor to report the side effect and ask for a re-evaluation of treatment.
Does your child make unusual movements and sounds that change from time to time? Are they worse under stress? Have they been present for a year or more? Do other family members have movement disorders?	**YES**	Tourette's syndrome, a neurological disorder.	Consult your GP, who will examine the child and may recommend consultation with a paediatric neurologist.
Is your child making involuntary jerking movements? Is she weak? Is she having mood swings? Did she have a sore throat weeks or months ago?	**YES**	Sydenham chorea, a complication of rheumatic fever.	Call your GP, who will examine the child and arrange a specialist assessment

Tics as signs of obsessive-compulsive disorder

In many cases, actions and habits thought to be tics are later recognized as signs of obsessive-compulsive disorder (OCD). While able to suppress the actions for a short time, a person with a compulsive disorder feels a buildup of emotional pressure that eventually erupts in a flurry of tics. A biochemical problem may be at the root of this disorder and, in many cases, other family members have similar symptoms.

Children with obsessive-compulsive disorder usually observe repetitive rituals as a protective mechanism. They may be obsessed with bodily wastes and contamination, or a need to keep things the same. Eventually, the ritualistic behaviour crowds out normal activities. Although distressed by their compulsions, children may try to get their parents to join in the rituals. Features of an obsessive-compulsive disorder are often present at the time tics first appear, and they become more pronounced in adolescence and early adulthood.

In recent years, several medications have been developed to help control tics, attention difficulties, and OCD. Medication generally needs to be taken for a while before real improvement can be seen. Occasionally, the symptoms of a tic disorder may emerge after a child has begun treatment with a stimulant medication for attention deficit/hyperactivity (see p. 93). At times, medication may need to be changed.

Urinary Incontinence

In General:

Many children have occasional wetting accidents for 6 months to a year after toilet training. By age 5, daytime accidents are rare, although some youngsters still wet the bed periodically at night (see Bed-wetting, p. 32). A few children over age 5 have wetting problems during the daytime. This daytime incontinence is much less common than nighttime wetting and usually requires your doctor's attention. When it recurs after a long period of being dry, the child may be under emotional stress or have an acute infection or other problem. The child should be seen by his doctor.

Consult your doctor if your child:

- Complains of pain on urination.
- Passes cloudy or pinkish urine.
- Is passing an unusually large volume of urine and looks thin, pale, and tired.
- Wets again after achieving a pattern of daytime and nighttime dryness.

Warning

Occasionally, swimming in chlorinated swimming pool water may irritate the urethra, making a child feel he has to urinate frequently.

Questions to consider	If answer is	Possible cause is	Action to take
Does your child often have a wetting accident when caught up in play or on outings?	**YES**	Excitement; distraction; putting off going to the toilet.	Train the child to take notice of his urge to urinate. Remind him to go to the lavatory at intervals and before outings. If he looks as if he needs to go, don't let him delay. If he's in an unfamiliar place, show him where the lavatories are.
Is your child wetting herself frequently after a long period of dryness? Is she having accidents or frequent dribbling of urine? Does she have pain or burning on urination?	**YES**	Urinary tract infection; emotional stress.	Consult your GP. A urinary tract infection must be treated promptly. If the family is under stress, discuss important changes with your child, but don't overload her with details. Try to uncover sources of stress at school. Encourage regular lavatory breaks.
Is your child urinating very often and/or having occasional accidents? Is he on medication for asthma?	**YES**	Side effect of medication.	Discuss this with your doctor, who may modify the treatment.
Is your child badly constipated in addition to having urinary troubles?	**YES**	Pressure on bladder due to full rectum. (See Stool Incontinence, p. 142.)	Consult your GP, who will examine the child and recommend a treatment plan. Dietary changes may include extra fibre and fluids.

QUESTIONS TO CONSIDER	IF ANSWER IS	POSSIBLE CAUSE IS	ACTION TO TAKE
Is there a constant dribbling of urine? Has your child previously been diagnosed with a spinal disorder or other chronic illness?	**YES**	Neurogenic bladder.	Discuss the problem with your doctor, who will suggest ways to keep your child's discomfort at the lowest possible level.
Is your child passing unusually large volumes of urine both day and night? Is he overly thirsty even though drinking plenty of fluids? Is he looking tired and thin?	**YES**	Diabetes mellitus.	Call your GP, who will examine the child and perform diagnostic tests. If diabetes is confirmed, your child will need lifelong treatment.

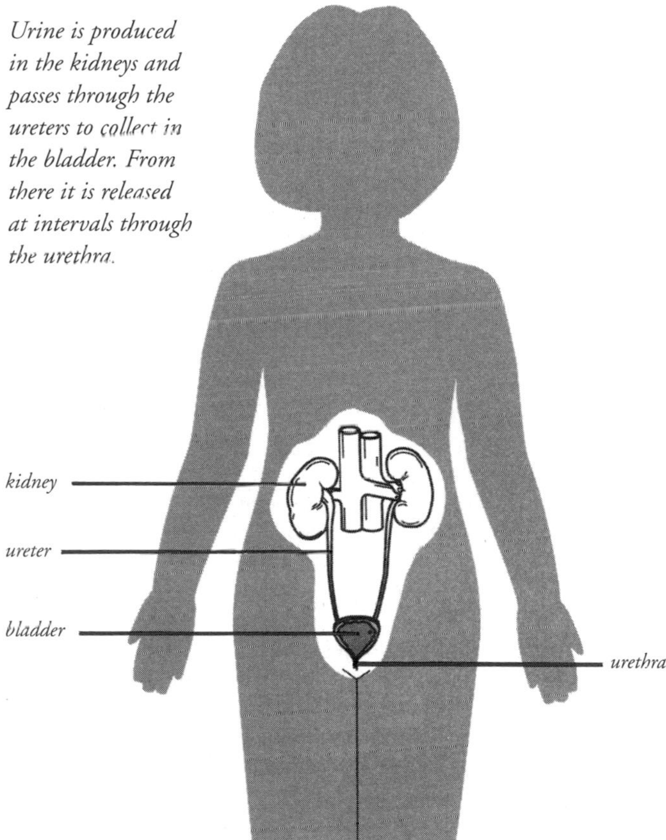

Urine is produced in the kidneys and passes through the ureters to collect in the bladder. From there it is released at intervals through the urethra.

Developing bladder control

Before they can learn how to control passing urine or bowel movements, children have to be able to recognize what a full bladder or rectum feels like. They also have to be able to hold on to the contents and control their release. It's very unusual for a child to develop this complicated skill until well into the second year; many do so quite a lot later (see Steps to toilet training, p. 33). Between the ages of 3 and 4 years most youngsters learn to control their bladder and bowel functions while awake, but accidents – especially wetting – should be expected occasionally. Nighttime control over passing urine usually develops between 2½ and 3½ years, but bed-wetting is fairly common up to age 5 and is not at all rare in normal, healthy youngsters for several more years (see Bed-wetting, p. 32).

Urinary Pain/Difficulty

In General:

Children usually need to pass urine more often than adults because their bladders are smaller and they tend to consume more fluids in relation to their size. In addition, young children may feel the need to pass urine more urgently because it takes a long time – several years – to develop mature control of the muscles that open and close the bladder. If a child has pain on urination, a urinary tract infection is probably the reason, but several other conditions may also be involved.

Warning

Some children who have pain due to recurrent urinary tract infections are in the habit of passing urine infrequently. They may also be severely constipated. Train your child to respond promptly when he or she feels the urge to use the lavatory.

☎

Call your GP immediately if your child:

- Cannot pass urine.
- Is passing bloody urine.
- Has a swelling in the abdomen and difficulty urinating.
- Has pain on urination.
- Is urinating with unusual frequency.
- Is having daytime or nighttime wetting after achieving a pattern of dryness.

Questions to consider	If answer is	Possible cause is	Action to take
Is your toilet-trained child urinating often or with greater urgency? Has she started wetting her bed or underclothes after a long dry period? Does she have abdominal pain? Does her urine smell bad? Is there blood in her urine?	**YES**	Urinary tract infection.	Consult your GP. If a bacterial infection is present, it must be treated promptly with antibiotics to prevent complications.
Does your baby's urine have an unpleasant smell? Is she feverish and fretful?	**YES**	Urinary tract infection.	Consult your GP, who will examine the baby, perform diagnostic tests including a urine culture, and prescribe appropriate treatment.
Is your daughter complaining of pain in the genital area? Is there a discharge or redness around the vaginal opening?	**YES**	Foreign object in the vagina. (Also see Vaginal Itching/Discharge, p. 156.)	Children sometimes push foreign objects into their vaginas, causing pain and irritation. Call your doctor, who will examine the child, arrange for the object to be removed,, and prescribe treatment if needed to prevent infection.
Does your son have signs of swelling or irritation at the tip of his penis? Is he having difficulty passing urine and emptying his bladder?	**YES**	Inflammation of the glans penis (balanitis); narrowing of the urethral opening (meatal stenosis).	Irritation can be caused by infection or, in circumcised boys, by the growth of scar tissue at the opening (meatus) of the urethra. Consult your doctor, who will examine the child and provide appropriate treatment.

Questions to consider	If answer is	Possible cause is	Action to take
Is your daughter having difficulty passing urine? Does she feel irritation in her vaginal area?	**YES**	Labial adhesions.	Occasionally, a girl's genital folds (labia) grow together and close off the vaginal and urethral openings. Consult your doctor, who will examine the child and provide any necessary treatment.
After a bath, does your child complain of a burning sensation when he urinates?	**YES**	Soap in the urethra.	Show him how to rub soap into a lather on his hands instead of rubbing it directly on his skin. Have him use a flannel and rinse thoroughly with clear water.
Is your child having difficulty passing urine? Can you feel a lump on one side of his abdomen? Is there blood in the urine? Does he have vomiting and/or pain?	**YES**	Wilms tumour (a type of kidney tumour) or another condition requiring diagnosis and treatment.	Call your GP at once for an examination and diagnostic tests. Your child will have to be hospitalized for more extensive tests and treatment.
Does your child have redness, bruises, or other marks around the anus or vagina? Are there unexplained marks elsewhere on the body? Is he or she either unwilling or too young to tell you where they came from? Are there signs of urinary infection?	**YES**	Sexual abuse.	Call your doctor who will examine the child, determine the likely cause of the condition, and advise a plan for management.

Preventing urinary tract infections

Pain on urination is most often due to infection. Girls are particularly susceptible to urinary tract infections because their urethras are very short and germs from the bowel can easily pass along this route to the bladder. To reduce the risk of infection, girls should always be taught to wipe from front to back after bowel movements. A popular home remedy for infections is drinking cranberry juice. Some studies have shown that this contains substances that make the urine more acidic and stop bacteria from growing. However, drinking plenty of plain water to flush out the bladder may be just as effective. Other helpful measures include the following:

- Wear cotton underpants and avoid very tight-fitting jeans and other trousers.
- Avoid bubble baths, perfumed soaps, and other substances that can cause irritation to the genitals and urethra.
- After swimming, change into dry clothes instead of sitting around in a wet swimsuit.
- Avoid foods and beverages that can cause bladder irritation. Common offenders include colas and other caffeinated drinks, chocolate, and some spices.

Vaginal Itching/Discharge

Vulvovaginitis

Consult your doctor if your daughter has:

- Recurrent vaginal itching, pain, and irritation.
- An unusual vaginal discharge.

In General:

The normal vaginal discharge is made up mostly of cells and secretions shed from the vaginal walls. It is white or colourless, has no unpleasant odour, and varies in consistency from watery to a thick mucus. This discharge increases in quantity as your daughter nears her first period and changes thereafter according to each stage of her menstrual cycle. In a girl of any age, vaginal itching or pain, along with a discharge of unusual odour or colour, indicates that she may have vaginitis. The condition should be investigated and treated.

School-age and adolescent girls sometimes have vulvovaginitis – inflammation of the vagina and external genitalia – because the vagina and the bladder opening can easily be contaminated with faecal bacteria from the anus. Young girls are especially susceptible to infections of the genital area because the mucous membranes of the vulva and vagina are immature, lacking the protection they will get when higher levels of oestrogen begin to be produced at puberty. Further insulation against injury is provided at puberty as labial fat pads and pubic hair develop over the external genitalia.

Common causes of vulvovaginitis include irritating chemicals or allergens in soaps and lotions, along with germs carried by ringworms (see Rectal Pain/Itching, p. 124). Irritation may be caused by foreign objects inserted in the vagina, including tampons that adolescent girls may forget to remove at the end of their menstrual periods. The overgrowth of yeasts may occur during a chronic illness such as diabetes. Antibiotics and other medications also can upset the normal vaginal environment and allow bacteria or yeasts to spread.

Warning

Do not buy over-the-counter antifungal or antiyeast medications to treat your daughter's vaginitis. These products won't help if her condition is either noninfectious or caused by a different type of germ. Your GP will prescribe appropriate treatment.

Questions to consider	If answer is	Possible cause is	Action to take
Does your newborn daughter have a clear, white, or blood-tinged discharge from the vagina?	**YES**	Effects of withdrawal of mother's hormones.	This is normal and will stop after a few days.
Does your daughter have redness around the vulva and vagina? Does she also have a thick, white, curdlike discharge?	**YES**	Yeast infection.	Consult your GP who will examine the child and prescribe treatment. Use only the treatment your doctor prescribes.
Does your infant daughter have a nappy rash? Is there a white discharge?	**YES**	Yeast (monilial) nappy rash.	Call your GP, who will examine the baby and prescribe treatment.

QUESTIONS TO CONSIDER	IF ANSWER IS	POSSIBLE CAUSE IS	ACTION TO TAKE
Does your daughter have a foul-smelling discharge from the vagina?	**YES**	Infection; foreign body in the vagina.	Call your doctor; your daughter may need treatment for an infection or removal of a foreign body.
Is your daughter passing urine more often than usual? Does she also have redness and irritation around her vulva and vagina?	**YES**	Vulvovaginitis.	Consult your doctor, who will prescribe any necessary treatment.
Has your daughter aged 9 to 10 complained of an increase in secretions from her vagina?	**YES**	Effects of hormones with approaching puberty.	This effect is normal provided the discharge is white or colourless and free of unpleasant odour. Talk to your daughter about the changes in her body she is about to experience.
Does your pre-adolescent daughter have a blood-tinged discharge?	**YES**	Foreign body in the vagina; infection.	Consult your doctor, who will examine the child and determine whether treatment is required.
Are there bruises or other marks in addition to redness and discharge around your daughter's vulva, vagina, and/or anus?	**YES**	Sexual abuse.	Consult your doctor, who will treat the symptoms and determine the cause, and may be able to draw your daughter out on a subject she is fearful of discussing.

Preventing vulvovaginitis

Girls should be taught basic hygiene for preventing vulvovaginitis and urinary tract infections. The rule is, 'Always wipe from front to back' in order to avoid contaminating the bladder and vaginal openings with traces of faeces.

Girls who often get irritations should use hypoallergenic soaps and avoid bubble baths and scented or deodorant soaps. Underwear should be changed daily, and perhaps more often during menstrual periods. Tight clothing – such as leotards, tights, or jeans – and underwear made of synthetic fabrics can form a warm, damp environment in which germs readily grow. Tight-fitting garments, including swimsuits, should be washed after each wearing, and girls should wear loose-fitting cotton underwear and tights with a cotton gusset.

In General:

Your health visitor or GP will check your child's eyes routinely at regular well-child visits. Provided the eyes are developing normally and you have no family history of serious eye disorders, formal vision testing is not usually done until 3 years of age, when children are capable of following directions and describing what they see. If screening tests at any age show defects in vision or signs of eye disease, your doctor will recommend further evaluation by an ophthalmologist.

Despite what many people believe, the common vision problems – shortsightedness, farsightedness, and astigmatism – are not made worse by reading too much or sitting too close to the television. Nor does wearing glasses weaken the eyes. A tendency to these vision problems usually runs in the family.

For problems with the alignment of the eyes or diseases affecting the eyes, see Crossed Eyes/Wandering Eye (p. 54) and Eye Problems (p. 70).

Consult your doctor if your child:

- Squints.
- Bends his head unusually close to his work.
- Complains of headaches, eyestrain, or blurring after reading or doing close work.
- Can't see close-up objects clearly.
- Twists his head to view objects.
- Sees distant objects in a blur.

Warning

Shortsightedness often emerges when the eye structures change in size and shape during the growth spurt at puberty.

Questions to consider	If answer is	Possible cause is	Action to take
Is your child having trouble seeing distant objects? Does she squint a lot? Does she hold a book very close to her face? Does she bend very close to the surface she's writing on?	**YES**	Shortsightedness (myopia).	Consult your GP, who will examine the child and determine whether referral to an ophthalmologist is warranted.
Does your child complain of sore eyes or headaches after reading? Do close objects look blurry to him?	**YES**	Farsightedness (hyperopia).	Most children are born with some degree of farsightedness which gradually resolves itself, but ask your GP to examine your child and determine whether he should be seen by an ophthalmologist.
Is your child complaining of blurry vision at any distance?	**YES**	Astigmatism, a condition in which the eye's refractive surfaces are curved in such a way that light is not sharply focused on the retina.	Your GP will examine the child and may provide a referral to an ophthalmologist for further examination.
Is your child seeing double? Does he cover one eye or tilt his head to focus on objects?	**YES**	Disorder requiring diagnosis and treatment.	Consult your GP promptly for an examination and possible referral to a specialist.

Dealing with colour blindness

Colour blindness is a common visual defect that is rarely a significant handicap, although people who are colour blind cannot pilot aircraft or hold other jobs where the inability to perceive colours could be hazardous. Those who are colour blind see colours, but not of the same hue or intensity as others. Most colour-blind people cannot tell red from green; some with a mild form of the condition have difficulty only in dim light. A more unusual defect is the inability to distinguish yellow and blue.

Colour blindness is inherited, usually passed from mother to son; few females are affected. Parents may suspect colour blindness when their child doesn't learn to name certain colours; other cases are diagnosed at about the time the child starts nursery or kindergarten. While the condition cannot be cured, wearing colour-filter glasses or contact lenses can improve some people's perception of contrasts, though it doesn't help them to see colours normally.

How the eye sees

Rays of light pass through the cornea and lens to the retina. From there, the light impulses are sent to the optic nerve and then to the visual cortex, the area of the brain that interprets what we see.

When our eye focuses on an object, the image is projected through the pupil (the black spot at the centre of the eye) to the retina, which is a multi-layered structure on the inside of the eyeball. The image is received upside down, but the brain's visual cortex interprets the message and lets us perceive the image correctly.

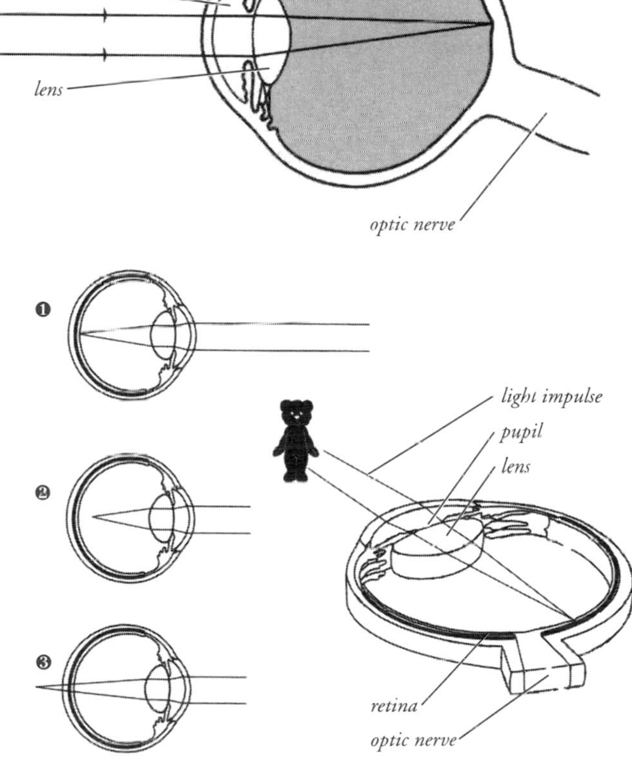

❶ *In normal vision, light rays focus sharply on the retina.*

❷ *In shortsightedness (myopia), light rays from a distance come to a sharp focus in front of the retina. Blurry vision caused by this condition can be corrected by wearing glasses with concave lenses.*

❸ *In farsightedness (hyperopia), light rays from close objects come to a sharp focus behind the retina. People with this condition can see clearly if they wear glasses with convex lenses.*

Vomiting

Emesis

In General:

In children, vomiting is a common response to a number of different events or stimuli, including illness, ingestion of toxic substances, or emotional stress brought about by pressure at school or tension at home. An isolated vomiting episode is not a cause for concern. Recurrent vomiting, however, may be a sign that your child needs medical attention, especially if there is also abdominal pain, fever, or headache.

Forceful vomiting in babies is quite different from the normal developmental phase of spitting up (p. 16). For the special problem of induced vomiting in adolescents, see Eating Disorders (p. 178).

Call your doctor immediately if vomiting is accompanied by:

- Swelling and sharp pain in the abdomen.
- Blood or bile (green material) in the vomit.
- Confusion, lethargy, or irritability.
- Diarrhoea for more than 12 hours.
- Signs of dehydration such as dry lips and scant urine.

Warning

Occasional vomiting is not a cause for worry, but if your baby vomits after every feed in a 12-hour period, call your doctor.

Questions to consider	If answer is	Possible cause is	Action to take
Does your toddler or older child who is vomiting also have diarrhoea and mild fever?	**YES**	Gastroenteritis; food poisoning.	Withhold solid foods but give clear liquids as soon as your child can keep them down. As symptoms improve, resume a normal diet. If symptoms last longer than 12 hours, call your doctor for advice.
Does your child have symptoms of an infection such as a sore throat, earache, or burning on urination?	**YES**	Infection.	Seek your doctor's help for treatment of the underlying infection. Vomiting will stop as symptoms improve.
Does your child seem tense or upset? Does he have no other symptoms of illness?	**YES**	Stress, anxiety.	Let your child talk about what's bothering him. If no cause is obvious and vomiting continues or becomes more frequent, consult your doctor.
Does your child feel nauseated and vomit when riding in cars, boats, or lifts?	**YES**	Motion sickness.	Ask your doctor how to prevent motion sickness. (Also see Dizziness, p. 64.)
Is your baby under 2 months? Does he vomit forcefully after every feed?	**YES**	Pyloric stenosis (a narrowing of the passage between the stomach and small intestine) or another condition requiring treatment.	Call your doctor, who will examine the baby and refer to hospital for treatment.

Questions to consider	If answer is	Possible cause is	Action to take
Is there blood or greenish bile in your baby's vomit? Is she crying, pulling her legs up, distressed, and in pain?	**YES**	Gastrointestinal blockage (e.g., intussusception or folding of the intestine) requiring diagnosis and treatment.	Call your doctor straightaway. Your baby needs urgent medical attention.
Did the vomiting follow a fall or head injury? Is your child increasingly sleepy or less responsive?	**YES**	Head injury.	Take your child to your local accident and emergency department.
Is your child irritable or drowsy? Has he complained of a headache? Does he have a fever?	**YES**	Meningitis or another serious disease of the nervous system.	Call your doctor immediately, or call 999 if there is any risk of delay.

Feeding a vomiting child

Vomiting is common and uncomfortable. Fortunately, it's usually not serious and quickly passes. While a child is vomiting, care should be taken to prevent dehydration due to fluid loss, especially if she also has a fever or diarrhoea. Before your child feels well enough to eat again, she will probably be able to drink fluids. Encourage her to drink frequently, even if she can manage only a few sips at a time.

Let your child choose the drinks she enjoys. For a toddler or pre-schooler, a commercial rehydrating solution is suitable, while a school-age child may prefer a 50-50 blend of a high-energy drink and water. Avoid drinks with a high sugar content and/or caffeine, which may make the fluid loss worse.

If your child vomits after drinking, the best course is an hour or two with no food or fluids – not even water. She may be able to take just spoonfuls of liquid or prefer to suck on crushed ice for a while. Call your doctor if the vomiting continues for more than 6 hours or the child has a stomachache and fever. Don't give any medications to stop vomiting except as prescribed by your doctor.

When your child hasn't vomited for several hours and can keep fluids down, let her try a small helping of any food she chooses from her usual diet. Good choices to begin with might be toast, porridge, bananas, applesauce or other cooked fruits, or a soft-boiled egg. Don't give milk, dairy products, or foods containing large amounts of insoluble fibre – such as raw fruits and vegetables and bran cereals – until your child's stomach feels settled. Get her back to a normal diet as soon as possible.

In General:

Youngsters generally take their first steps around their first birthday, although a few normal children don't walk independently until about 17 months of age. The developmental stages leading up to the first steps follow a recognized sequence, starting with rolling over and progressing through sitting up, crawling, and cruising to walking unaided (see Developmental Milestones for the First Three Years, p. 60). A few independent souls, however, skip over the crawling stage; they go directly from scooting about on their bottoms to walking. No matter what style of locomotion your baby prefers, what's important is that he uses each arm and leg equally, and coordinates the two sides of his body.

At first, the toddler plants his legs wide apart, points his toes out, holds his arms bent at the elbows, and rocks from side to side as he moves along. Although he trips and falls a good deal at the beginning, once he's been walking for a few months he'll be confident enough to carry out complicated manoeuvres, such as stepping sideways and backwards, stooping to pick up and carry a toy, or throwing a ball while on the move.

Consult your doctor if your child is:

- Not walking by age 17 months.
- Still walking on the balls of his feet by age 3.
- Not using both arms and legs symmetrically.

Warning

Baby walkers are a serious safety hazard. They often put youngsters in danger of falling down open steps and stairways and get them into dangerous places that would otherwise be out of their reach. It is also possible that they slow down general development.

Questions to consider	If answer is	Possible cause is	Action to take
Is your 15-month-old showing no signs of getting ready to walk? Does she show little interest in moving about?	**YES**	Developmental delay.	Consult your doctor or health visitor for an evaluation of the child's development.
Does your child turn his toes noticeably inward or outward when he walks?	**YES**	Normal developmental stage.	This tendency usually disappears as the child matures. It rarely interferes with mobility. (See Bow Legs, Knock Knees, Pigeon Toes, p. 42.)
Is your child limping? Is she complaining of pain?	**YES**	Injury; infection; arthritis; or another condition requiring treatment.	If you can't see and remove an obvious source of pain, such as a splinter, ask your doctor to determine the cause of the limp.
Does your child limp but is not complaining of pain? Does he walk with a waddling gait?	**YES**	Neuromuscular weakness; hip joint disorder.	Consult your doctor, who will examine the child and determine whether he should be seen by a specialist.

Questions to consider	If answer is	Possible cause is	Action to take
Does your child still always walk on the balls of her feet after many months of walking?	**YES**	Habit; neuromuscular problem.	Although normal during early walking, toe-walking after age 2 years should be evaluated. Ask your doctor to determine whether your child has a problem requiring treatment.
Does your toddler have difficulty walking? Does he fall a lot and have trouble getting on his feet again? Does he use his hands to 'climb up' his legs when trying to stand? Does he tend to waddle when he walks?	**YES**	Muscular dystrophy or another neuromuscular condition requiring diagnosis and treatment.	Call your doctor, who will examine the child and may refer you to a specialist. If the diagnosis is confirmed, your child will need long-term treatment. Your doctor will also help you find support groups for children and parents.

Shoes for active toddlers

In the early months, babies' feet develop best if they're not confined in shoes; socks or bootees are all that's needed to keep the feet warm. Once youngsters start walking outdoors, however, they need shoes for protection. Look for comfortable shoes with nonskid soles, such as canvas lace-ups, that will help keep your toddler steady on slippery floors. Buy well-made shoes but don't spend a lot of money. At this stage, the feet grow so rapidly that the first pair of shoes won't last more than 2 or 3 months. You should check the fit about once a month; it's better to have no shoes at all than shoes that are too tight.

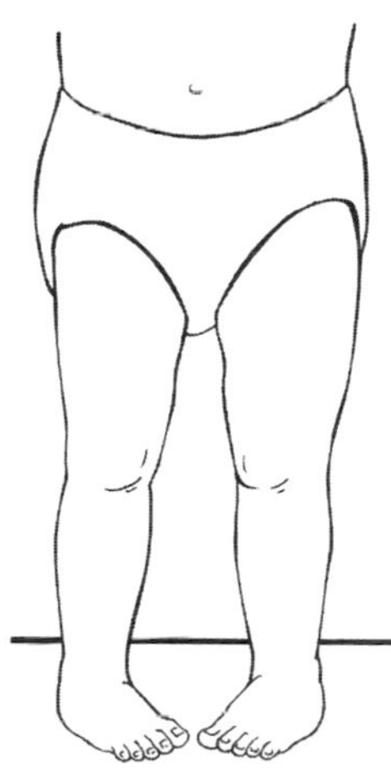

The typical bow legs and pigeon toes (in-toeing) of the early months gradually straighten out over the first 3 years. As the child begins to walk, however, the inward curve of the lower leg (left) may turn to mild knock knees between ages 2 and 3 (right). The legs generally straighten out by about 10 years without treatment. Braces and corrective shoes are rarely helpful. Most youngsters have straight legs by adolescence, although a tendency to in-toeing or out-toeing may run in some families.

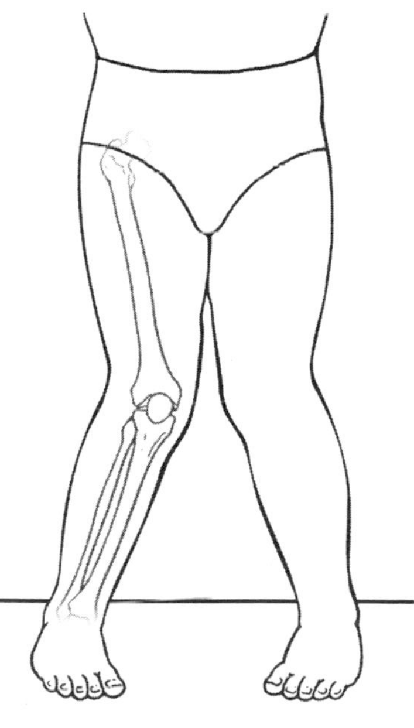

In General:

Illness may leave a child feeling weak and shaky, especially if the youngster had a fever and stayed in bed for a few days. She'll quickly get her strength back once she's on her feet again, eating and exercising normally. Weakness that doesn't go away or gets worse, however, requires medical attention.

Congenital conditions that affect muscle strength and movement may be detected at or shortly after birth. Others appear only later, after the child has begun to walk. Certain forms of muscle weakness are progressive; the child gradually loses strength and mobility and may eventually be confined to a wheelchair. Others come on acutely – possibly due to infection or other illness – but get no worse provided treatment is available.

The outward appearance of a child's muscle is not always a good indicator of strength. Children with certain forms of muscular dystrophy, a progressive weakness, have calf muscles that look large and overdeveloped although they are actually weak. On the other hand, many youngsters with scrawny-looking limbs have normal strength.

Your doctor determines whether weakness is present by evaluating your child's muscle strength and motor function. He checks muscle bulk and tone (the resistance of the resting muscle), as well as the child's posture (see p. 120), movement, and reflexes. He looks, too, for abnormal, involuntary movements that may indicate a problem in the nervous system. In particular, your doctor will examine the child for subtle signs in the eye muscles, the tongue, and the intercostal muscles between the ribs, which are used in breathing.

Consult your doctor if:

- Your baby uses the arm and leg on only one side to crawl.
- Your child is increasingly clumsy and fatigued.
- Your child lacks energy despite plenty of food and rest.

Warning

Do not use honey in preparing food for your infant under 1 year of age. Honey may harbour Clostridium botulinum *spores, which can cause life-threatening food poisoning (botulism), with severe muscle weakness and difficulties in breathing and feeding.*

Questions to consider	If answer is	Possible cause is	Action to take
Is your baby slower than others his age in reaching his movement (motor) milestones (see p. 60)? Do his limbs and muscles feel oddly soft and 'mushy'?	YES	General hypotonia (low muscle tone, i.e., floppiness or lack of resistance to movement); benign hypotonia; developmental delay; hereditary muscular dystrophy.	Consult your doctor, who will evaluate the child's development and may refer you to a specialist, if necessary.
Does your baby feel weak and listless? Is she falling behind in developmental milestones (see p. 60)? Does she get tired quickly? Does her face look swollen?	YES	Thyroid disorder.	Babies are generally checked at birth to make sure their thyroid glands are working properly. Consult your GP, who will examine your child and order laboratory tests if a thyroid problem is suspected.

Questions to consider	If answer is	Possible cause is	Action to take
Is your son having difficulty walking or standing again after he falls? Does he use his hands to 'climb up' his legs when trying to stand? Does he fall unusually often, or have a waddling walk? Have other family members had muscular dystrophy?	**YES**	Muscular dystrophy (a genetic disorder passed from mothers to sons) or another neuromuscular condition requiring diagnosis and treatment.	Call your GP, who will examine the child and may refer you to a specialist. If the diagnosis is confirmed, your child will need long-term treatment. Your doctor will also help you find support groups for parents and children.
Has your child been unusually tired since recently having a sore throat?	**YES**	Infectious mononucleosis (glandular fever)	Consult your doctor. There is no specific treatment for mononucleosis and most children are back to normal in a month or 6 weeks. Your doctor will evaluate the child's general health and advise you about rest and recovery.
Is your school-age child or adolescent lacking energy as the day wears on? Do her eyelids droop in the morning? Does she seem to get weaker each day?	**YES**	Myasthenia gravis (a disease affecting the immune system, which causes weakness in certain muscles).	Call your doctor, who will examine the child and provide a referral, if needed, to a neurologist.
Does your child have weakness that began in the legs and is gradually working upward? Has she had a viral (respiratory or gastro-intestinal) infection in the last 10 days or so? Are her muscles sore? Is she irritable?	**YES**	Guillain-Barré syndrome (a nerve condition that may follow a viral illness).	Call your doctor, who will examine the child and may recommend hospitalization. Most children get better in 2 to 3 weeks, but a few may have long-term effects.

Diagnosing muscular dystrophy

If a child is born with a birth defect or other family members have a genetic disorder, parents are usually anxious to know whether the condition may affect future children. Duchenne muscular dystrophy, an inherited disorder, is a progressive muscle weakness that begins in infancy and is usually fatal by the second or third decade. For the moment no cure has been found, but doctors are continually researching possible treatments.

Like haemophilia (see p. 39) and colour blindness (see p. 159), Duchenne muscular dystrophy is passed from mothers to sons. Only boys are affected. Thanks to our expanding knowledge of genetics, a woman with a family history of muscular dystrophy can find out whether she is a carrier and what the risk is that she will pass it on. Genetic counselling can help to prepare a couple for the extra care an affected child will require, or they may decide on adoption to complete their family.

In General:

Your child's exact weight is less important than the rate at which she is growing and gaining weight. Still, loss of weight or failure to gain is worrying at any stage of childhood, except in the first week of life, when most healthy babies lose up to 10 percent of their birth weight. Babies generally start to gain weight on the fifth day of life and are back to their birth weight by about 10 to 14 days old. From then on, weight gain should continue until growth is completed. It's essential that babies have good nutrition in their first year, as that's when the rate of growth is greatest. An unusual slowing down in a baby's or toddler's growth rate may signal failure to thrive (see p. 82), which may have both physical and emotional roots. This condition requires a doctor's attention to determine the cause and treatment.

The rate of weight gain is not steady; children typically grow in spurts, with a marked gain in height often followed by a consolidation phase when their weight catches up to their height.

The intense growth of the first 12 months is succeeded by a relative slowing of the growth rate offset by a noticeable decrease in the child's appetite during the following year. This cycle recurs to some degree throughout childhood, culminating in the growth spurt, voracious appetite, and final filling out of adolescence. Both obesity and unhealthy weight loss due to eating disorders are growing health problems in the United Kingdom, especially in adolescent girls (see p. 178).

Consult your doctor if your child is:

- Losing or failing to gain weight.
- Gaining weight out of proportion to his height.

Warning

Overweight children often are troubled by their weight problem, but find it impossible to slim down without professional help. It's hard for a child to diet if his parents are overeating, and crash diets can be physically and emotionally harmful. Sensible family eating habits and exercise are the keys to successful weight control.

Questions to consider	If answer is	Possible cause is	Action to take
Is your baby lethargic or fretful? Is she feeding exceptionally slowly? Does she seem to be ill?	**YES**	Underlying illness.	Call your doctor, who will evaluate the baby's health.
If your baby is breast fed, is he losing or failing to gain weight, despite feeding eagerly?	**YES**	Insufficient calories.	Consult your health visitor or doctor promptly. If your baby is 4 to 6 months old, he may be ready for solid foods.
If your baby is formula fed, is she losing or failing to gain weight? Does she drain every bottle?	**YES**	Insufficient calories.	Consult your health visitor or GP. Be careful to mix formula according to instructions. Increase the amount you offer in the bottle and let your baby stop when she's ready. If your baby is 5 months or older, ask whether it's time to try solids. Avoid large servings of juice.

QUESTIONS TO CONSIDER	IF ANSWER IS	POSSIBLE CAUSE IS	ACTION TO TAKE
Is your bottle-fed baby gaining weight too fast?	**YES**	Overfeeding.	Discuss your concerns with your health visitor. Don't offer food every time your baby cries; she may simply want attention, changing, or distraction. The crying may also signal a change in sleep pattern or indicate that your baby is ready for solid foods.
Is your school-age child overweight? Has she always been chubby?	**YES**	Excess weight in this age group is frequently due to physical inactivity and overeating, which is often a family problem.	Cut down on fats and don't serve a lot of sweets and other high-calorie, low-nutrient foods. Encourage more physical activity. Serve meals at the dining table, not in front of the television. Watch your child's juice intake; juices contain calories. If your child is grossly overweight, ask your doctor for diet and exercise guidelines.
Has your toddler or school-age child lost weight? Is she pale or unusually tired?	**YES**	Illness requiring diagnosis and treatment.	Call your doctor without delay for an examination.

Helping your child to lose excess weight

Obesity is a complex problem that doctors do not fully understand. Genes appear to play a role; so too do cultural attitudes. We do know, however, that obesity for medical reasons is rare. Even if a child is genetically predisposed to be overweight, he does not need to become fat. Children become overweight because they eat more than they need to make up for the amount of energy they expend. Although most children are adept at adjusting the amount of food they consume to match the energy they burn, the body's inborn mechanism for regulating appetite can be thrown off by family habits of eating too much, particularly high-calorie foods such as sweets and fats. Likewise, parents who insist that children clean their plates whether they're hungry or not are encouraging overeating. And some children eat for comfort as a reaction to stress and anxiety.

You can help your child lose excess weight by ridding the family diet of foods that contain many calories but have little nutritional value. Tops in this category are cakes, biscuits, sweets, ice cream, and sweetened drinks. Cut down on the amount of fat you use in preparing food, avoid rich sauces, and spread butter and margarine very thin. Serve fresh fruits and low-fat yoghurts for dessert. Offer your children water or unsweetened juices instead of fizzy drinks. And encourage exercise for the whole family to burn up the excess calories instead of storing them as body fat.

Wheezing/Noisy Breathing

In General:

Children breathe silently and effortlessly when their airways are working normally. But if the airflow is blocked, a high-pitched sound can be heard as air is forced through the narrowed tubes. Wheezing is a term for the whistling sound you hear when your child breathes in and out through constricted airways. Common causes of airflow obstruction include swelling due to infection, blockage by a foreign body, or inflammation and bronchial muscle spasms due to asthma. In some conditions, children make noise or wheeze only as they breathe in; this sound, called stridor, is a feature of croup (see Dealing with croup, p. 53).

Call 999 immediately if wheezing is accompanied by:

- Severe difficulty in breathing.
- Bluish colour around the lips.
- Abnormal drowsiness.
- Inability to speak or make normal sounds.

Warning

A child may suddenly start wheezing when a hazardous object lodges in the airway. Isolated bouts of mild wheezing may be caused by a minor respiratory infection. But if your child is wheezing all the time, bring it to your doctor's attention.

Questions to consider	**If answer is**	**Possible cause is**	**Action to take**
Does your infant make quite loud wheezing sounds as she breathes in? Is she feeding and growing normally?	**YES**	A temporary, incomplete firmness of the windpipe (tracheal) structures which is normal in young babies (laryngomalacia, tracheomalacia.)	As long as the baby is feeding, growing, and playing well, no action is necessary. The sounds will lessen and taper off altogether by about 18 months of age as the cartilages become firmer. Bring the wheezing to your doctor's attention.
Does your child also have symptoms such as a runny nose or cough?	**YES**	Common cold.	Give liquids to thin secretions and keep your child comfortable. If symptoms get worse or don't clear up within a week, ask your GP's advice.
Is your baby also coughing? Did wheezing come on 3 to 4 days after a cold? Is she breathing fast? Is she having difficulty feeding?	**YES**	Bronchiolitis (viral infection).	Viral infections can occur at any time but are very common in winter and spring. Keep your baby comfortable and, if symptoms get worse or do not improve in 3 days, call your GP.
Does your child cough repeatedly or have difficulty breathing, especially at night? Is there a family history of allergies or asthma?	**YES**	Asthma.	Call your doctor, who will examine the child. If the diagnosis is confirmed, treatment will be prescribed.

QUESTIONS TO CONSIDER	IF ANSWER IS	POSSIBLE CAUSE IS	ACTION TO TAKE
Is your child having trouble catching his breath? Does he have a barking cough and hoarseness? Are symptoms worse at night? Has he recently had a respiratory infection?	**YES**	Croup (laryngotracheobronchitis, see p. 52).	Give paracetamol to relieve discomfort, and use a cold vaporizer at night. If symptoms persist, call your doctor. (Also see Dealing with croup, p. 53.)
Is your child having severe difficulty breathing? Did wheezing come on suddenly? Could your child have choked on a bit of food or a small object?	**YES**	Foreign body in airway (most common in children between 6 months and 2 years).	This may be an emergency: if your child is under 1 year, follow the first aid guide for choking (p. 201) or, for an older child, try the Heimlich manoeuvre (see p. 203) to dislodge the object. If child is turning blue or having trouble breathing, have somebody call 999 while you keep trying to clear the airway.
Does your child have a deep, chesty cough? Is there fever? Is he breathing rapidly? Does the space between the ribs appear to suck in every time your child takes a breath?	**YES**	Pneumonia.	Call your doctor. (See Breathing Difficulty/Breathlessness, p. 44.) Paracetamol may soothe discomfort.
Does your child snore? Does he breathe through his mouth? Does he have a runny nose? Does he sometimes get an earache? Is his voice nasal? Has he had these symptoms since getting a respiratory infection? Or does he always breathe this way?	**YES**	Enlarged adenoids (adenoidal hypertrophy); blocked nose due to allergy.	Consult your doctor, who will examine the child and determine whether treatment is needed. (Also see Runny/Stuffy Nose, p. 126.)

Why small children wheeze more

Wheezing is particularly noticeable in children under 3 years old. This is because their airways are small, and blockage caused by muscle spasm, inflammation leading to swelling of the mucous membranes, and buildup of secretions is proportionately greater than in older children.

Environmental pollution, including cigarette smoking by members of the household, is one of the factors known to cause airway disease and wheezing in young children. If any of your family members smoke, try to get them to stop. At the very least, don't let anyone smoke in the house.

Wind

Flatulence, eructation

IN GENERAL:

Wind is a common symptom of intestinal disorders, but it's rarely a sign of a serious problem. Young babies who are eager to feed often gulp down air, which builds up as wind in their intestines. Some doctors believe that discomfort due to wind is one of the factors that can aggravate colic. (See Crying/Colic, p. 6.)

A certain amount of wind is normally produced as food is digested. Children as well as adults, however, often have excess wind because their diet is too high in certain types of insoluble fibre, which ferments in the intestine. Many infants and toddlers also swallow air when crying or breathing through the mouth because of a stuffy nose. Older children gulp air when eating or chewing gum. Carbonated drinks may also be a factor. A few children over the age of 4 have wind because they gradually lose the ability to digest lactose, the sugar in milk; this inborn trait is seen mainly in those of African or Asian descent. Older children often seek attention with the deliberately noisy belching and flatulence that youngsters find so entertaining. And some children just produce more wind than others, no matter what they eat.

Call your doctor if your child has wind in the stomach or intestine with:

- Severe abdominal pain.
- Nausea and vomiting lasting for 12 hours or longer.
- Diarrhoea persisting for more than 3 days.
- Bulky, unusually foul-smelling stools.

Warning

Don't treat wind in your child with over-the-counter indigestion remedies. If wind is troubling enough to be a concern, ask your doctor's advice.

QUESTIONS TO CONSIDER	IF ANSWER IS	POSSIBLE CAUSE IS	ACTION TO TAKE
Does your new baby pass a lot of wind during colicky crying periods? Does she tend to gulp in her eagerness to feed?	**YES**	Swallowing air (aerophagia) during feeding.	Take time to burp your baby at more frequent intervals during each feeding and afterward. (See Burping your baby, opposite.)
Does your pre-schooler or older child have wind, along with frequent colds, sniffles, and a stuffed-up nose?	**YES**	Swallowing air during mouth breathing.	Consult your doctor, who will examine the child and may recommend treatment.
Does your school-age child have a long history of wind with intermittent diarrhoea, bloating, and discomfort?	**YES**	Intolerance to lactose or another food substance; coeliac disease (gluten sensitivity) or another malabsorption disorder; food allergy (rare); irritable bowel syndrome.	Consult your doctor, who may recommend that you keep a food diary (see Allergic Reactions, p. 26) to track daily food consumption and symptoms, or an elimination diet to identify suspect food(s). If your child thinks a certain food causes the discomfort, omit it from the family meals for a week or two, then reintroduce it to see if symptoms recur.
Has your child suddenly developed bloating, cramping, and diarrhoea with excess windiness?	**YES**	Infectious diarrhoea; parasitic infection such as giardiasis.	Consult your doctor, who will examine the child and prescribe treatment depending on the cause of the diarrhoea. (See Diarrhoea, p. 62.)

Flatulence, eructation

Questions to consider	If answer is	Possible cause is	Action to take
Has your child had excess wind and an upset stomach since taking an antibiotic or another medication?	**YES**	Medication side effect.	Call your doctor, who may substitute another medication or recommend measures (such as taking medication at mealtimes) to keep side effects to a minimum.
Does your youngster belch and pass wind noisily and often?	**YES**	High-fibre diet; carbonated beverages; attention-seeking behaviour. In general, your child's daily intake of fibre should equal his age plus 5 grams (for an 8-year-old, 8+5 = 13 grams).	Reduce the amount of bran and other insoluble dietary fibre and add more soluble fibre from fruits and vegetables. Provide noncarbonated beverages. Encourage moderate exercise, especially after meals. If passing wind is your child's way of seeking attention, let him know his behaviour is unacceptable (but take care that your disapproval doesn't spur him on).

Burping your baby

The right way to burp your baby is the way that makes her comfortable. Don't interrupt a feed if it will upset the baby, but take advantage of natural pauses during a bottle feed or when she switches breasts while nursing. Whatever position she prefers, protect your clothing with a towel or nappy in case she spits up.

Burping is not essential. In many cultures, parents never burp their children.

❶ *Hold your baby upright with her head on your shoulder. Support her head and back while you gently but firmly pat her back.*

❷ *Support the baby on your lap in a sitting position with one hand and pat her back with your other hand.*

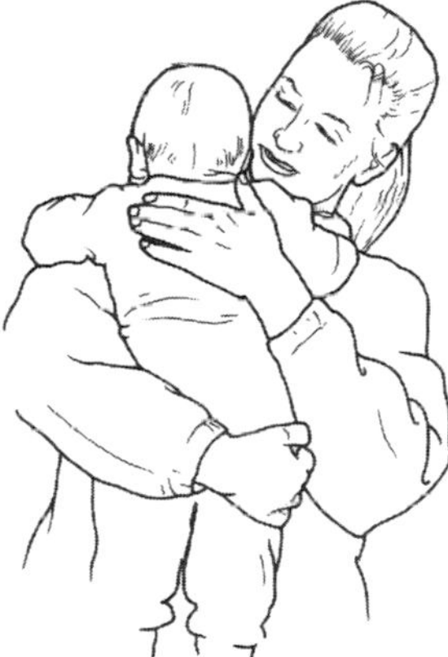

❸ *Lay the baby face down on your lap. Use your knee to support her head a little higher than her chest and gently rub her back.*

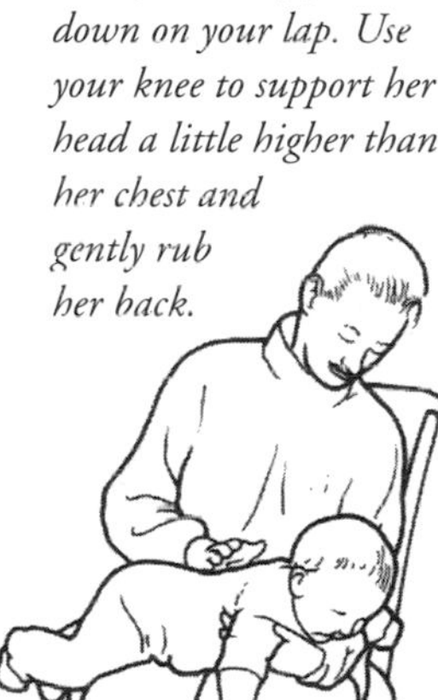

CHAPTER 3 COMMON SYMPTOMS IN ADOLESCENTS

While most teenagers are brimming over with health, energy, and strength, several disorders tend to make their first appearance or reach a peak frequency during these years. The physical changes of puberty may have a bearing on the development and progression of various illnesses. On the other hand, the presence of a disease may affect the timing of puberty.

Teenagers are also prone to a number of stress-related conditions. Pressure to perform at school, among peers, and within the family can lead to anxiety and tension which emerge in the form of physical ailments or worsen symptoms already present.

As your teenagers grow up, they may be less open to sharing concerns about their health with you. During this phase, they can benefit from the open, trusting relationship they established in earlier years with their family doctor.

Several of the following symptoms may appear at any time during childhood but, on the whole, they are more likely to be seen among youngsters in transition from children to young adults. Your doctor will be glad to help your adolescents understand the changes they are going through, and offer guidelines for health and diet to avoid problems farther down the road.

In General:

Every youngster has occasional anxiety, when apprehension may be intensified by symptoms such as dry mouth, racing pulse, sweating, tremors, and 'butterflies in the stomach'. In the very young, a period of separation anxiety is a normal developmental stage (see Fears, p. 72). In later years, anxiety often occurs in anticipation of stressful situations. Luckily, the anxious feeling evaporates and may turn into relief as soon as a taxing event is over.

A few youngsters suffer anxiety even when there is no precipitating event. Free-floating anxiety may be the result of a chronically stressful situation, such as family tension, financial strains, alcoholism, or illness. Viewed in this light, anxiety looks like an understandable response to events beyond a child's control. For some, anxiety becomes a chronic condition that interferes with school, friendships, and work.

Severe anxiety can take on various forms and cause serious difficulties in daily living. Attacks of panic disorder, a common manifestation, may come on several times a day without warning. During an attack, fearfulness is worsened by symptoms such as a pounding heart, clammy skin, trembling, diarrhoea, and nausea. Many victims hyperventilate (breathe fast and shallowly, leading to light-headedness or fainting) and some actually fear that they are about to die. A few adolescents develop panic disorder when faced with the normal challenges of growing up. Your doctor may recommend referral for psychological therapy for an overanxious adolescent. A course of medication may occasionally be helpful. Regular aerobic exercise has physical effects that help to reduce anxiety, as do meditation and biofeedback techniques.

Consult your GP if your adolescent:

- Refuses to go to school.
- Avoids family activities and spends his time alone.
- Becomes upset if kept from a set routine or doing things his own way.
- Has a noticeable weight loss or gain along with a change in behaviour.

Warning

Certain medications used to relieve anxiety may produce additional symptoms, especially if not used exactly as prescribed. Follow your doctor's instructions and call immediately if new symptoms appear during therapy.

Questions to consider	If answer is	Possible cause is	Action to take
Is your teenager complaining of palpitations or chest pain? Does she have vague symptoms such as a headache or stomachache? Does she use them as an excuse to avoid difficult tasks?	**YES**	Anxiety; hyperventilation syndrome; physical illness such as prolonged QT syndrome, a type of irregular heartbeat (see p. 92); manipulative behaviour.	Question your adolescent about situations that may be bothering her. Consult your doctor, who will rule out physical illness and suggest ways to help your youngster change her behaviour.
Is your teenager refusing to go to school or playing truant?	**YES**	Anxiety (school phobia); boredom; negativism.	Consult your child's teachers to identify school-related problems and suggest ways to deal with them. Ask your GP to refer to a counsellor if needed. Enlist your child's cooperation in making and implementing decisions that affect him.

Questions to consider	If answer is	Possible cause is	Action to take
Has your adolescent abruptly developed signs of anxiety? Is she having problems at school? Has her behaviour changed for the worse? Do you think she may be using drugs?	**YES**	Effects of illegal drugs.	Talk to your child about the legal and health implications of drug use; let her know where you stand on this issue. Consult teachers to identify school problems. Ask your doctor's advice about dealing with the situation.
Is your adolescent having attacks of rapid breathing with other symptoms? Is she intensely fearful during episodes?	**YES**	Panic attacks.	Ask your teenager whether specific situations or people are the source of her worry. Your doctor may recommend referral for psychological therapy and possibly medication to relieve the anxiety.
Is your adolescent having problems with schoolwork? Is he disruptive in class? Does he fail to hand in assignments? Does he act the class clown?	**YES**	Learning difficulty; behaviour problem; performance anxiety/ procrastination (see below).	Consult your child's teachers to identify specific problems. Help him to organize his study space and work habits at home. Your doctor may recommend counselling.
Is your child also having symptoms such as frequent urination, fatigue, weight loss, or eye problems?	**YES**	Physical illness mimicking anxiety, such as diabetes mellitus or thyroid disorder.	Consult your doctor, who will examine your child to determine whether a medical problem exists and prescribe appropriate treatment.

Procrastination and performance anxiety

'Stubborn, lazy, inattentive, puts everything off until tomorrow': A youngster who hears himself described in these harsh terms often enough will eventually incorporate them into his own self-image. He fails to try because that's what he thinks others expect. The effects can be disastrous.

The procrastinating adolescent may fail to hand in his homework because he was afraid to ask how to go about it. Chores don't get done because he'd rather be called lazy than fail to reach the standards he thinks his parents expect. Because he has a poor sense of organization, he can't break a task down into manageable components. When he fails to begin, then, he is accused of not trying or caring.

A youngster can benefit from help with organization: an orderly space where he can keep articles used for school, sports, and free time; a desk or table that is kept clear for homework; a daily checklist of essential tasks and a calendar marked with future assignments. Steady encouragement is essential: parents should show they're pleased if a job is done – not perfectly, but well enough and on time. What's important is that parents help their youngster to see that major journeys are only a matter of putting one foot in front of the other.

In General:

Children, like their elders, have mood changes; they can be elated today but down in the dumps tomorrow. There is an important difference, however, between feeling sadness (reactive depression) and having the emotional illness that is called clinical depression. If occasional periods of low spirits (especially after a temporary setback) lift after a few days, there is no cause for concern. But youngsters who persist in feelings of hopelessness, worthlessness, futility, and anger need help to find their way out of their misery.

Although clinical depression strikes all age groups, adolescents are particularly vulnerable. Among teenagers, the rate of suicide – the most serious consequence of depression – has trebled in the last 25 years and continues to rise.

☎

Consult your GP Immediately if your youngster:

- Is preoccupied with death or expresses a wish to end his life.
- Seems to rally from depression by giving away treasured possessions or setting his affairs in unusually good order.
- Hints he has the means to end his life, should he decide to do so.

Warning

Depression tends to run in families. The causes may be rooted in both brain chemistry and behaviour. If you recognize symptoms of depression in any family members, try to persuade them to seek medical help. Although depression tends to recur, people with depression usually respond well to treatment.

Questions to consider	If answer is	Possible cause is	Action to take
Is your adolescent extremely solitary and withdrawn virtually all the time? Is she overconcerned about any aspect of her appearance?	YES	Adolescent behaviour; shyness; self-consciousness about a perceived physical or social problem.	Provide opportunities for socializing to extend but not overtax her capabilities. Consult your doctor to determine what can be done to cope with a problem such as acne or obesity. Reassure but don't patronize.
Has your child's behaviour undergone a marked change since a major family upheaval, such as a death or divorce? Or does your child have a chronic illness?	YES	Reactive depression; anxiety.	Talk about the situation. Be patient but not overindulgent while your child adjusts to conditions. Keep teachers informed to help them cope with unusual behaviour. If your child is ill, let him take part in decisions affecting his treatment. If there's no improvement in a month, consult your doctor.
Does your teenager complain of vague symptoms such as headaches or stomachaches? Does he sometimes miss school? Does he drive or handle dangerous items carelessly? Do you suspect he is using drugs or alcohol? Is he sullen or childish?	YES	Depression; acting out; anxiety over school or social problems; family tension.	Consult your GP who will determine whether your child should be referred for counselling.

Questions to consider	If answer is	Possible cause is	Action to take
Is your child often bored? Has his interest in school-work, sports, or hobbies declined? Is his concentration poor? Does he often express feelings of worthlessness?	**YES**	Depression; depressive reaction to unsatisfactory family dynamics or other overpowering situation.	Consult with teachers to identify specific difficulties. Ask your GP to evaluate your child's overall health. Your GP may recommend therapy for the child and, if advisable, the family.
Has your child had a marked change in appetite, with weight loss or gain? Is he sleeping much more or less than usual? Does he lack faith in his ability to succeed? Has he lost interest in pleasurable activities?	**YES**	Severe clinical depression.	Call your doctor for advice and referral to a mental health specialist.
Is your adolescent acting erratically? Is she unusually talkative or having trouble sleeping? Are her activities (overspending, unrealistic plans) a source of concern? If she has had a similar episode, was it followed by a slump?	**YES**	Bipolar disorder/ manic depression; substance abuse.	Consult your GP, who will evaluate your youngster and may refer her to a mental health specialist.

Coping with depression

Depression is often triggered by an event such as academic failure, death in the family, or romantic disappointment. Certain medications may cause depression as a side effect, and it's not uncommon for a short-lived period of depression to follow a viral illness. In many cases, however, there is no identifiable cause.

Ask your doctor to evaluate your adolescent if any of the following signs of depression are present:

- Reduced interest in normal activities; lack of pleasure in daily life.
- Fatigue, restlessness, trouble concentrating.
- Withdrawal, lack of sociability.
- Change of appetite; marked weight loss or gain.
- Sleeping much more or less than usual.
- Dwelling obsessively on minor problems.
- Acting out, reckless behaviour.
- Vague but troubling physical symptoms.

While depression sometimes lifts by itself, it is never helpful to tell a depressed person to 'snap out of it'. Physicians use medications and psychological support to relieve the suffering caused by depression. Once the mood improves, the person's energies may be channelled into constructive activities. Regular, moderate exercise is beneficial because it stimulates the production of endorphins, the brain's natural mood enhancers, which can help keep depression at bay.

In General:

In recent years, eating disorders have emerged as a disturbing problem among adolescents in the United Kingdom and other affluent countries. Although teenage girls are by far the most often afflicted, youngsters of either sex and in all age groups may develop an unhealthy preoccupation with food, dieting, and body image. Eating disorders range from picky eating to self-starvation (anorexia nervosa), and from occasional overeating and weight problems to the binge eating characteristic of bulimia. Of these, the three abnormal eating patterns that demand medical attention are: anorexia nervosa, bulimia, and bulimarexia, a combination of the two.

Anorexia nervosa is characterized by an obsession with weight loss and a grossly distorted body image in which the youngster perceives herself as being fat when in reality she may be dangerously emaciated. Although these young women are often preoccupied with food and prepare elaborate meals, they refuse to eat. Despite increasing emaciation, anorexic girls often exercise for hours on end to burn up the few calories they consume. By contrast, a teenager with bulimia (the so-called binge-purge syndrome) appeases her constant craving for food by gorging on huge quantities of high-calorie foods then ending the binge with laxatives and self-induced vomiting or occasionally excessive exercise, to avoid gaining weight. Bulimics usually maintain a fairly normal weight, although frequent variations of 5kg (10lb) or more are not uncommon. Many youngsters combine the two disorders in bulimarexia, eating less than they need to maintain their weight with periods of bingeing and purging. This dangerous practice satisfies the desire to eat while at the same time getting rid of dreaded calories.

An eating disorder has many serious effects on a youngster's health. Anorexic girls often fail to menstruate and risk long-term effects including premature bone loss (osteoporosis). Bulimics who force themselves to vomit have a high rate of dental caries as regurgitated stomach acids erode their tooth enamel. Both starving and binge-purging can be life-threatening. Without professional help, it is almost impossible to get anorexic or bulimic youngsters back to healthy eating and sound nutrition. For many, admission to hospital for intravenous feeding is necessary, and counselling must involve both the child and her parents.

For Feeding Problems involving babies and young children, see pp. 9 and 74.

Consult your doctor at once if your child has previously been diagnosed with an eating disorder and has any of the following:

- Rapid or irregular heartbeat.
- Chest pain.
- Faintness or loss of consciousness.
- Continuing weight loss despite treatment.
- Cessation of menstrual periods.

Warning

Ask your doctor's advice if your pre-adolescent or teenager insists on an extreme diet that may be deficient in important nutrients.

Questions to consider	If answer is	Possible cause is	Action to take
Is your child refusing to eat with the rest of the family? Does she seem overconcerned about losing or gaining weight? Are you worried that she's not eating enough?	**YES**	Anorexia; adolescent preoccupation with diet and appearance.	If your child's weight, appearance, or diet is causing worry, discuss your concerns with your doctor.

Questions to consider	If answer is	Possible cause is	Action to take
Is your son refusing family meals because he's following his own diet, whether for sports or another reason? Is he trying to gain or lose weight for a sports competition? Has he lost weight? Are you concerned about his nutrition?	**YES**	Normal behaviour; personal preferences; food fads.	Review training with your son's coach to make sure his advice is sound; discuss any concerns with your doctor. As long as your teenager's diet is healthy, respect his preferences.
Does your child spend long periods in the bathroom after eating? Does she tend to skip family meals and, instead, fix snacks for herself? Does she complain that her weight goes up and down?	**YES**	Binge-purge syndrome (bulimia); bulimarexia (combination of anorexia and bulimia).	Consult your doctor, who may want to examine your child; with sensitive questioning, your doctor may be able to obtain information that your child is uncomfortable discussing with those close to her.
Has your daughter lost a lot of weight in a short time? Does she look gaunt? Is her hair thin? Has she developed downy hair on her face and arms? Does she try to cover up her thinness with bulky clothing?	**YES**	Anorexia nervosa; metabolic disorder; depression.	Consult your doctor without delay; your daughter's condition should be diagnosed and treated promptly.
Has your daughter started exercising for hours to control her weight? Does she have food fads or follow a strict diet?	**YES**	Exercise anorexia.	Evaluate your child's diet over several days to assess her calorie and nutrient intake. Discuss your concerns with your doctor.

Identifying those at risk for eating disorders

Experts haven't yet found a way to predict which youngsters are likely to develop an eating disorder. In many cases, however, the eating problem develops after a girl embarks on a stringent weight-loss diet. Those affected often, though not always, come from a demanding, perfectionist home environment where achievement or external appearances are overemphasized. Often, the mothers are also overly concerned with weight. In some cases, sexual conflicts also seem to play a role. Youngsters involved in highly competitive athletic activities, where attention is focused on weight and form, are especially prone to eating disorders. Girls who practise ballet and gymnastics, for example, have a high incidence of delayed menarche (first menstrual period), which is also a prominent feature of anorexia. Boys who wrestle competitively sometimes try to meet their weight groups by fasting, dehydration, and bingeing.

Continued on next page

Feeding teenagers

Teenagers, already highly susceptible to peer pressure, face daily pressure to conform to artificial standards of appearance and behaviour that are dreamed up as marketing ploys. Waif-thin models in fashion magazines make poor role models for adolescents, who need a balanced diet to support the many changes of puberty along with exercise for healthy bones and strong muscles.

Many teenagers diet to lose weight. Idealistic youngsters also often renounce meat and poultry for humanitarian reasons, while other sensitive teenagers may reject particular foods because of a heightened fastidiousness related to conflicting feelings about entering the adult world. Omitting meat or another specific food will not take away essential nutrients as long as the overall diet is well balanced and the adolescent is getting enough daily calories: about 3,000 for a boy and 2,400 for a girl at the peak of the growth spurt.

Nutritionists recommend that complex carbohydrates – whole-grain cereals and breads, pasta, beans and other legumes – make up 50 to 60 percent of a teenager's daily calories. Not only are these foods good sources of energy, but they also provide protein and important vitamins and minerals. Vitamin supplements are rarely needed. With plenty of fresh fruits and vegetables and low-fat dairy products, the diet should provide adequate nutrients for growth metabolism. If a teenager dislikes milk or has trouble digesting it, yoghurt, cheese, lactose-free milk, and soya milk can supply essential calcium and vitamins.

Even if a teenager's busy schedule means that many meals are hamburgers or pizzas eaten on the run, there needn't be any nutritional problems. Fast foods are not necessarily junk foods. A diet that includes lots of fast foods can still be based on the right proportions of carbohydrates, protein, and fats, and include dairy products, fruits, and vegetables for calcium, folic acid, and other vitamins, and other essential nutrients.

Usually rich in fat, sugar, and salt, 'junk' foods – chips, potato crisps, sweets, colas and other sugary soft drinks, among others – contribute little that's useful other than calories and may actually interfere with the absorption of essential nutrients. For example, the essential minerals calcium and phosphorus compete with one another in the digestive process. Both are needed for healthy bones and teeth, but too much of one in the diet means that less of the other is absorbed. A teenager who drinks lots of fizzy drinks, which are high in phosphorus, may decrease the amount of calcium her body absorbs.

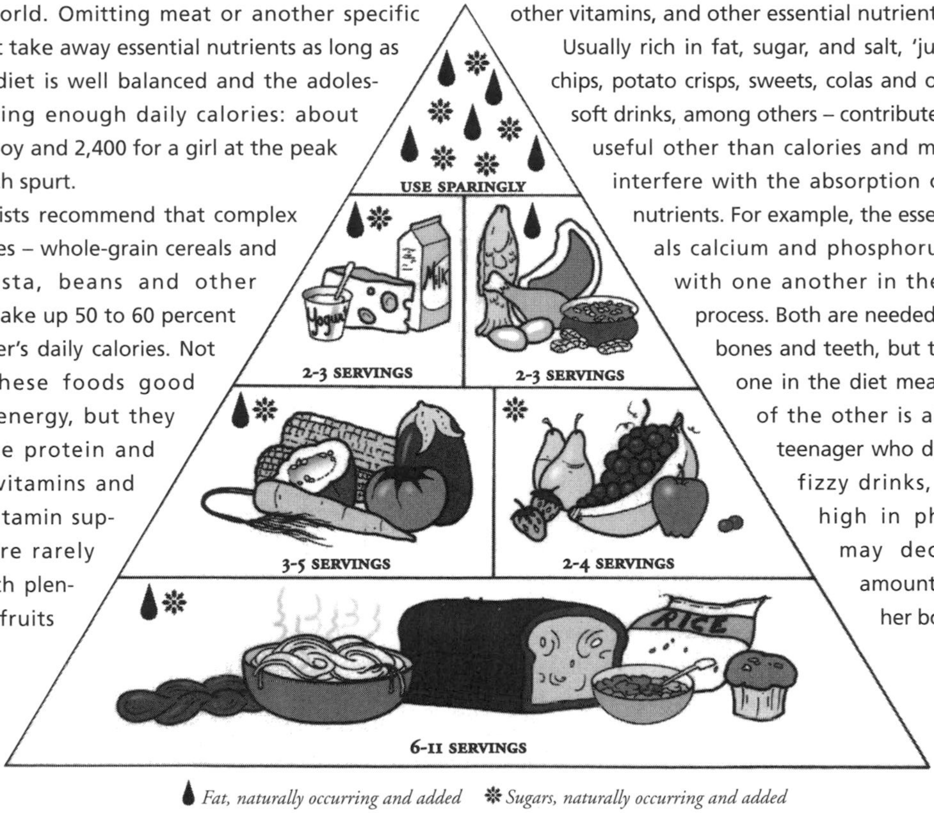

Fat, naturally occurring and added *Sugars, naturally occurring and added*

RECOMMENDED SERVING SIZES: Bread: 1 slice • Cereal, pasta, rice: 30g (1oz) • Vegetables: 60g (2oz) Fruit: 1 medium piece, e.g.1 apple • Milk, yoghurt: 230ml (8oz) • Cheese: 45g (1½oz) • Meat, poultry, fish: 60–90g (2–3oz)

The Food Guide Pyramid is an outline to follow so that a week's food intake averages out on a daily basis to the servings shown. The Food Pyramid number of servings for each food group is calculated for a theoretical average person.

In General:

Fainting is brought on by a sudden fall in the flow of blood to the brain. This may occur for a number of different reasons, but the result is that the blood pressure rapidly drops and the brain is temporarily deprived of blood and oxygen. The affected youngster feels light-headed and perhaps nauseated; her skin feels cold and clammy and she passes out. Fainting is in some ways the body's protective mechanism: when the fainting person lies flat, blood can flow more easily to the brain, so she quickly recovers consciousness. Within a minute or less, in almost all cases, she's awake again and aware of her surroundings, although she may continue to feel weak and wobbly for a while longer.

Fainting is unusual in a child under about age 10 years. The breath-holding spells that cause children to pass out during the terrible twos (see p. 41) are different from fainting, although the underlying reflex mechanism is similar. It's fairly common, however, for adolescents to faint, and girls tend to do so more often than boys.

An occasional fainting spell is not usually a sign that something is seriously wrong. The triggering stress is commonly excitement, overexertion, fear, hunger, or being confined in a hot, stuffy atmosphere. Certain odours may cause faintness. A surprising number of youngsters and adults faint at the sight of blood, such as when a sample is drawn for a routine test. This is not a cause for concern and the person generally recovers quickly. Even so, if a fainting spell occurs in a child who has never had one before, you should consult your GP. He will examine the child to make sure that the loss of consciousness was caused by fainting and not a more serious, treatable condition such as a seizure (see Convulsions, p. 50) or an irregular heartbeat (see Heartbeat Irregularities, p. 90).

☎

Call 999 immediately if your child has fainted and:

- She isn't breathing.
- Her limbs, face, and body are jerking.
- Her skin is turning bluish.
- Her breathing is shallow and her pulse is weak.
- She is still unconscious after more than 2 minutes.

Warning

If a youngster feels faint, don't splash cold water on her face. Have her lie on her back, if possible, with her legs and feet slightly raised. In this position, the blood can flow more easily to the heart and brain. If she cannot lie down, tell her to sit with her head lowered. Loosen any tight clothing and make sure she can breathe freely. She should rest for at least 5 minutes or until she feels well enough to get back to normal activities.

Questions to consider	If answer is	Possible cause is	Action to take
Does your teenager complain of feeling faint when she stands up suddenly? Is she tired and pale at times?	YES	Orthostatic hypotension (a momentary drop in blood pressure when abruptly changing position); iron deficiency anaemia.	The faint feeling is not unusual or serious; it just means that the reflexes controlling your child's blood pressure are acting slowly. If your child is unusually tired and pale, your doctor will examine her to determine whether treatment is needed.

Continued on next page

Questions to consider	If answer is	Possible cause is	Action to take
Was your child breathing rapidly before becoming faint? Was it during an emotional upset? Has she had other episodes of anxiety with rapid, shallow breathing?	**YES**	Hyperventilation (rapid, shallow breathing); panic attack; anxiety (see p. 174).	Consult your doctor, who can suggest ways to deal with anxiety and may recommend counselling.
Has your teenager fainted after standing a long time in strong sunshine? Or has he been confined in a warm, stuffy environment such as a crowded school assembly or church? Is he usually active and healthy?	**YES**	Heat exhaustion; dehydration; lack of fresh air.	Let your youngster rest until he feels well enough to resume his activities. Offer water or a drink containing sugar as soon as he's well enough to take it. If this was his first fainting episode, your GP may want to examine him.
Has your child fainted during a coughing bout? Does he often cough and wheeze, especially at night? Has he been diagnosed with asthma?	**YES**	Asthma.	Call your doctor, who will examine the child and adjust his medication or prescribe different treatment.
Is your child feeling weak, faint, and shaky? Has it been several hours since he ate? Or did he eat a large amount of sugary food such as sweets on an empty stomach?	**YES**	Low blood sugar.	Give the child food or a drink that contains sugar for immediate energy. Call your GP for an examination. Encourage your child to eat regularly to maintain a steady supply of energy; provide a balance of starches, protein, and a small amount of fat at each meal.
Has your child previously been diagnosed as diabetic?	**YES**	Diabetes mellitus.	If your child has diabetes mellitus and has had several spells of faintness, call your doctor. Your child's medication may need to be adjusted.
Did your child suddenly become ill and faint? Does he have swelling around the mouth? Is he having trouble breathing? Could he have been stung by a bee or other insect? Is he allergic to a food? Or is he taking a medication such as an antibiotic?	**YES**	Severe allergic reaction (anaphylaxis).	Call 999 at once; this is an emergency. Give CPR (see p. 205) if necessary while you're waiting for help.

QUESTIONS TO CONSIDER	IF ANSWER IS	POSSIBLE CAUSE IS	ACTION TO TAKE
Has your adolescent had one or more fainting spells after exertion or emotional upsets? Does she ever complain that her heart is racing or skipping beats?	**YES**	Prolonged QT interval (a type of irregular heartbeat, see p. 92).	Consult your GP, who will perform a physical examination to determine whether treatment is warranted.
Has your teenage daughter been faint and nauseated several days in a row? Does she seem worried or withdrawn? Do you believe she may be sexually active?	**YES**	Pregnancy.	Talk calmly to your daughter. If you have reason to think she could be pregnant, consult your doctor without delay.

The phenomenon of teenage group fainting

Most teenagers have an overwhelming need to feel part of a group – to have what their friends have, to do what their friends do. Sometimes this need extends beyond clothes, buzzwords, and the latest music craze to illness. It sometimes happens, for example, that almost every member of a secondary-school class falls victim to mysterious, identical symptoms. While real enough, the symptoms are vague and not specific to any known illness. They invariably include hyperventilation and fainting, and may involve nausea, dizziness, and stomachache as well. The symptoms typically appear within a short period ranging from hours to a few days. Just as typically, they vanish as quickly as they came. The victims have no abnormalities on physical examination or laboratory testing. They never appear seriously ill and the illness never recurs. Youngsters most often involved in these outbreaks are teenage and pre-adolescent girls.

Interestingly, symptoms are always restricted to a single group of students and do not affect the members of another class using, say, the same gym. Teachers and school staff don't become ill. One feature that is always present is 'line of sight transmission.' In other words, girls feel faint when they see others fainting and don't get ill unless they can see others developing symptoms.

Researchers who have investigated numerous outbreaks of mass fainting in adolescents call it 'mass sociogenic illness'. In earlier times, it might have been termed mass hysteria or 'the vapours'. Even when the symptoms appear to have no physical cause, however, every effort must be made to inspect the school or other premises for safety and cleanliness. The youngsters and their parents should be assured that no hazardous conditions are present.

In General:

Fatigue includes feeling tired and sleepy, but also a temporary loss of energy and heaviness in the muscles. Fatigue can be a warning to slow down and let the body repair itself. Thus, it's normal to feel fatigued after physical activity or a period of intense pressure at school. Fatigue is also a common symptom of illness. Even a mild cold may temporarily rob a teenager of energy and make him want to sleep longer than usual. Healthy youngsters rapidly get back to normal once an illness is over. When fatigue is unusually severe or prolonged, however, it may be because of a chronic disorder such as iron-deficiency anaemia or reflect an emotional problem such as depression (see p. 176).

The tendency to sleep more than they did a few years earlier is normal in adolescents. Also, teenagers tend to be their most sleepy in the morning, making it difficult for them to concentrate during early morning classes. This sleepiness is due in part to the rapid growth rate and hormonal changes that come with adolescence.

A sudden attack of extreme drowsiness may indicate that a youngster needs medical attention, especially if there are other symptoms such as fever, vomiting, and confusion. In very rare cases, irresistible daytime drowsiness that occurs with certain other symptoms is caused by narcolepsy, a rare condition that can be managed with medication. You should consult your GP if your adolescent has fatigue that isn't relieved by rest, complains of muscle weakness, or hasn't recovered his energy weeks after the end of an illness.

Consult your GP if your adolescent's fatigue lasts more than a week or two or is accompanied by:

- Fever, a persistent sore throat, muscle and joint aches, and swollen glands.
- Constant thirst and nagging hunger, frequent urination, weight loss, numbness or tingling in the hands or feet, blurred vision, and anxiety.
- Unusual pallor, bruising in places not normally injured, loss of appetite and weight, bone pain, night sweats, swollen glands, and fever.

Warning

Unusual fatigue may be a signal that your youngster is abusing substances, particularly if she is taking little part in family activities, her grades have slipped, and she evades your questions about the time she spends with friends. It may also be a symptom of pregnancy.

Questions to consider	If answer is	Possible cause is	Action to take
Has your adolescent been tired since having a sore throat and swollen glands?	YES	Glandular fever; other viral infection.	Consult your GP who will examine the youngster and advise on treatment.
Does your adolescent feel tired all the time? Does she have trouble falling or staying asleep? Is she irritable?	YES	Adolescent insomnia; depression; boredom.	Try to eliminate sources of stress. Encourage your teenager to eat properly and exercise regularly. If insomnia persists, talk to your doctor.
Has your child been feeling unusually tired since starting medication for allergies or another condition?	YES	Medication side effects.	If your youngster takes an antihistamine, give it at night so he sleeps well but isn't tired in the daytime. If he is taking another medication, tell your doctor about the side effects and ask whether the prescription should be changed.

QUESTIONS TO CONSIDER	IF ANSWER IS	POSSIBLE CAUSE IS	ACTION TO TAKE
Does your teenager feel nervous or anxious for no reason? Is she pale? Has her weight changed noticeably?	**YES**	Iron-deficiency anaemia; thyroid disorder; crash diet; pregnancy; other conditions requiring diagnosis and treatment.	Consult your doctor, who will examine your adolescent and perform diagnostic tests as necessary. If your youngster wants to lose weight, ask your doctor to recommend a plan for steady weight loss.
Is your youngster often fatigued starting 3 or 4 hours after waking? Does he snore? Does he awaken often during the night? Is he having difficulties at school?	**YES**	Sleep apnoea; oversleeping (hypersomnia).	Consult your doctor, who will examine your child's nose and throat and determine if diagnostic tests and treatment are needed.
Does your adolescent often fall asleep during the daytime? Does he have a short attention span? Does he feel weak when he's upset? Does he always see vivid visual images while falling asleep? Is he having problems at school?	**YES**	Narcolepsy.	Consult your doctor, who will examine the youngster and may recommend referral for investigation.
Do your child's eyelids look droopy? Does she have fatigue that gets worse as the day goes on? Is she having vision problems?	**YES**	Myasthenia gravis (a disorder of the immune system) or another condition requiring diagnosis and treatment.	Consult your doctor, who will examine the youngster and order diagnostic tests.

Myalgic encephalomyelitis (ME)

A variable pattern of symptoms that always includes severe fatigue has become known as ME. Long-lasting fatigue that gets worse with effort is always a major part of the picture. (In contrast, healthy people can often beat fatigue with regular, moderate exercise.) The cause is unknown. ME is not infectious, although it may follow a viral illness. Those affected often report having felt nonspecific symptoms such as sore throat, fever, swollen lymph glands, muscle pain, and diarrhoea weeks or months before. Increasingly, they lack energy, have trouble concentrating, and lose interest in activities they used to enjoy, but there is no sign of physical illness and laboratory tests are normal. To confirm a diagnosis of ME, symptoms must be present for 6 months or more. Though not a children's disorder, ME occasionally affects older teenagers and young adults.

Time seems to be the only proven treatment. A regular schedule for sleep, rest, exercise, and meals is usually beneficial. Recovery may be helped along by medications to relieve specific symptoms such as depression and muscle aches.

High Blood Pressure

Hypertension

In General:

The long-term effects of high blood pressure (hypertension) are serious and include heart attacks, strokes, and kidney failure. Fortunately, treatment to lower even mildly elevated blood pressure can reduce the risk. The sooner treatment is started, the better the preventive effect. That's why doctors keep a check on blood pressure, looking at two measurements. The systolic pressure is the highest pressure in the arteries as the heart pumps blood out to circulate around the body. The diastolic pressure is the lowest pressure in the arteries when the heart relaxes to take in blood between beats. If the pressures are above an acceptable level, treatment – including dietary changes, regular exercise, and medication, if necessary – will be started. The cut-off point between normal and high blood pressure levels in adults is 140 (systolic) over 90 (diastolic), measured in millimetres on a mercury gauge; children's blood pressure, however, is lower and doctors evaluate it according to a youngster's age, height, and weight.

Hypertension is very unusual among young children but sometimes develops during adolescence. Young people whose blood pressures are in the high-normal range are more likely to develop hypertension during adulthood. Children of hypertensive parents are also more likely to develop high blood pressure later on. High blood pressure is more common in those with African ancestors than in those of other races. It becomes more severe with age and is worsened by a high-salt diet.

When no medical cause for high blood pressure can be identified, the condition is known as primary or essential hypertension. Many factors, such as heredity, salt consumption, emotional stress, and obesity, play a part in the development of essential hypertension, which accounts for more than 95 percent of all cases. High blood pressure due to an underlying illness is called secondary hypertension. A small number of children – usually adolescents – have high blood pressure, mostly mild to moderate in severity. Severe hypertension in children is usually caused by an illness such as kidney disease or a tumour.

Youngsters with hypertension rarely have symptoms unless their blood pressure is extremely high, usually because of an underlying condition. High blood pressure is sometimes discovered during routine pre-athletics examinations at school. A flushed face or racing heart following exercise is not an indication of hypertension; the only way to identify the condition is by using a blood pressure gauge.

Call your doctor immediately if your child has high blood pressure and develops any of the following:

- A persistent or severe headache.
- Dizziness.
- Shortness of breath.
- Visual disturbances.
- Unusual fatigue.

Warning

Help your children avoid unnecessary sodium by seasoning dishes with herbs and spices instead of salt. Keep salt off the table. Don't buy heavily salted snacks; if you're buying commercially prepared foods, look for unsalted and low-salt versions. Learn to recognize sodium in all its forms as another name for salt when reading labels.

Questions to consider	If answer is	Possible cause is	Action to take
Is your child's blood pressure in the high-normal or mildly elevated range? Is there a history of high blood pressure on either side of your family?	**YES**	Essential hypertension (high blood pressure without an obvious physical cause).	Monitor your child's weight and food intake. Encourage regular exercise. Ask your doctor to check your youngster's blood pressure at regular visits and find out whether any further action is advisable.

QUESTIONS TO CONSIDER	IF ANSWER IS	POSSIBLE CAUSE IS	ACTION TO TAKE
Has your child been diagnosed with hypertension? Are there symptoms of a kidney disorder? Is the blood pressure higher in the arms than the legs?	**YES**	Kidney disease (causing renal hypertension); coarctation of the aorta (an inborn condition affecting the artery that arises from the heart); tumour; hyperthyroidism.	Your doctor will carry out tests to determine the cause and recommend treatment accordingly.
Is your child overweight? Has your doctor diagnosed high blood pressure?	**YES**	Obesity-related hypertension.	Ask your doctor's advice about helping your child to lose weight while providing the calories and nutrients necessary for growth. Discourage eating salty foods.
Has your youngster become unusually irritable but with no other apparent symptoms? Or has he suddenly developed headaches, dizziness, or a change in vision?	**YES**	Severe hypertension.	Call your doctor at once. Your child must be evaluated and diagnosed.

How salt affects the blood pressure

Table salt is a compound of sodium and chloride, two chemicals that are essential for health, but only in small amounts. In fact, sodium and chloride occur naturally in so many foods that we don't need to add them. Salt is hardly needed to preserve foods any more since refrigeration and newer technologies now do this job better. The real reason we keep on adding salt to foods is habit; we've developed a taste for it. We eat a lot of salt: on average, one to three teaspoons a day, containing 2,300 to 6,900 milligrams of sodium. Health and nutrition experts calculate that a healthy adult needs only about 500 milligrams of sodium a day and that a single daily teaspoonful of salt is more than adequate. Children need even less than adults, and baby foods should always be prepared without salt. Overconsumption of salt is an important factor in raising the blood pressure in people who are extra sensitive to sodium.

In a healthy person, the kidneys retrieve sodium from the blood, conserving and recycling the element as a valuable resource. Salt concentrations help to regulate the amount of water in the body. In people who are sodium sensitive, the kidneys retain more sodium than the body needs, throwing the sodium-water concentration off balance. The body tries to dilute the sodium by increasing the amount of fluid circulating in the bloodstream; the excess fluid shows up as puffiness, especially in our hands, feet, and legs. The increased fluid volume makes the blood vessels oversensitive to nerve stimulation and they constrict, thus raising the blood pressure. (Picture how the water pressure changes when you partly choke off a garden hosepipe.) In consequence, the heart has to work harder to keep the blood moving through tight vessels. The constant high pressure weakens the blood vessel walls. This effect is often first noticeable in the vessels of the eyes and kidneys. Cutting down on salt consumption helps to lower the sodium concentration and ease the pressure on the heart, kidneys, and blood vessels.

If you have hypertension or know you are salt sensitive, cut down on salt in your family's diet now to help your children avoid high blood pressure later.

In General:

On occasion, childhood knee pain can be caused by serious conditions such as arthritis, auto-immune diseases, infections, tumours, and blood disorders. Most often, however, knee pain in children is due to minor bumps or overuse.

The kneecap (patella) is linked to the thighbone (femur) at the patellofemoral joint. This joint is kept stable by the combined force of ligaments and muscles, as well as the fit of the bony structures. The base of the kneecap is V-shaped and slides through a matching groove (trochlea) in the thighbone. The kneecap does not slide straight but shifts slightly sideways as it moves, as force is exerted on it by the muscles and tendons. A slight irregularity in the bone or unevenness in the strengths of the muscles, tendons, and ligaments can make the kneecap track abnormally. This causes knee pain that gets worse with strenuous activity.

Injuries to the knee ligaments are common in adults but less so in children. This is because children's immature ligaments are stronger than the bone they're attached to. On forceful impact, the bone will break before the ligament can tear. As the bones harden during adolescence, however, injuries to the knees and ligaments become more like those that occur in adults. Skiers, tennis players, in-line skaters, and basketball and football players are particularly vulnerable. Knee injuries in girls are becoming more common as increasing numbers take up competitive sports. Young athletes who play contact sports should always wear protective gear for games and practice.

Consult your GP if:

- Knee pain or swelling last more than 3 days.
- Pain and/or swelling follow an injury to the knee.
- The knee joint is tender, red, and warm to the touch, whether or not an injury has occurred.
- Your child complains of weakness or instability in the knee.

Warning

Although conditions directly affecting the knee are the usual cause of pain there, knee pain may also be a symptom of a hip disorder.

Questions to consider	If answer is	Possible cause is	Action to take
Does your child have tenderness, redness, warmth, and/or swelling over the knee?	**YES**	Infection; trauma; arthritis.	Call your doctor, who will examine the child and determine whether referral to a specialist is necessary.
Does your child have pain and tender swelling at the top of his shin? Have symptoms come on since he started taking part in a sport?	**YES**	Bruising; muscle strain; Osgood-Schlatter disease (a common, painful, but benign condition in adolescents).	Ask your doctor to examine the child. If Osgood-Schlatter disease is confirmed, treatment usually involves rest, decreased participation in sports, and pain medication as required.
Does your child have the feeling that her knee is 'out of joint'? Does the feeling follow an injury?	**YES**	Dislocation of the kneecap; ligament tear; chondromalacia patellae (softening of the kneecap cartilage).	Call your doctor, who will determine whether the knee has been injured. Treatment may involve rest followed by isometric exercise. Children rarely need surgery.

QUESTIONS TO CONSIDER	IF ANSWER IS	POSSIBLE CAUSE IS	ACTION TO TAKE
Does your son limp from pain after strenuous activity? Does he complain of stiffness, buckling, or locking in the knee joint? Does the knee make an audible click? Is it swollen?	**YES**	Osteochondritis dissecans (possibly due to trauma; much more common in boys).	Your doctor will examine the child and advise on management of this common condition, which results from separation of a small bone section and causes inflammation and splitting of the cartilage. Your doctor may refer the child for evaluation by an orthopaedic specialist.
Is your child complaining of vague pain in the knee, especially after vigorous activity? Does the knee look normal? Does it seem to function without locking or giving way?	**YES**	Patellar maltracking; knee pain of unknown cause; slipped capital femoral epiphysis (dislocation of the head of the thighbone).	Consult your GP, who will examine the child to rule out serious causes of knee pain and may recommend isometric exercises to improve strength and flexibility. Ice packs can be used to relieve discomfort. The pain usually disappears with time. Slipped capital femoral epiphysis may require surgical pinning.
Is there a swelling at the back of your child's knee?	**YES**	Popliteal cyst (Baker's cyst), a benign condition in school-age children.	Ask your GP to examine the child. The recommended approach to a popliteal cyst is to leave it alone, as these benign swellings normally disappear without treatment. Surgery is necessary only if there is severe discomfort or the swelling increases.
Does knee pain awaken your child from sleep?	**YES**	Overuse; tumour; blood disorder; or another systemic condition.	If the child has pain in the daytime or is limping, or if pain lasts more than a few days, call your doctor.
Is your child's knee painful and slightly swollen? Is there a loud click or 'clunk' as the knee is bent?	**YES**	Discoid lateral meniscus, a rare condition where the meniscus, a pad of cartilage at the top of the shinbone, is round instead of half-moon shaped.	Consult your doctor who may recommend a consultation with an orthopaedic specialist.

Preventing knee injuries

The most common cause of knee pain is overuse, in which repeated, low-grade injury causes a progressive loss of strength in the entire limb. Conditioning exercises are essential for preventing joint and muscle injuries in children. Coaches and school athletics directors should stress the importance of warm-ups and stretching exercises before sports.

Most acute, minor muscle injuries can be managed by applying cold compresses immediately after the injury, giving paracetamol or ibuprofen for pain, and having the child rest for 1 to 2 days. If your child has severe or persistent pain related to exercise, call your GP for an evaluation. Your doctor will suggest exercises to improve strength and function. The youngster should not play sports again until your doctor gives the go-ahead. Pain caused by injury to a joint may require a consultation with an orthopaedic specialist.

Mood Swings

Consult your doctor if your child:

- Has a noticeable weight change due to either lack or increase of appetite.
- Has lost interest in activities she formerly enjoyed.
- Is sleeping much more or much less than usual.
- Expresses feelings of worthlessness or guilt.
- Has a marked change in energy level, becoming either listless or overactive.

In General:

Youngsters at either end of childhood are the most vulnerable to mood swings. During the terrible twos, children are buffeted by complicated feelings towards their parents: love, jealousy, frustration, fear of a parent's displeasure or abandonment. A pre-schooler's moods may switch from sunny to thunderous and back again in the space of a few minutes until she develops verbal fluency and outgrows tantrums (see p. 148). The middle years are relatively free of emotional ups and downs. Adolescence, however, unleashes a new set of mood swings due partly to hormonal changes and partly to the anxieties and uncertainties of the teen years (see Anxiety, p. 174).

Many parents insist that sugar consumption affects their children's energy level and behaviour, although studies have failed to show any connection between children's diet and moods. There is a link, however, between mood and exercise. People who exercise regularly maintain a steady output of endorphins – the brain's natural mood-enhancers – which may help promote a balanced emotional state.

Warning

Don't ignore severe mood swings, especially if they involve cycles of deep depression and extreme elation, and hope that your adolescent will 'snap out of it'. Your child may need medical help.

Mood swings particularly affect youngsters with chronic illnesses. Especially vulnerable are those with hormonal disorders, such as diabetes mellitus or thyroid problems, and those with motor disabilities, which at times lead to feelings of frustration and helplessness. Counselling and participation in a peer support group may help a teenager to see that others share her difficulties and are overcoming similar problems. Extreme emotional volatility may indicate poor impulse control, an underlying personality disorder, or drug or alcohol use. In a very few teenagers it may signal the onset of mental illness. At the very least, an adolescent who has extreme, unpredictable mood swings is hard to get along with at home and is likely to run into difficulties with schoolmates, teachers, and other authority figures such as employers. Such a youngster needs help, whether or not she admits to a problem.

Emotional problems sometimes become apparent with a gain or drop in weight (see Depression, p. 176 and Eating Disorders, p. 178). Be alert to danger signals: if your child gets careless about his appearance and hygiene, if he stops seeing friends, if his school performance takes a nosedive, or if he is just acting differently, you may be able to head off trouble by talking with your doctor. When mood swings interfere with family life, social relationships, and school performance, ask your doctor to refer your child to a specialist in emotional disorders for an evaluation of the problem and recommendations for management.

Questions to consider	If answer is	Possible cause is	Action to take
Is your teenager sometimes moody, feeling up one minute and down the next? Is she generally well and happy?	**YES**	Normal adolescent behaviour.	Try to keep your sense of humour in dealing with teenage moods. This behaviour is a normal phase.

QUESTIONS TO CONSIDER	IF ANSWER IS	POSSIBLE CAUSE IS	ACTION TO TAKE
Does your teenage daughter become tearful, oversensitive, and moody for several days each month?	**YES**	Premenstrual syndrome (PMS or perimenstrual dysphoric disorder).	Explain to your daughter that the feelings are part of the natural hormonal cycle. PMS isn't disabling and she can learn to anticipate it and plan her activities accordingly.
Has your child been irritable and moody since a recent viral illness?	**YES**	Gradual recovery from viral illness.	Irritability is not unusual following a viral illness. If the child isn't back to normal in a week or two, talk to your doctor.
Over a period of days or weeks, has your adolescent become sad, tearful, irritable, and withdrawn? Was the change set off by an identifiable event?	**YES**	Reactive depression, a normal response characterized by feelings of sadness. (See Depression, p. 176.)	Discuss the event as well as practical solutions to problems. If the mood lasts longer than 3 weeks or is getting worse, consult your doctor, who may recommend counseling and/or medical therapy.
Does your child have low moods lasting weeks at a time, alternating with normal moods? Is there a family history of depression?	**YES**	Mild chronic depression (dysthymia).	If the low moods are interfering with family life, schoolwork, or the child's happiness, consult your doctor. Your child may need further evaluation and treatment.
Does your child have a chronic illness? Are you concerned that he may neglect to take medication or perform monitoring tests?	**YES**	Anxiety, resentment, and denial related to chronic illness; effects of the illness.	Consult your doctor, who may refer your child to a counsellor as well as a peer support group.
Do your child's low moods alternate with periods when she is erratic, hyperactive, argumentative, and sleeping little?	**YES**	Bipolar disorder (manic depression).	Consult your doctor; your teenager may need medication to settle her moods and psychotherapy to deal with confused feelings.

Temperament and moodiness

Children are often characterized as having an easy, withdrawn, or difficult temperament. An easy child has a positive outlook, takes changes and new situations in his stride, and meets challenges with good humour and minimal anxiety. A withdrawn child adapts more slowly, is less outgoing, and tends to be more anxious when confronted with new people and situations. The difficult child may have tantrums and adjustment difficulties. Within these categories, children are adaptable according to activity level, regularity of habits, sensory threshold, and mood (the degree of pleasantness in communications and actions). Parents shouldn't hurry to label a child as difficult or moody if the child has had stresses that can temporarily affect behaviour. What's more, a child may seem difficult only when his personality and behaviour differ from those of his parents and teachers. Be sensitive to your child's emotional makeup in dealing with conflicts. Help your child to make the best of his basic characteristics. Your doctor can offer advice and referral.

In General:

Adolescence is a time of transition between childhood and adult independence. Although parents often find this a trying time, about 80 percent of youngsters manage to cross over into adulthood with only minor problems or none at all. But for some, outside forces block the way. And for a few, the transition is hampered by emotional or physical problems.

Youngsters having a difficult adolescence may become seriously depressed. Others seek escape in self-destructive behaviour or physical symptoms that cover up clinical depression (see p. 176). For many parents, the first clue that their teenager needs professional help is a change in his personality. Different from the normal ups and downs of adolescence, the change is a deep-rooted shift in attitude and behaviour. A change in personality shouldn't be written off as teenage moodiness. Occasionally, a personality change follows serious accidental head injury, or results from a rare physical condition such as a metabolic disorder or brain tumour. In many adolescents, a marked personality change is a signal that they are taking part in risky behaviour such as substance abuse and other self-destructive acts. Also in this category is irresponsible sexual activity, which all too often leads to pregnancy, sexually transmitted diseases including AIDS, and long-term emotional problems.

Because the results of risky behaviour are potentially tragic, parents should be alert to warning signs of personality change indicating that a teenager needs help. Whether the personality change is a symptom of depression, a conduct disorder (see Behaviour Problems, p. 34), a physical condition, or emerging mental illness, the adolescent needs to be evaluated. Your doctor will guide you in choosing suitable treatment and may recommend family therapy advice.

Consult your doctor (and talk to your child) if your youngster's personality has changed and:

- He has missed school repeatedly or his grades have dropped.
- You believe he may be using alcohol or illegal substances.
- He is withdrawn, reclusive, and uncommunicative.
- He is usually hostile and aggressive.
- He is acting in a way that may endanger life or risk confrontation with the law.
- He also has symptoms suggesting a physical illness.

Warning

If your teenager makes off-hand remarks about suicide, don't ignore them. Direct questioning may show you that he wants to talk over his problems. He should be evaluated by your doctor without delay.

Questions to consider	If answer is	Possible cause is	Action to take
Is your adolescent hostile and aggressive? Is he having problems at school?	YES	Learning problem; behaviour problem.	Consult your doctor, who will evaluate your child and may recommend treatment or referral.
Is your adolescent secretive about how he spends his time? Does he have money or possessions he can't account for?	YES	Substance use, including dealing in illicit drugs.	Discuss your concerns with your GP, who may suggest how to approach the youngster.

Questions to consider	If answer is	Possible cause is	Action to take
Is your child missing school? Have her grades plummeted?	**YES**	Truancy; school difficulties; substance use; acting out; pregnancy.	Talk to your child's teachers to identify specific problems and get recommendations. Consult your doctor about counselling.
Is your teenager's erratic behaviour interfering with family life? Does she have mood swings, with prolonged ups and downs? Is she having difficulties at school?	**YES**	Emotional disorder; mental illness.	Consult your doctor immediately for an evaluation.
Does your adolescent have bouts of trembling? Is she panicky and short of breath during attacks? Does her heart race? Is she having trouble concentrating?	**YES**	Anxiety attacks; early sign of diabetes.	Consult your GP, who will perform an examination to rule out physical conditions and may prescribe treatment.
Has your teenager become aggressive or forgetful? Does he get headaches that are worse when he lies down? Does he have double vision, muscle weakness, or nausea and vomiting?	**YES**	Tumour or another condition requiring diagnosis and treatment.	Consult your GP immediately.

Teenage suicide

Tragically, suicide is one of the most common causes of death in teenagers in many Western countries. The rate is increasing yearly. Although girls attempt suicide more often, boys outnumber girls in suicide deaths because boys are more likely to choose a lethal method.

Adolescents try to kill themselves primarily because of undiagnosed or untreated depression, serious conflicts with family and friends, physical and sexual abuse, sexual identity crises, and problems with school and the law. Many youngsters attempt suicide while under the influence of drink or drugs. And it's impossible to draw a clear line between some accidents and suicide attempts because many fatal accidents occur when teenagers use alcohol or drugs. The substance loosens their inhibitions and lets them flirt with self-destructive behaviour such as driving while intoxicated or performing dangerous stunts on a dare. Experts calculate that only about a third of those who attempt suicide really intend to destroy themselves. The others are looking for attention, love, or escape from an unbearable situation.

A youngster who can't shake off depression or anger over problems in the family, at school, or with the community may be harbouring ideas of suicide. At the very least, he may be risking injury to himself or others through irresponsible behaviour. Your doctor should evaluate him as soon as possible to rule out physical problems and determine whether he should be referred to a psychiatrist or another mental health professional.

In General:

As puberty approaches, boys and girls should get straightforward information about their bodily changes and health-related issues. They need to know about erections, nocturnal emissions ('wet dreams'), masturbation, the menstrual cycle, intercourse, and pregnancy, as well as abstinence, contraception and sexually transmitted diseases (STDs), including AIDS. Schools teach the biology of sex, but parents should make sure youngsters understand that sexuality is also tied to emotions, responsible behaviour, and moral choices based on respect for themselves and others. To have a healthy influence on adolescent development, sexual activity must fit within the religious and moral framework of the family.

Economic and social shifts have blurred some of the guidelines for dating and sexual behaviour. Teenagers are taking part in sexual activity at progressively younger ages. For instance, in the United States slightly more than half of all adolescents have had intercourse at least once by the age of 17 years, and 80 percent of boys and 70 percent of girls have engaged in sexual activity by age 19. If you find the trend towards earlier sexual activity disturbing, be sure that you let your teenager know what your views are and what standards of behaviour you'd prefer to see. While you can educate, however, you cannot always enforce your rules. If your teenager chooses differently, let him or her know you'll always be ready to listen when he or she needs to talk.

Early sexual experience in teenagers tends to be associated with other high-risk behaviour, including promiscuity, alcohol and drug use, school problems, and delinquency. Youngsters need guidance in developing self-control, commitment, and responsible sexual attitudes. Many parents are uncomfortable discussing sexual issues. Your doctor can provide impartial advice, suggest reading material, and refer your youngster for further help and advice if needed.

Talk to your doctor if you find it difficult to communicate with your adolescent and you are concerned that he or she is:

- Having unprotected intercourse.
- Taking part in high-risk behaviour including sexual activity, drug and alcohol use, or truancy.

Warning

If your adolescent is involved with a partner who is much older or in a position of relative authority, you should question whether the relationship may be abusive. Direct action may only drive a wedge between you and your child. Your doctor may recommend consultation with a family counsellor.

Questions to consider	If answer is	Possible cause is	Action to take
Do you have reason to believe your adolescent is sexually active?	**YES**	Adolescent development and peer pressure.	Let your teenager know your views on commitment and respect. Make sure he or she understands the importance of contraception, as well as the prevention of STDs. If you find it hard to talk to your teenager, discuss this with your doctor.
Does your adolescent daughter have pain on urination? Does she urinate frequently or have blood in the urine? Is she sexually active?	**YES**	Inflammation of the bladder (cystitis).	Consult your GP. Your daughter may need antibiotic treatment. She may also need advice about contraception and disease prevention.

QUESTIONS TO CONSIDER	IF ANSWER IS	POSSIBLE CAUSE IS	ACTION TO TAKE
Has your teenager asked you for contraceptives?	**YES**	Sexual activity.	If you do not approve, say so. But if you believe she'll continue without your approval, suggest that she consult your GP or practice nurse, who can give impartial advice..
Has your teenager suggested that he or she is physically attracted to members of the same sex?	**YES**	Developmental stage; homosexuality.	It's not unusual to question one's sexual orientation during adolescence. Your local library will have age-appropriate books on this issue. If your teenager wants to discuss these concerns in depth, your doctor will recommend resources.
Has your sexually active daughter missed a period? Is she having nausea or faintness?	**YES**	Pregnancy.	Discuss your concerns with your daughter. If you have reason to think she may be pregnant, consult your doctor promptly.
Is your daughter unusually upset or withdrawn? Did the upset happen after she accepted a date or a ride with someone? Or has she abruptly broken up with a boyfriend?	**YES**	Unwelcome pressure to take part in sexual activity; date rape; rape.	Try to get the facts without making your daughter overanxious. Give her tips about resisting pressure; tell her you support her and she can always call you for a ride. If she has been forced into sex, call your doctor immediately for advice about taking legal action, if necessary.
Does your child insist he or she is of the other sex? Has he or she expressed a desire for treatment to change his or her body? Have these ideas been present since early childhood?	**YES**	Gender identity disorder.	Consult your doctor. Those with this rare condition believe they are trapped in the wrong body. They are physically normal; many marry and have children before seeking help. Some undergo sex reassignment, but the results are not always satisfactory.

Abstinence has an important place in sexual activity

Numerous surveys show that many people would like to see the entertainment media portray sex more responsibly. Yet movies and television continue to send the message that everyone is sexually active and there is no need to worry about such consequences as unplanned pregnancy or sexually transmitted diseases. Your best approach is to counter these pervasive messages with sound sex education. Your GP can provide information to help you teach your youngsters effectively about sex, in a way that communicates factual knowledge, your family values, and your behavioural expectations. Youngsters should be aware of all the facts, including the responsibilities and risks of sexual behaviour and the importance of abstinence as a healthy preference.

Although the media rarely portray abstinence among teens in a positive fashion, adolescents should be encouraged to postpone sexual intercourse until they are physically and emotionally mature. They should not feel compelled to be sexually active just because others are. Sex education should include the information that abstinence and celibacy are valid and praiseworthy choices. The teenager who makes up his mind to abstain from sexual intercourse should always be supported in his decision. An adolescent who is sexually active, or who intends to be, should be actively educated about the inherent safety of abstinence, as well as contraception and protection against sexually transmitted diseases.

In General:

Skin problems are so common in adolescents that it's rare to find a teenager with a perfect complexion. About 85 percent of adolescents have acne to some degree. The lucky ones – about three-quarters of those with acne – have nothing more troubling than a few blackheads, known medically as comedones, caused when sebaceous glands become blocked. These glands are attached to the hair follicles, through which they secrete a greasy substance, called sebum, to lubricate and protect the hair and skin. Mild acne blemishes generally clear up with little or no scarring, provided they are left alone and don't become infected. In severe cases, inflamed pustules and cysts may disfigure the face, back, and chest. This severe form, known as cystic acne, is more common in boys and is generally managed by dermatologists.

A tendency to acne runs in families, but skin eruptions are triggered by increases in the levels of male hormones – androgens – that occur in both sexes at puberty. Under the influence of these hormones, the sebaceous glands enlarge and increase their output of sebum. Girls who have acne often break out due to a surge in hormone levels in the week or so before each menstrual period.

Acne can be very upsetting to teenagers, who are often self-conscious and concerned about making the right impression on their friends. In many cases, however, parents are more concerned than their children. Safe, effective treatment is now available. Your GP may recommend an over-the-counter lotion or cream to deal with minor problems. Many teenagers find they have fewer blemishes if they avoid soaps (which are harsh and alkaline) and use a water-rinsable cleansing lotion or soap substitute (which is mildly acidic and less irritating) to wash their faces at least twice every day. Avoid overwashing and vigorous scrubbing, however; these can irritate the skin and worsen acne. For more severe outbreaks, treatment may include a prescription medication as well. Teenagers with acne should avoid oil-based skin creams and cosmetics.

Consult your GP if your adolescent:

- Has several painful, warm, reddened swellings with pus visible at the peak (they may be boils, see Skin Problems, p. 132).
- Compulsively picks at skin blemishes (she may benefit from counseling for an underlying emotional problem).

Warning

Picking at blemishes can make the skin vulnerable to infection, which may result in permanent scarring. Left alone, most acne lesions heal and don't leave a permanent mark.

Questions to consider	If answer is	Possible cause is	Action to take
Is your adolescent getting occasional blackheads or pimples?	**YES**	Adolescent acne.	To reduce skin oiliness, encourage your youngster to clean his face at least twice a day with a nonalkaline soap substitute. If pimples are troubling, your GP may recommend an over-the-counter cream or prescribe a benzoyl peroxide-based treatment.
Does your teenager have acne spreading over his face, shoulders, chest, or back?	**YES**	Cystic acne (acne conglobata).	Consult your doctor, who will examine the youngster and will be able to prescribe treatment, usually with antibiotics. Left untreated, this condition can lead to unsightly scarring and severe distress.

Questions to consider	If answer is	Possible cause is	Action to take
Does your teenager have a burning or itching feeling in her feet? Is the skin between her toes whitish and moist? Do her toenails look yellow?	**YES**	Athlete's foot; fungal infection (tinea pedis).	Consult your GP, who may recommend an antifungal treatment. Encourage your adolescent to dry thoroughly after baths and showers, use cotton socks, and wash trainers.
Does your teenager have itching in his crotch area?	**YES**	Dhobi itch (tinea cruris); intertrigo (inflammation in skin creases and folds); crab (pubic) lice.	Consult your GP, who will evaluate the problem and recommend appropriate treatment. Encourage your son to wear loose-fitting cotton underwear, avoid tight trousers, and dry thoroughly after baths and showers. Crab lice are eradicated with special shampoos, creams, or lotions that contain chemicals to kill the parasites. Consult your GP for advice on which one to use.
Has your adolescent developed a rash with pale reddish, scaly spots over her trunk and upper arms?	**YES**	Pityriasis rosea; fungal infection.	Pityriasis rosea is common in teenagers and generally clears up in 6 to 12 weeks. Its cause is unknown. The rash is itchy but harmless and leaves no scars. Consult your GP, however, to make sure that the rash is not due to a fungal infection.

Effects of diet on acne

Despite old wives' tales, there is no proven link between acne outbreaks and a diet that includes liberal amounts of chocolate, sweets, and fried foods. Nor is acne caused by sexual activity or constipation. Nevertheless, some acne sufferers find that pimples regularly appear after they have eaten certain foods. Researchers theorize that in such cases, it's not the foods themselves that trigger the outbreak. Instead, they suspect that the real culprit may be stress. It's well known that stress can trigger or worsen acne, perhaps by altering hormone levels. In some people, hormonal changes seem to stimulate food cravings, especially for chocolate and other sweets. So the person may mistakenly blame sweets for the acne, when the real cause is stress. Exercise – coupled with a diet that balances carbohydrates, protein, and a small amount of fat with plenty of fresh vegetables and fruits – benefits the entire body, including the skin.

The only known cause and effect between diet and acne is an acnelike flare-up that some people get after eating foods with a high iodine content. Kelp supplements sold in health food shops have been linked to acne. The levels of iodine in fish and shellfish are unlikely to cause acne in teenagers. High doses of some of the B-complex vitamins sometimes can cause acne. Finally, a number of medications – especially steroids and other hormone preparations, anticonvulsants, and lithium – can cause acne.

PART 2

Illustrated First Aid Manual and Safety Guide

CHAPTER 4 BASICS OF FIRST AID

ADMINISTERING FIRST AID

First aid involves giving immediate, often lifesaving care to a child who is injured or has a sudden illness. It demands fast thinking and action to provide needed care until medical assistance can be obtained. Train yourself to stay calm in emergencies: count slowly or breathe deeply if it helps keep you steady. You will be able to think more clearly and your child will be less likely to get upset. Read this chapter several times so you'll know what to do in an emergency. Keep this book where it's easy to find.

Make sure there's an up-to-date list of emergency numbers (GP, dentist, hospital accident and emergency department, next-door neighbour) next to every phone in your home. Include any information your baby-sitter might need. Top the list with the 999 emergency number and your own address and phone number: your memory can play tricks in crisis situations.

LIFESAVING TECHNIQUES

Every parent and care-giver should know how to do three critical lifesaving techniques: cardiopulmonary resuscitation (CPR), the infant CPR/choking procedure, and the Heimlich manoeuvre. The Red Cross and St. John's Ambulance Brigade offer courses on these techniques.

THE IMPORTANCE OF PREVENTION

Each year tens of thousands of British children need medical care to deal with injuries.Unintentional injuries are the leading cause of death in children under 5. While automobiles are involved in a large number of injuries and deaths, most events occur around our homes, even on furniture and play equipment designed specially for children. It's not enough to be ready to deal with injuries as they occur. To keep your children safe, you must be alert to hazards in everyday objects, your environment, and your youngsters themselves. The Guide to Safety and Prevention, beginning on page 221, can help you recognize potentially dangerous situations in your home. Refer to it frequently; you'll need to revise your safety procedures from time to time as your children grow older and face new risks.

First aid kit

You will find it easier to cope with an emergency if you know that a few essential supplies are to hand. Prepare for sudden injury or illness by assembling two sets of basic items – one for your home, the other for your car – and keep each set in a marked container out of the reach of young children. Chemists also stock prepacked first aid kits.

Check the supplies from time to time and replace dated items; replace other items as you use them. If any family member has a condition requiring special medication, keep a supply in each first aid kit.

The following should be in every first aid kit:

✓ Roll of 7.5cm (3 in) wide gauze bandage.

✓ Packet of sterile, nonstick dressings, 10cm (4in) square, individually packaged.

✓ Adhesive bandage strips.

✓ Butterfly sutures and thin adhesive strips.

✓ Roll of 2.5cm (1in) surgical tape.

✓ Scissors.

✓ A 7.5cm (3in) elastic bandage.

✓ Packet of cotton buds.

✓ Roll of cotton wool.

✓ Aspirin or another over-the-counter painkiller for adults.

✓ Paracetamol tablets or syrup for children. (In children, aspirin is associated with an increased risk of Reye syndrome, a rare but serious illness that may follow a viral infection; as in adults, it can also cause side effects such as stomach upset and intestinal bleeding. Ibuprofen is a safe alternative in most children.)

✓ Oral thermometer.

✓ Small jar of petroleum jelly.

✓ Tweezers, safety pins.

✓ Calamine lotion.

✓ Antiseptic cream.

✓ Bar of soap.

✓ Torch.

✓ Antihistamine tablets or liquid.

CHOKING

Choking, the most common preventable cause of death in children under 1 year of age, occurs when something other than air enters the windpipe. The gagging, gasping, and coughing that happen when a drink goes down the wrong way are rarely harmful, and the child recovers as soon as the passage is cleared. But choking is an emergency when food or a foreign object cuts off the flow of air to the lungs. The choking child cannot speak, cry out, or cough. His face rapidly becomes flushed then turns blue.

Prevention

Parents must be especially watchful with young children who are sampling new foods; food is the most frequent cause of choking (p. 223). Small toys are also a common hazard. (For further guidelines, see Guide to Safety and Prevention, p. 221.)

What You Can Do

If your infant or child is choking and unable to breathe, you must act immediately; you may not have time to call for help. If possible, have someone nearby call for emergency assistance while you administer emergency help for choking.

Don't use the Heimlich manoeuvre to help a choking infant under 1 year old; you may damage the delicate internal organs.
If you can't see the object, don't try to remove it with your fingers; you may push it farther down and close off the windpipe.

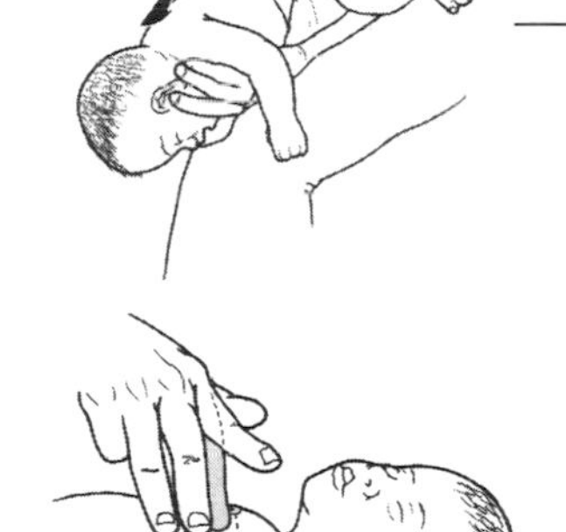

Place your baby face down on your arm. Hold his head and neck steady, and brace your forearm against your thigh.

Use the heel of your hand to give five quick, firm blows between the infant's shoulder blades.

If this fails to dislodge the object, position the infant face up on a firm surface. Place your index, third, and fourth fingers below an imaginary line between the nipples and in the middle of the breastbone. The position of the third and fourth fingers is the area for chest compression.

Use two fingers to give five firm, rapid chest thrusts near the centre of the breastbone, pushing the breastbone in about 1cm (½in).

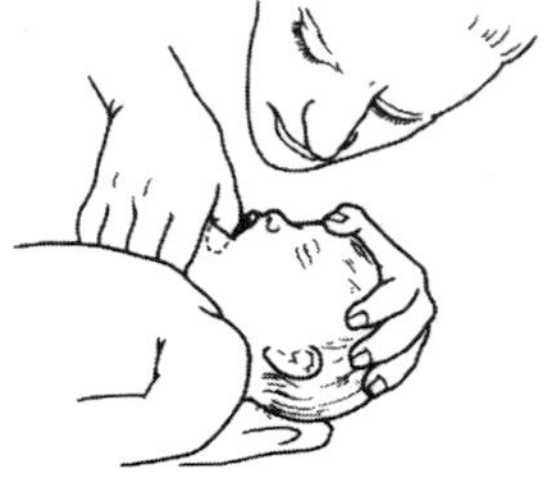

If your baby becomes unresponsive or unconscious, lift the jaw and tongue forward by grasping the chin and gum with your thumb or index finger. If you can see the foreign object, sweep it out with your other index finger. (If you can't see it, don't fish for it.)

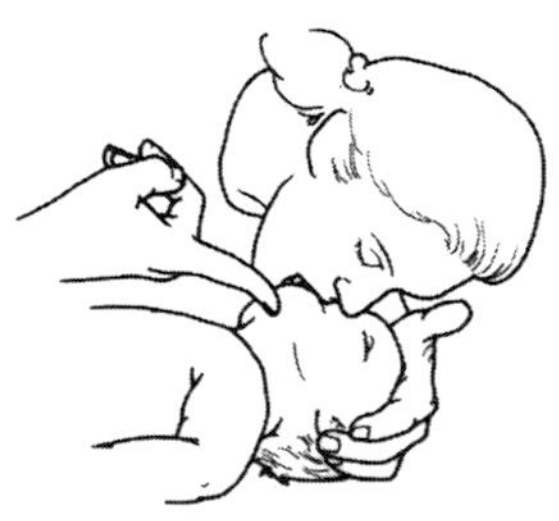

If your child is not breathing, tilt his head back, cover his mouth and nose with your mouth, and try to give two breaths. If the infant's chest doesn't rise, the blockage is still present.

Repeat steps 1 through 6 until the object is coughed up, the infant starts to breathe, or help arrives.

If your child is choking and can't breathe, have somebody call 999 while you begin the following emergency measures. If the child is coughing, crying, or speaking, however, do any of the following; instead, call 999 or your doctor for advice.

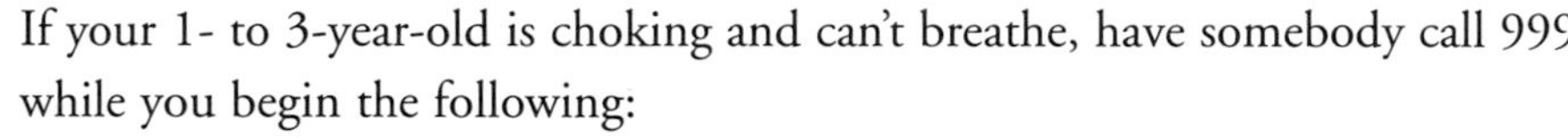

If your 1- to 3-year-old is choking and can't breathe, have somebody call 999 while you begin the following:

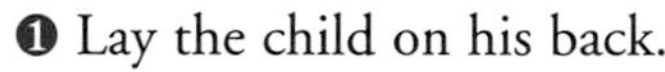

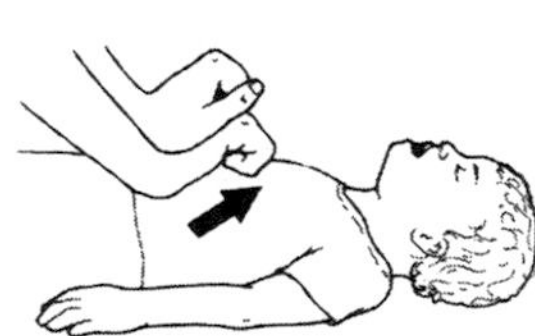

❶ Lay the child on his back.

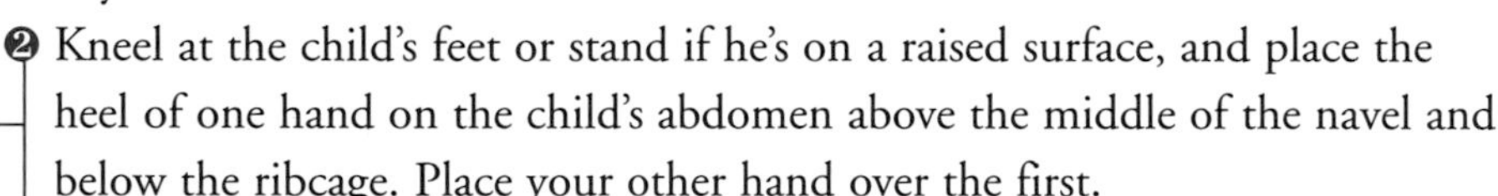

❷ Kneel at the child's feet or stand if he's on a raised surface, and place the heel of one hand on the child's abdomen above the middle of the navel and below the ribcage. Place your other hand over the first.

❸ Press into the abdomen with up to five rapid upward thrusts. Keep thrusts gentle in a small child.

❹ Lift jaw and tongue with your thumb and index finger. If you can see the object, sweep it out with your other index finger.

Repeat steps 2 and 3 until the child coughs up the object, starts to breathe, or becomes unconscious. If the child becomes unconscious, give mouth-to-mouth resuscitation until emergency help arrives.

❶ Treat a choking *older* child standing, sitting, or lying down.

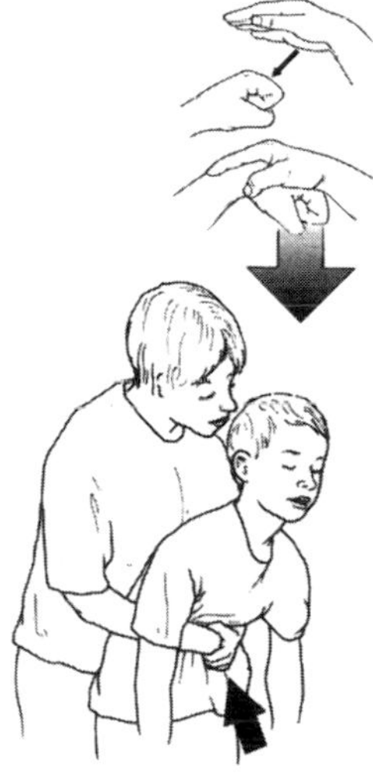

❷ Place the thumbside of a fist against the middle of the child's abdomen, just above the navel. Grasp the fist with your other hand.

❸ Give up to five firm, rapid, upward thrusts into the abdomen.

Repeat steps 2 and 3 until the object is coughed up, or until your child starts to breathe or becomes unconscious.

If your child becomes unconscious, give mouth-to-mouth resuscitation until emergency help arrives.

Professional Help

Once a blockage is cleared, most children are soon back to normal. A child who breathes on his own within 2 or 3 minutes is unlikely to have long-term damage.

- If your child is not breathing by the time help arrives, the emergency team will attempt to dislodge the blockage with the Heimlich manoeuvre. At the same time, they will prepare your child for transport to a hospital for further treatment, such as insertion of a breathing tube.
- If your child keeps on coughing, gagging, or drooling, or has difficulty in swallowing or breathing after a choking incident, it may mean that some of the foreign material is still partly blocking the airway. The emergency physician will take action to remove the blockage.

To be used when a child is unresponsive or unconscious, or when breathing or heartbeat stops.

Try to rouse your child by shaking him gently and calling his name. If he fails to respond and is not breathing or you can't feel a pulse, call for help, then begin to give CPR.

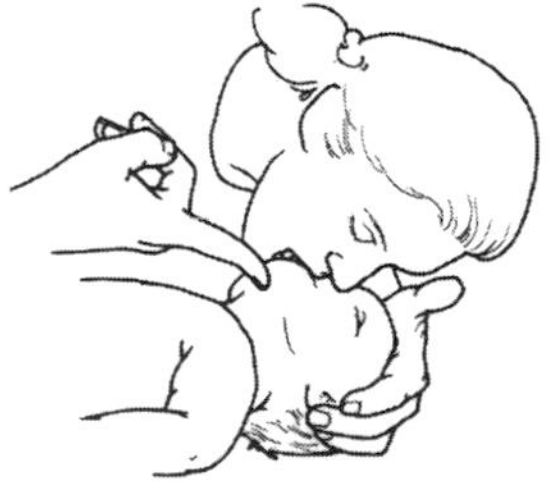

❶ Call for help immediately.
❷ Tilt the infant's head back. Seal your lips tightly around his mouth and nose.
❸ Give two slow breaths until his chest gently rises.

If air goes in:

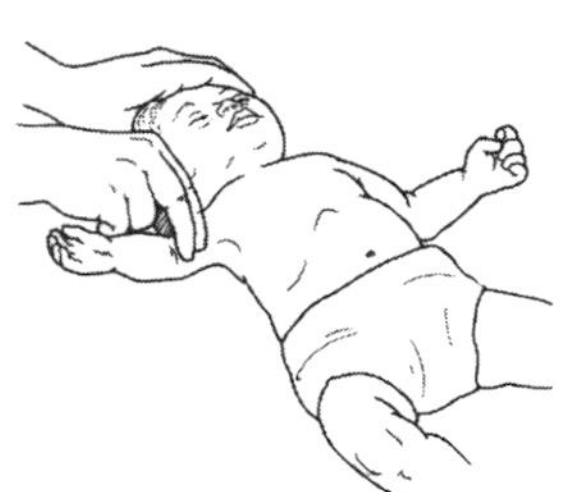

❹ Briefly check for a pulse.

If there is a pulse:

❺ Give one slow breath every 3 seconds for about 1 minute (20 breaths).
❻ Recheck the pulse about every minute.

Continue rescue breathing as long as a pulse is present but the infant is not breathing.

If there's no pulse:

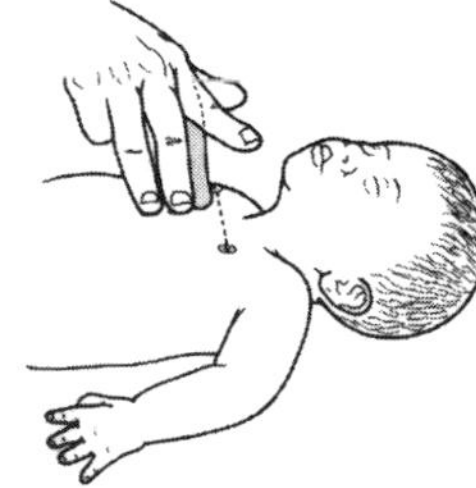

❼ Position the infant face up on a firm surface.
❽ Place your index, third, and fourth fingers below an imaginary line between the nipples and in the middle of the breastbone. The position of the third and fourth fingers is the area for chest compression.
❾ Compress the child's chest five times.
❿ Give one slow breath.
● Repeat cycles of five compressions to one breath until you feel a pulse or help arrives.

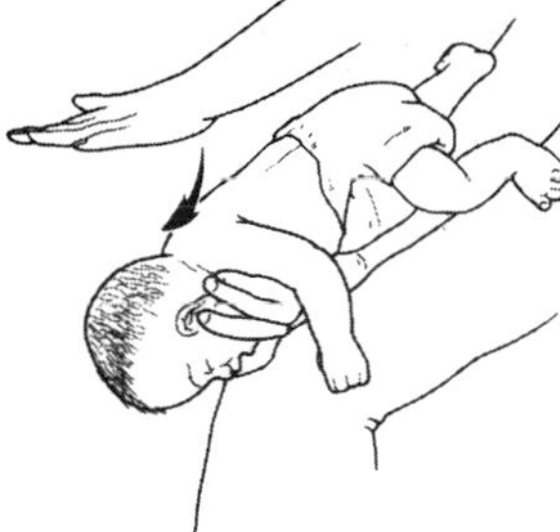

If air won't go in, the airway may be blocked.

❶ Re-tilt the infant's head back. Try to give two breaths again.

❷ If air still won't go in, position your baby face down on your arm, with your hand supporting his head.

❸ Give up to five back blows with the heel of your hand between the infant's shoulder blades, as before.

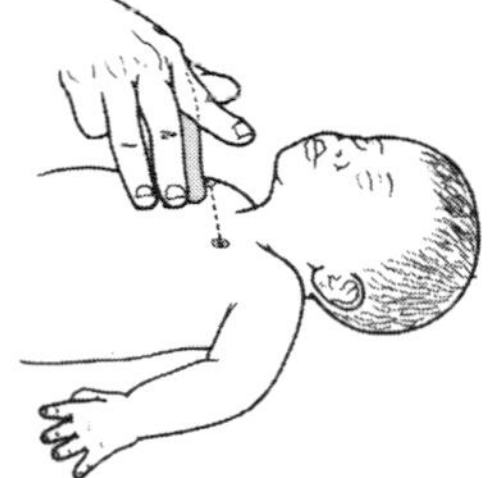

If there is still no pulse:

❹ Reposition the infant face up on a firm surface and place your index, third, and fourth fingers below an imaginary line between the nipples and in the middle of the breastbone. The position of the third and fourth fingers is the area for chest compression.

❺ Give up to five chest thrusts near the centre of the breastbone.

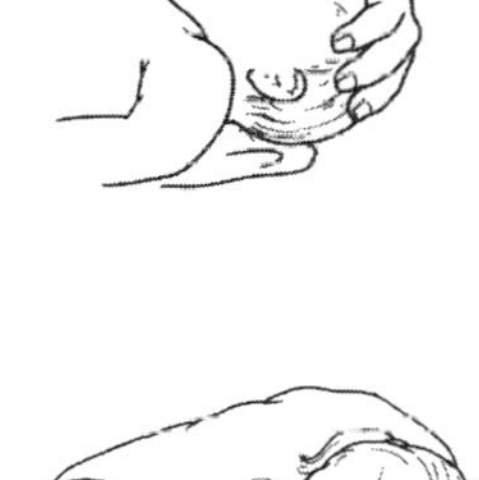

❻ Lift the child's jaw and tongue. If you can see the foreign object, sweep it out with your finger.

Repeat steps 1 through 6 until breaths go in or the infant starts to breathe on his own.

To be used when the child is unresponsive and breathing or heartbeat stops.

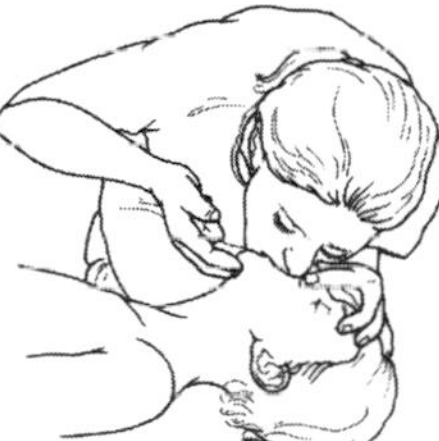

❶ Call for help.

❷ Tilt the child's head back. Seal your lips tightly around his mouth; pinch his nose shut.

❸ Give two slow breaths until his chest gently rises.

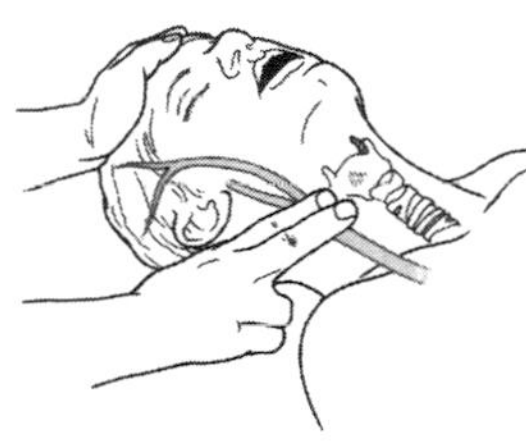

If air goes in:

❹ Apply gentle pressure to feel for a pulse.

If there is a pulse:

❺ Give one slow breath every 3 seconds for about 1 minute (20 breaths).

❻ Recheck the pulse about every minute.

Continue rescue breathing as long as a pulse is present but the child is not breathing.

If there's no pulse:

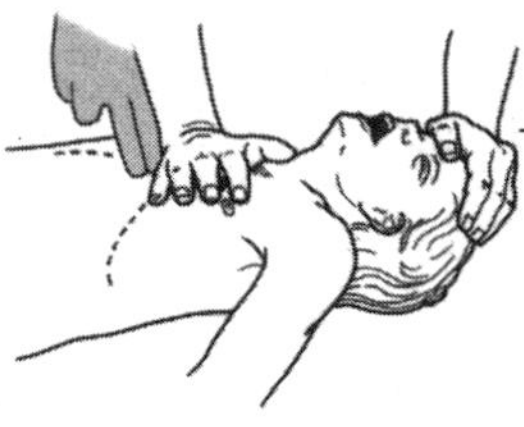

❹ Find the hand position near the centre of the breastbone.
❺ Position your shoulders over your hands.
❻ Compress the child's chest five times about 1–3cm (½–1 in).
❼ Give one slow breath.
❽ Repeat cycles of five compressions to one breath until you feel a pulse or help arrives.

If air won't go in and there's still no pulse there may be an airway obstruction. To clear the airway:

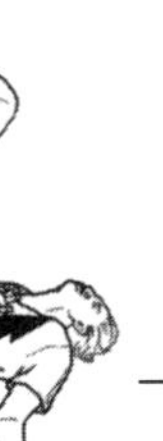

❸ Re-tilt the child's head back. Try to give two breaths again.
❹ Kneel over the child and place the heel of one hand on the child's abdomen above the middle of the navel and below the ribcage.
❺ Give up to five quick, firm, upward abdominal thrusts.

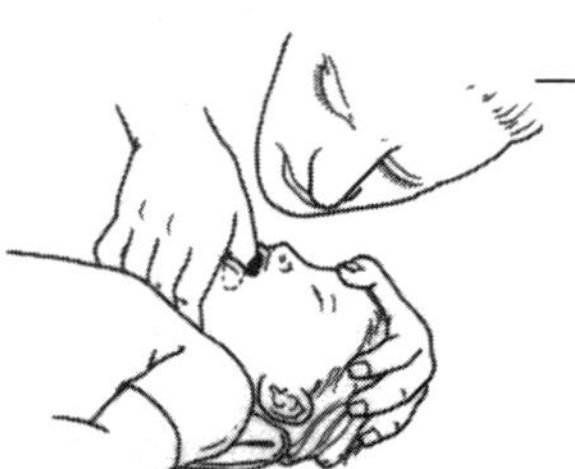

❻ Lift the child's jaw and tongue. If you can see the foreign object, sweep it out with your finger.

Continue CPR until help arrives or the child starts to breathe on his own.

DROWNING

A child can drown in only a few centimetres of water, whether on a lakeshore or in a bathtub, toilet, or bucket of water. A child drowns either because he ventures into water that is too deep, or because he is trapped in a position where his face is held in water. A child drowns when he inhales water and suffocates.

If a child is rescued before death occurs, the event is referred to as near-drowning. Recovery from near-drowning depends on how long the child was deprived of oxygen. A child who was submerged only momentarily is likely to recover completely. Every child who has escaped drowning must be examined by a doctor, even if he seems to have suffered no ill effects. A child who stopped breathing, inhaled water, or lost consciousness should remain under medical observation for 24 hours to make sure his respiratory and nervous systems are undamaged.

Prevention

See pp. 226, 228, 231–232.

What You Can Do

- As soon as the child is out of the water, check to see if he is breathing. If not, begin CPR at once (see pp. 204–206).
- Ask anyone nearby to call for emergency help, but don't waste time looking for someone.
- Give CPR until emergency help arrives or the child is breathing on his own and has a pulse of 80 to 100 beats per minute.
- Once emergency help arrives, the team members will give oxygen and continue CPR, if necessary.

POISONING

Iron pills and over-the-counter medications, including chewable vitamins, are the most common causes of childhood poisonings. Alcohol, household cleaners, and pesticides are other common sources of preventable poisonings.

Prevention

Store all medications and hazardous materials in locked cupboards out of children's reach. Keep all medications in containers with child-resistant caps, and discard unused prescription medications as soon as the illness they were needed for is over. (For more detailed guidelines, see p. 222.)

What You Can Do

- Suspect poisoning if you find a child with an open or empty container of medicine, vitamin pills, a liquor bottle, or other potentially hazardous substance. *Look for:*
  - Stains on clothing.

- Stains or burns around the mouth.
- Drooling and an unusual breath odour.
- Nausea, vomiting.
- Abdominal pain without fever.
- Breathing difficulties.
- Sleepiness, irritability, jitteriness.
- Convulsions or unconsciousness.

Everyday items that are hazardous to young children

- ✓ Detergents.
- ✓ Drain cleaners.
- ✓ Furniture and metal polishes.
- ✓ Petrol, kerosene, lamp oil.
- ✓ Poisonous house plants (e.g., African violet).
- ✓ Insect sprays and pest repellents.
- ✓ Mouthwash.
- ✓ Nail varnish remover.
- ✓ Paints, thinners.
- ✓ Rubbing alcohol.
- ✓ Spot removers.
- ✓ Tobacco products.
- ✓ Vitamins, including antenatal vitamin pills.

- Take the toxic material from the child; clear it out of his mouth; keep it to show the paramedic, casualty officer, or your GP.
- If your child has stopped breathing, start CPR immediately and have someone else call an ambulance.
- If you think your child has ingested poison, call your doctor's surgery immediately and follow their advice. If necessary, call 999, or have someone drive you to the nearest hospital emergency department. **Take the poison and its container with you.**
- If your child is exposed to toxic fumes, take her into fresh air immediately (outside or next to a wide-open window). Call 999 if she has difficulty breathing, is vomiting, or has decreased responsiveness.
- If the child has splashed a toxic substance in his eye, hold the eyelid open and pour a steady stream of lukewarm water into the eye for at least 15 minutes. Wrap a struggling child firmly in a towel or sheet and clamp him with one arm, or have another adult hold him. Call your doctor.
- If there is continuing eye pain or severe injury, call 999. Any eye injury should be seen by a doctor.
- If your child spills a hazardous chemical on her body, put on rubber gloves and brush off dry material. Remove contaminated clothing. Wash her skin with large quantities of soap and water. Call your doctor for instructions. Do not apply ointments or salves.

Professional Help

- Depending on the toxic substance and the child's condition, the child may be hospitalized for treatment and observation. Most children don't need to be hospitalized.

FREQUENTLY USED FIRST AID MEASURES

There are dozens of situations that may demand first aid; those covered in the following alphabetical section are among the more common. Because there is no time to consult a book when an emergency arises, it's a good idea to review the steps described here frequently so you'll know what to do if the need arises.

ANIMAL BITES

Most animal bites are inflicted by animals familiar to the child, including household pets. Even if damage is minor, infection is a risk whenever the skin is broken. Some animal bites may cause serious damage – especially those on the face – as well as emotional trauma.

Prevention

See Preventing injury from animals, p. 232.

What You Can Do

- If the wound is bleeding, press firmly for 5 minutes or until bleeding stops.
- Wash the wound with soap and rinse with plenty of water. Call your doctor.
- Always call your doctor if a bite breaks the skin; he or she will determine whether your child is adequately protected against tetanus and rabies or needs to be seen.
- Capture or confine the animal only if you can do so without danger to yourself or others. Do not destroy the animal; call the police to handle it.
- In the days following the bite, call your doctor if you see any of the following signs of bacterial infection:
  - Pus or drainage from the wound.
  - Increasing swelling or tenderness around the wound after the first 8 to 12 hours.
  - Red streaks or an increasing red zone spreading out from the bite.
  - Swollen glands above the bite.
- If your child has suffered a snake bite, call 999 or take the child immediately to a hospital emergency department. If the snake has been killed, carefully place it in a container and bring it with you. Do not apply ice or a tourniquet to the bitten area. Splint it and keep it immobile in a position level with the heart.

Professional Help

- A large wound may need stitches to promote healing and reduce scarring.
- The doctor may prescribe an antibiotic to prevent bacterial infection in an open wound.

BURNS

Hot liquids, including drinks and tapwater, are the most common causes of burns in children. Children may also incur serious burns from the sun, as well as from everyday household items, such as electrical appliances including clothes irons or hair-styling combs, cleaning products, and barbecues. Burns are painful; they also carry a high risk of infection. Severe burns may be life-threatening, and can cause permanent injury and scarring.

Prevention

See Fire injury prevention, p. 235.

What You Can Do

- Soak the burn in cold water straightaway. Do not wait to remove clothing. If possible, run cold water from the tap as long as it takes to cool the area and relieve pain, or cover the burned part with a cold, wet towel for at least 15 minutes. Do not use ice; this can cause skin damage and, in more extensive burns, a sudden drop in body temperature may even cause shock.
- While soaking the burn with cool water, remove clothing from the burned area unless it is stuck to the skin. If so, cut away as much as you can of the free clothing.
- If you have a sterile pad, lightly cover the burn. If no sterile pad is available, leave small wounds open, or for large burns use a clean sheet. Do not break blisters.
- If the burn is oozing, cover (as above) and call your doctor immediately.
- Never put butter, ointments, or powder on a burn; these home remedies may make the injury worse and increase the risk of infection.
- When caring for a burn at home, call your doctor if you see signs of infection, such as increased redness or swelling, or a discharge or unpleasant odour.

Burns are classified according to the depth and extent of tissue damage they cause

✓ Burns limited to the outer layer of the skin (epidermis) cause redness, tenderness, and swelling, but no blistering. They are not usually serious. Mild sunburn is a good example.

✓ Partial-thickness burns involve both the epidermis and the skin layer immediately underneath, called the dermis. These deeper burns cause redness, tenderness, significant pain and blistering, and are more serious, especially if they cover a large area or become infected.

✓ Full-thickness burns penetrate all skin layers and may destroy underlying tissue as well. The injured skin may be white or charred; the third-degree burn victim often does not suffer severe pain immediately after the injury because the burn destroys the nerve endings.

Professional Help

Always call your doctor if your child has partial- or full-thickness burns. Call 999 if burns are large and your child is becoming ill from the burn.

Consult your doctor if the burn goes deeper than the superficial skin, or if pain lasts longer than a few hours. Call the doctor immediately if your child has suffered an electrical burn, a large burn, or burns to the face, hands, feet, or genitals.

- If your doctor thinks you can manage the burn at home, he or she will tell you how to take care of it with medications and dressings.

Most doctors will admit a child to hospital:

- When the child has full-thickness burns.
- When burns cover 10 percent or more of the child's body.
- When the face, hands, feet, or genitals are injured.
- If the child is very young and too difficult to treat initially at home.

COLD INJURY

Cold injury may be a general lowering of the body temperature, known as hypothermia or frostbite, which occurs when exposure to extremely low temperatures causes ice crystals to form in skin and tissue fluids. Toes, fingers, nose, and ears are the parts most often frostbitten.

Prevention

- Make sure children are properly clothed for winter sports.
- Layering several light-weight pieces of clothing provides more protection against cold. Attach gloves with clips; never use strings. Use hats and cover ears.
- Limit time outside during periods of low temperature and high wind chill.
- Provide warming drinks at the end of outdoor play in winter.
- Take your child into a warm environment when he complains of feeling cold.

What You Can Do

- While still outside, cover frozen parts with clothing or any available cloth. Tuck frostbitten fingers, or the feet of a very young child, in your armpits while carrying the child to shelter.
- Do not rub the frostbitten part with snow or anything else.
- Once inside, remove wet clothes and wrap the child in warm blankets or any available cloth.
- Place the child's frostbitten part in warm – not hot – water, between 38° and 40°C (100–104°F; this temperature feels warm to the touch). Give warming drinks, such as hot milk, soup, or cocoa.

- If water is not available, wrap the frostbitten part in a blanket or other warm material. Do not use a heat lamp, hot water bottle, or heating pad. Ask your child to exercise the fingers or toes as soon as they feel warmer.
- Separate frostbitten toes or fingers with sterile gauze dressings.
- Do not place your child near a hot stove or radiator; the frostbitten part may be burned before feeling returns.
- Don't break blisters.
- Stop the warming process when the child's skin becomes pink and feeling begins to return.
- Seek medical attention straightaway.

Professional Help

- A child who has suffered hypothermia or frostbite should be examined by a doctor.

CONVULSIONS

High fever may trigger convulsions or seizures in young children. Most are brief, lasting only a minute or less, but they can be frightening. Febrile seizures rarely occur after 7 years of age. Most children who have one episode never have another. Febrile seizures usually stop on their own and do not require emergency medical attention. A small percentage of these children develop epilepsy, or non-fever-related seizures.

Prevention

- Give children's paracetamol in the recommended dose to reduce fever.
- Sponge a very feverish child (temperature above 38.5°C [102°F]) with cool – not cold – water to lower his temperature.
- Seizures due to a chronic condition such as epilepsy can usually be well controlled by anticonvulsant medication, which must be taken regularly and never stopped abruptly.
- If a child has epilepsy, provide information to help his friends, teachers, and caregivers understand his condition and how to cope with seizures, should they occur.

What You Can Do

- Place a convulsing child on his back with his head turned to the side, or on his side, on a carpeted floor or bed, and stay with him. Do not place anything in his mouth.
- If the convulsion continues for more than 3 to 5 minutes, the child has several seizures one after another, or the child vomits, call 999. Do not leave the child alone. If the child stops breathing and looks blue, begin rescue breathing and call 999.

- When the seizure stops, call your doctor immediately and get further instructions. If your child has a fever, the doctor may advise giving paracetamol and sponging with cool water to reduce the temperature.

Professional Help

- If your child has fever, your doctor may wish to examine him to find and treat the source of fever.
- If your child has previously had seizures and is on anticonvulsant medication, your doctor may adjust the dosage.

CUTS AND SCRAPES

Most minor cuts and scrapes can be treated by gentle, thorough cleaning with water and soap, and reassurance. Young children often invest adhesive bandages with healing powers; parents may find that a bandage works wonders, even on unbroken skin.

Keep your children's immunizations, including tetanus, up to date. If your child isn't fully immunized or it's been longer than 5 years since her last tetanus shot, ask your doctor if a booster is needed.

Cuts, or lacerations, penetrate the tissues beneath the skin. Bleeding may be heavy, and a cut may damage nerves and tendons.

Prevention

Active, curious children suffer minor cuts and scrapes in the course of their explorations. Parents can't expect to prevent every mishap, but they should take sensible measures to reduce the risk of serious injury.

- Keep dangerous items (such as sharp knives) and breakable items (such as glassware) out of young children's reach.
- Keep toys and outdoor play equipment, such as swings and climbing frames, in good repair. If toys can't be repaired, discard or dismantle them. Don't let unsupervised children play on hazardous equipment, such as swings or climbing bars.
- Make sure children wear protective pads and helmets for sports that involve hazards, such as skateboarding, bicycle riding, and in-line skating.
- Show children how to use knives and scissors properly, to pass them safely to others, and to respect them as tools, not toys.
- Warn children never to run while carrying breakable objects or sharp instruments such as pens, pencils, and scissors.

What You Can Do

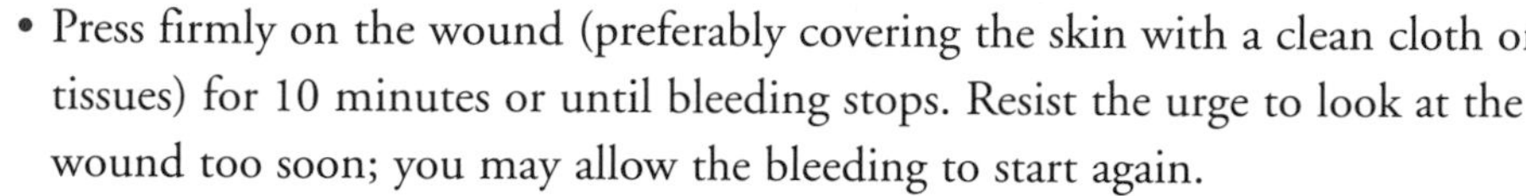

- Press firmly on the wound (preferably covering the skin with a clean cloth or tissues) for 10 minutes or until bleeding stops. Resist the urge to look at the wound too soon; you may allow the bleeding to start again.

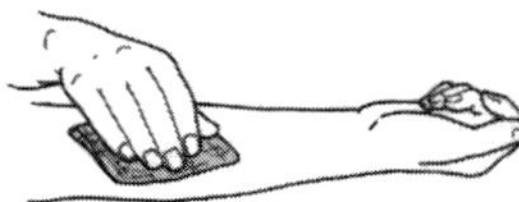

- If the wound bleeds again after 10 minutes of continuous pressure, call your doctor and then reapply firm pressure continuously. Do not apply a tourniquet unless you have had special training; it can cause severe damage.
- When bleeding stops, gently wash the wound with plain water and examine it to make sure it's clean.

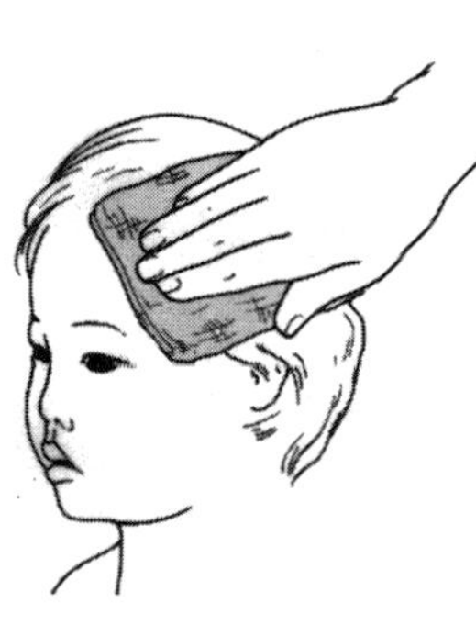

- Treat short, minor cuts at home, provided the edges come together by themselves.
- Cover the cut with a sterile dressing.
- Applying an antiseptic cream before putting on the bandage will help prevent infection.
- It's safe to wash the wound at least daily after the first 24 hours. Dry gently but thoroughly.
- As the wound heals, look for increased redness and swelling or pus drainage, which may indicate infection. If these symptoms are present, call your doctor.

Professional Help

- Call your doctor for advice about any cut that goes right through all layers of the skin or is more than 1cm (½in) long, even if bleeding is not severe. Deep cuts may require treatment to repair damaged nerves and tendons.
- Seek your GP's attention for cuts to the face, chest, and neck, or long lacerations. For best results, wounds should be stitched within 8 hours.
- Ask your doctor to examine a laceration if you believe foreign matter, such as glass or dirt, may be trapped in it or if the child is too distressed to let you examine the wound thoroughly. Your doctor can administer a local anaesthetic to make examination, cleaning, and treatment easier.

In scrapes, or abrasions, the outer layer of skin is ground away, resulting in a raw, red appearance, although the amount of bleeding is very small and there is little risk of scarring. Properly cared for, abrasions quickly form a protective scab and heal without further treatment. They must be kept clean to prevent infection.

What You Can Do

- Rinse the wound under running water to flush away contaminants and debris, then wash thoroughly with soap and water. Antiseptic creams have some protective value.
- Lightly cover a large oozing wound with a sterile dressing after applying an antiseptic cream to prevent the dressing from sticking to the wound surface.
- Make sure that dressings and surgical tapes around fingers and toes are loose enough to allow free circulation.
- Change the dressing routinely each day or whenever it becomes wet or dirty. If the dressing sticks, soak it off in warm water. Dressings are not usually needed after 2 or 3 days. Wash the wound at least daily.
- Leave the wound alone once a scab forms; don't pull off the scab.
- Be alert for pus, increased redness and tenderness, or fever, which may indicate that infection is present.

- Call your doctor if you need help cleaning a wound or if the injury occurred against a highly contaminated surface.
- If infection develops, your doctor should examine the child.

DENTAL EMERGENCY

Teeth that are knocked out can often be re-implanted if you act promptly.

Prevention

- Provide properly fitted mouth guards for children involved in contact sports such as hockey or rugby.

What You Can Do

- If a permanent tooth has been knocked out, place it in a container of milk.
- Fold a clean piece of gauze or a tissue into a pad and place it over the wound. Have your child hold his jaws together gently but firmly to keep the pad in place and stop the bleeding.
- Place a cold cloth or ice pack on the lip to relieve swelling and pain.
- Give paracetamol if your child is in pain.

- Take your child and the tooth to the dentist or the hospital emergency department straightaway.

Professional Help

- A child who has sustained a heavy blow to the face or jaw may need to be x-rayed to determine the extent of damage.
- The dentist will try to re-implant the tooth if possible.

ELECTRICAL INJURY

Electric shock can cause injury ranging in severity from a pinprick sensation to death. Young children often suffer severe shocks when they chew on appliance cords or poke metal objects into unprotected outlets or appliances.

Prevention

See Child-proofing Your Home, p. 223.

What You Can Do

- Disconnect the power supply before you touch an injured child who is still receiving current: pull the plug or turn off the mains switch.
- Never touch a live wire with your bare hands. If you have to lift a live wire from a child, use a dry stick, a rolled-up newspaper, thick clothing, or another sturdy, dry, nonmetallic object that won't conduct electricity.
- Move the child as little as possible, because severe electric shock may have caused injury.
- If you can't remove the source of the current, try to move the child, but don't use your bare hands. Insulate yourself with rubber or with any of the nonconductive items suggested for lifting a live wire, so that the current doesn't pass from the child's body to yours.
- Once the current is off, quickly check your child's breathing, pulse, skin colour, and alertness. If your child is not breathing or there is no heartbeat, begin CPR immediately (see pp. 204–206) while someone else goes for help.
- Once your child is safely removed from the current, check him for burns and call 999 or your doctor.

Professional Help

- A child who has received an electric shock should be seen by a doctor, since shock may cause internal damage that cannot be detected without a medical examination.
- Your doctor will clean and dress surface burns and order tests for signs of damage to internal organs.
- Mouth burns (such as from biting an electric cord) are often much deeper

than they appear. Your child may require surgery after the initial healing. Parents must be alert to the possibility of bleeding from mouth burns hours or even days after the injury. If bleeding occurs, apply a clean pad and call your doctor immediately.

FRACTURES

A fracture is a broken bone, and broken bones are a common type of childhood injury. Most are caused by falls and sports injuries; the most serious breaks are usually the result of automobile crashes. Because children's bones are more flexible than those of adults, they absorb shock better and heal more quickly.

Prevention

- Make sure your child has properly fitted footwear, headgear, and protective pads when needed for sports.
- On all car rides, pre-schoolers must be properly strapped into approved car seats or booster seats in the rear. All children should ride in the rear seat, properly buckled into safety belts or child passenger seats.

What You Can Do

- If your child has a neck or back injury, call 999 immediately. Don't move her yourself, as it may cause serious harm to the spinal cord.
- Contact your doctor at once if you suspect a broken bone. It can be difficult to recognize a fracture, especially in a very young child. Look for swelling, pain, unwillingness to let anyone touch it (guarding), limping, and loss of movement. A bone may be broken even though the child can move the limb.
- If your child has a broken leg, call an ambulance and wait for the emergency team to transport her; don't try to move her yourself.
- If the hand or foot below the injury is blue or cold, call 999 immediately.
- Protect the limb from unnecessary movement by using a scarf for a sling or a rolled-up newspaper or magazine for a splint, until your doctor or emergency physician can see the child. If it is a sports injury, a pair of shin guards wrapped around the suspected injury works well.
- Don't give drinks or pain relievers without asking your doctor; if your child requires immediate surgery or other treatment, fluids may increase the risk of anaesthesia and pain relievers may interact with other necessary medications.
- For an older child, place a wrapped ice pack or cold towel over the injury to relieve pain. Do not use ice on infants and toddlers; extreme cold can lead to further injury.

- If the wound is open, press firmly to stop bleeding; use a tourniquet only if you have been trained to do so. Cover the wound with a sterile dressing. Don't try to push broken bones back into the wound; call 999 at once.
- In the days after a fracture has been treated, watch your child for signs of fever, which may signal infection.
- While the limb is in a cast, contact the hospital where the cast was applied if your child complains of pain when moving fingers or toes, feels numb, or has pale or blue fingers or toes; this may indicate severe swelling underneath the cast, which could permanently damage nerves, muscles, and blood vessels.
- Contact the hospital if the cast breaks or loosens.

Professional Help

- Your doctor will order x-rays to assess the injury and may recommend an orthopaedic consultation.
- A plaster or fibreglass cast, or a splint, will be applied to immobilize the bone; surgery may be needed for extremely complicated fractures.
- If the bone has broken through the skin surface, your child may need to take an antibiotic.

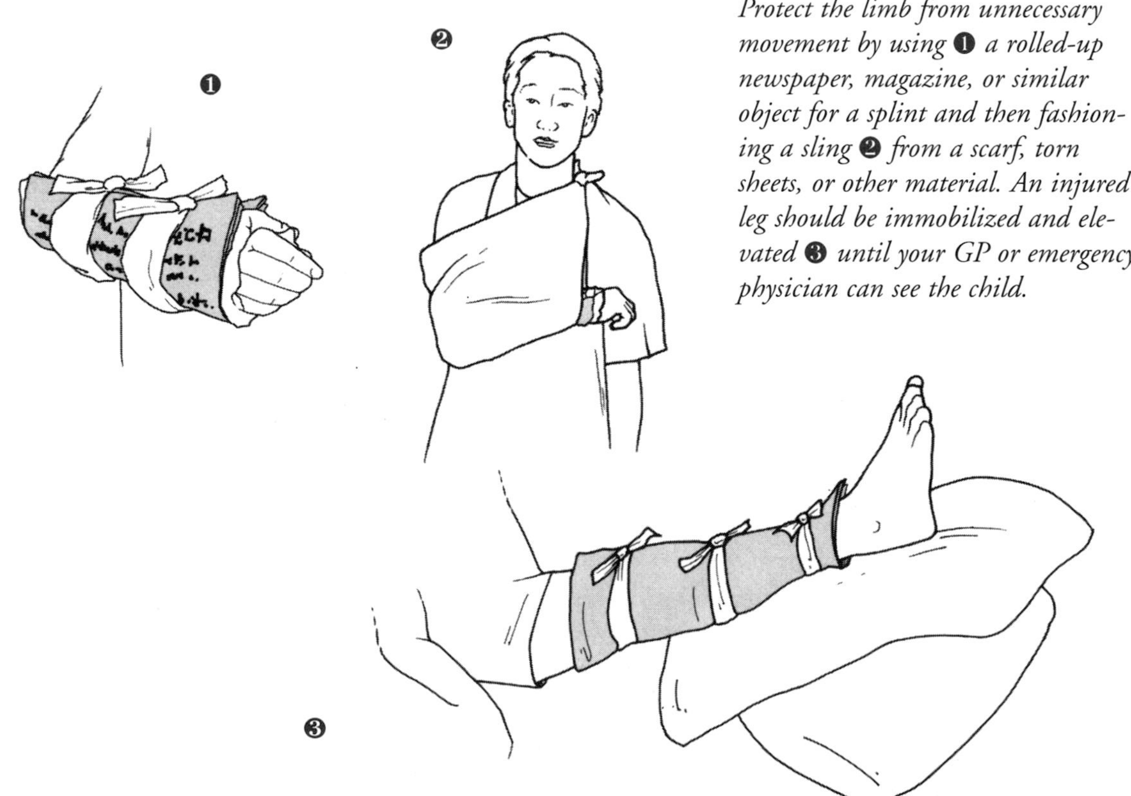

Protect the limb from unnecessary movement by using ❶ a rolled-up newspaper, magazine, or similar object for a splint and then fashioning a sling ❷ from a scarf, torn sheets, or other material. An injured leg should be immobilized and elevated ❸ until your GP or emergency physician can see the child.

HEAD INJURIES

Babies recover quickly from the bumps and collisions they experience while becoming independently mobile. Although after-effects of minor bumps are very rare, parents and care-givers must be able to recognize signs that a child's head injury warrants a doctor's attention.

Prevention

- Don't use baby walkers; they're a common cause of childhood face and head injuries.
- Pad fireplace hearths and keep your home free of hazards that could trip an inexperienced walker.
- Install window guards, and place gates at the top and bottom of all steps until your toddler has mastered them under your supervision.
- Stabilize unsteady items of furniture or store them until your child is older.
- Never allow youngsters to ride bicycles unless wearing helmets that meet safety standards. Set an example by wearing a bike helmet yourself while riding a bicycle.
- Always keep one hand on your baby when he or she is lying on a changing table. Never leave your child unattended on a changing table.
- Don't place bouncing chairs on raised surfaces.
- On all car rides, pre-schoolers must be properly strapped into approved car seats or booster seats in the rear. All children should ride in the rear seat, properly buckled into safety belts or child passenger seats.

What You Can Do

- Clean and dress superficial wounds. Apply a cold compress to reduce swelling. Keep an eye on your child for 24 to 48 hours to make sure there are no signs of more serious injury. Give children's paracetamol if your child complains of headache.

  Call your doctor or 999 immediately if your child:
  - Is unusually lethargic or irritable.
  - Has a headache that persists even after taking paracetamol.
  - Vomits twice.
  - Has muscle weakness, clumsiness, slurred speech, or problems with vision.
  - Becomes unconscious, has a seizure, or breathes irregularly.
  - Has bleeding or discharge from the nose or ear.

Professional Help

- If you think your child may have a neck or back injury, or serious head injury, don't move him. Call 999 for transport to the hospital.

CHAPTER 5 GUIDE TO SAFETY AND PREVENTION

INTRODUCTION

Preventable injuries are the leading cause of death in children over 1 year old. Each year, one out of every four children suffers an injury that requires medical attention. Even the most vigilant parents have moments, such as when the telephone rings or they are in the middle of preparing dinner, when their attention is divided. The likelihood of injury also increases during times of family stress – for instance, an illness, a death in the family, a pregnancy or birth, or change in environment – and during the summer break and other school holidays, when children spend more time around the house.

Of course, injuries vary in severity. Minor scrapes and spills go along with a child's exploration and learning process. Your child must touch, taste, feel, smell, and investigate in order to learn. Hazards that adults avoid by second nature, such as a hot stove or a sharp knife, are especially threatening to children, who are just learning to navigate through our perilous world and don't understand such dangers. Remember, to a small child, everything is new and equally interesting. Sharp is no different from dull, hot from cold, heavy from light, and dangerous from safe. 'Child-proofing' reduces the chances of an injury to your child by making an environment as safe as possible.

GENERAL GUIDELINES

Ideally, child-proofing should begin even before the birth of your baby. With a conscious effort, you'll soon be in the habit of searching the floor for small objects, putting breakables away, and latching doors shut. Certainly, by the time your child can sit on his own and use his hands for exploration (about 6 months), your home should be completely child-proofed. Reassess your safety measures as your child grows. How far and fast he can move, where he can reach, and what attracts his attention change constantly.

- *The first few months.* Be sure all toys are 'mouth-safe'. As soon as a baby masters putting things in her mouth, this will be her favourite way to learn about objects for months or even years. Toys should be too big to fit entirely in her mouth, nontoxic, durable, lacking small or pointed parts, and without ribbons or strings. Never hang a dummy or anything else around a baby's neck. A string or ribbon could catch on something and strangle the child.

- *6 to 18 months.* Your baby's improved coordination, ability to sit on his own, and rapidly increasing mobility require increased and constant watchfulness. Frequent room-by-room checking for possible hazards is extremely important at this age. Your baby's curiosity has extended beyond himself to the world around him and his ability to explore that world increases daily. When your baby grabs for an object you don't want him to play with, such as your handbag, offer a permitted object as a distraction.
- *Toddlers.* A toddler's mobility and curiosity, and the fact that a child at this stage will eat or drink even the worst-tasting substances, make poison prevention a critical priority. (See Poison prevention, below.) Use a firm 'no' for really dangerous situations, such as a hot radiator, and explain why – 'NO! The radiator is HOT!' At the same time, physically remove the dangerous object or move the child to reinforce the idea that 'no' means 'Stop right now.'

Poison prevention

Every year, large numbers of children under the age of 6 suffer accidental poisoning. Parents' personal care products, cosmetics, and household cleaning products are common causes of childhood poisoning, with over-the-counter medications at the top of the list. Although they are generally safe for adults, over-the-counter products such as vitamin and mineral supplements (especially those with iron), aspirin, paracetamol, and laxatives cause serious, even life-threatening, reactions in children because of children's smaller size and their tendency to ingest the entire contents of the bottle.

- Keep all medications and vitamins safely locked up high out of sight and reach. Put them away immediately after use. Don't leave medicines in handbags or pockets – children have an uncanny way of finding them, even in unusual places.
- Buy products with child-resistant caps and always use the caps.
- Never call medicine or vitamins 'sweets' when giving them to your child.
- Never leave cleaning fluids or the rags you clean with lying out.
- Many cosmetics and personal-care products are potentially toxic; put them away up high in child-proof cupboards.
- Certain house plants, such as philodendrons and dieffenbachias, are toxic. Check with a book on poisons to find out what plants are safe around small children. Teach children never to sample wild berries and other plant parts unless an adult says they are safe.
- Alcohol should be kept up high in locked cupboards. Glasses should always be emptied and rinsed immediately after a party where alcohol is served.
- You should never smoke near a child, whether in a house, car, or restaurant, because second-hand smoke is harmful to children. If you do smoke, make sure cigarettes and other tobacco products are out of a child's reach. Almost any amount of tobacco product may poison a child who eats it. This includes cigarettes, cigars, smoked butts, pipe and chewing tobacco, snuff, and nicotine gum, patches, and sprays.
- Never store cleaning products and other toxic substances in old food containers or other harmless-looking containers.
- Keep all insecticides, petroleum products, and fertilizers up high in a locked cupboard in the garage.

- *The pre-school years.* Make safety rules, repeat them often, and apply them consistently. Explain why these rules must be obeyed.

CHILD-PROOFING YOUR HOME

Try to see the world through your child's eyes: get down on your hands and knees and search for small objects, dangling cords, electrical sockets, breakable objects, and dangerous corners. It is important to remember that these safety precautions are not intended to be restrictive to your child. On the contrary, they can help your child explore her world freely and safely.

- Keep a list of emergency phone numbers next to every phone. Your memory may fail you in a crisis, so put the emergency 999 phone number and your address and phone number at the top of the list. Include the numbers of your doctor, hospital emergency department, next-door-neighbour, and a responsible relative or friend. Be sure to list any numbers your baby-sitter might need, such as work or bleep numbers.
- Install smoke detectors on every floor and check them every month. Keep a fire extinguisher in the kitchen and one by each stairwell. Practise your fire escape plan every few months. Have your children practise 'stop, drop, and roll' in case clothing catches fire.
- To prevent children from falling, install window guards that can be removed in case of a fire. Screens will not support a toddler's weight. Don't put furniture that can be climbed on underneath or near windows.
- Tie cords of venetian blinds or curtains up out of reach or cut them off.
- Get down on all fours and search the floor for tiny objects, such as safety pins,

Preventing choking

- Cut or break food into child's bite-sized pieces, and encourage children to chew food thoroughly. Chop foods with a resistant texture – such as sausages, bacon, or boiled potatoes – into smaller than bite-sized pieces.
- Don't give young children hard, smooth foods such as nuts which must be chewed with a grinding motion; children can't chew this way until about age 4. Keep peanuts away from children under 7 years.
- Don't let children eat while playing or running; teach them to chew and swallow before talking or laughing.
- Avoid foods that can slide into the windpipe, such as grapes, raw carrots or celery sticks, and boiled sweets.
- Choose toys and playthings carefully. Toys sold for children under 3 should not have parts smaller than 3cm (1¼in) in diameter and 6cm (2¼in) long. If there are older children in the household, make sure that toys with small parts, such as construction kits, are well out of a toddler's reach.
- Keep rubber and latex balloons away from young children; they may inhale them when they try to blow them up or choke on a scrap of broken balloon. Teach youngsters never to put balloons in their mouths.
- Keep coins out of young children's reach.

buttons, needles, and paper clips. Do this before setting your child down to play. Vacuum rugs frequently. If you have hobbies that involve small pieces, such as sewing or model building, limit your work to a specific area and clean up thoroughly.

- Search the undersides of tables and chairs for nails that stick out and rough surfaces that can cause splinters.
- Place gates at the top and bottom of staircases. Do not use concertina-style gates; they can trap a child's head and limbs. You may want to leave a few steps in front of the bottom gate so your child can practise climbing.
- Put safety guards in all unused electrical outlets.
- Do not let cords from appliances or lamps dangle within your child's reach.
- Put soft guards on the corners of sharp tables.
- Store glass and marble tables in the attic or basement until your child is older.
- Remove breakable knickknacks from low tables.
- If the floor is slippery, do not put socks on your child once he can pull himself to his feet.
- Make sure that all rugs are taped down and carpets securely tacked.
- Test the stability of all furniture. Be sure it will not tip over when a child who is learning to walk leans on it.
- Latch all doors either open or closed. Swinging doors are especially dangerous. You may want to remove them until your child is older.
- Put stickers or tape on glass doors at a toddler's eye level.
- Enclose radiators, floor registers, and other heat sources with wooden ornamental covers.
- Lock rooms that are not baby-proof.

As the place where your child will sleep and play, the nursery should be extra-safe. Be sure that all furniture, especially hand-me-down and previously owned furniture, complies with up-to-date safety requirements and is age appropriate. Test construction and stability and regularly inspect furniture for hazards caused by wear and tear. All fabrics in your child's room – pyjamas, sheets, curtains – should be flame retardant.

Extra care should be used when selecting a cot.

- There should be no more than 6cm (2¼ in) between the bars.
- The mattress should fit snugly within the cot and should be very firm. It should not sag when your child is on it. The top cot rail should be at least 65cm (26in)

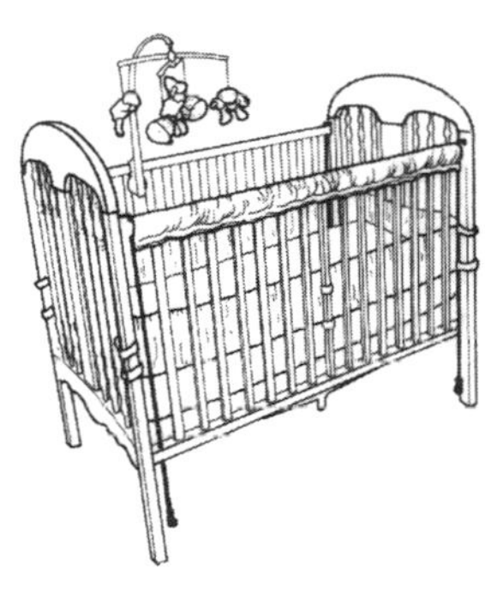

from the top of the mattress; continually lower the mattress as your child grows.

- Always check that the side-rail release mechanism is locked and cannot be accidentally released. Never leave your baby in the cot when the side rail is lowered.
- The headboard and footboard should be solid, with no cutouts. Any corner posts that can catch clothing should be removed.
- Place the cot away from windows where sunlight and draughts can make your child uncomfortable.
- Do not place fluffy duvets, heavy blankets, stuffed animals, or pillows in the cot with an infant. These can cause smothering.
- Mobiles and cot gyms should be removed once your child is able to pull herself to her hands and knees.
- As your baby gets bigger, do not place large toys or stuffed animals in the cot because they can make it easy for him to climb out.
- Cot bumpers, a good idea for infants, should be removed once your child can pull up to a standing position.
- Once your child is about 90cm (3ft) tall, she should start sleeping in a bed.

- Be sure that the changing table has a guard of at least 5cm (2in) on all sides.
- Always strap your child to the changing table and never leave your child unattended on the table or even turn your back – even when she's strapped on.
- Keep supplies – powders, oils, wipes, and nappies – within your reach but well out of the reach of your child.
- Never let your child play with baby product bottles. They may open or break.
- If you use powders, don't shake them near your baby. It's best to put some powder in your hand and smooth it on your baby. If possible, avoid powders that contain talc. Talc has particles that can damage the baby's lungs. Cornflour is a safe alternative.
- Place nappy pails out of reach of toddlers. Be sure lids are not the type that open with a pedal, and that they fit tightly.

Although bunk beds are extremely popular, they are not safe for all ages. Small children can easily roll off the top bunk or may not have the coordination to climb up and down. Wait until your child is a good climber (4 to 5 years of age) to purchase one. Or buy the type that can be separated into single beds and reassembled when your child is older. The following precautions may help prevent injury if your child has a bunk bed.

- Check to make sure the beds are sturdy and well constructed; wobbly, poorly constructed units can collapse, letting the top bunk fall onto the bottom one.

- Place the bed in a corner of the room. Put a guard, which your child cannot roll under, on the side that is not against the wall.
- Put a nightlight by the ladder for middle-of-the-night lavatory trips.
- Be sure there are supports under the top mattress. The bed frame is not enough.
- Don't allow jumping or climbing on bunk beds.

- If the playpen is mesh, the holes should be small enough that your child cannot use it as a toehold and it will not catch buttons. If the playpen has slats, they should be no more than 6cm (2¼ in) apart.
- Never leave your child in the playpen when the drop side is down.

The bathroom is a fascinating place for a child – filled with mirrors, a flushing toilet, taps, and interesting bottles, tubes, and gadgets. It is also an extremely dangerous place. Never leave a toddler unattended in the bathroom: it takes only a few inches of water and 1 or 2 minutes for a child to drown.

- Keep bathroom doors latched when not in use and, if the door locks from the inside, keep a key handy. It's easy for a toddler to lock himself in.
- Never leave an infant or young child unattended in the bath even for a second. Bathe your infant in only 5 or 7cm (2–3in) of water.
- Place skid-free mats inside and next to the bathtub.
- Keep medicines, razors and other sharp objects, and toiletries – including toothpaste and mouthwash – inside a locked medicine cupboard. Shampoo, conditioner, and other liquid products should be placed up high out of reach.
- Cushion the tub tap to prevent injury if a child falls against it.
- Keep toilet lids latched closed; locking devices are widely available. Teach older siblings to do this, too, as soon as they learn to use the toilet.
- Be sure the waste bin has a lid that closes securely. Place razor blades up high and out of reach, and dispose of them and other dangerous objects in a bin where there is no chance of a child getting into it.
- If you use electrical appliances in the bathroom, always unplug them and put them away (preferably in another room) when you are finished.
- Try not to use electric wall heaters. If you have one, tape over the controls.
- Set the immersion heater thermostat to 49°C (120°F) or lower. Young children suffer burns at lower temperatures than do older children and adults because their skin is thinner.

For most families, the kitchen is where all the action takes place and your child will want to be there with you. This room is filled with dangerous objects and appliances, so pay extra attention when baby-proofing and working there.

- When cooking, use back burners whenever possible. Turn pot handles inward so that they do not stick out over the edge of the hob.
- If you can, remove the stove knobs when not in use.
- Remove dangerous items, including cleaning products, plastic bags, and sharp utensils, from low cupboards and drawers, and put them somewhere that's not accessible to your child. Install child safety locks (available from hardware shops and department stores). Leave some 'safe' cupboards unlocked, so your child can bang pots and pans or plasticware around.
- Unplug and put away appliances when they are not in use. Be sure cords are tucked safely out of reach and sight.
- Be aware of your child's whereabouts when carrying hot liquids. Never carry your child in one arm and a hot liquid in the other. A trip could cause a nasty burn.

- Put all electronic equipment, such as the television and stereo, in closed cupboards or on shelves at adult height. Don't let appliance cords hang down.
- Use nonskid backing under throw rugs.

Preventing falls

THE HIGH CHAIR High chairs can be extremely dangerous. Be especially wary of restaurant high chairs. Many do not have a suitable restraint system.

- Never leave your child unattended in the high chair.
- Do not begin using a high chair until your child can sit securely on his own and is eating solids.
- Always strap your child in securely, using both the waist and crutch straps.
- Position the high chair far enough from walls and tables that your toddler cannot reach them and push off.

WALKERS Baby walkers present a serious safety hazard, causing a large number of injuries each year. Children in walkers are more likely to fall downstairs and get into dangerous places that would otherwise be beyond their reach. It is best not to use mobile baby walkers. They provide no benefit to children and are responsible for many injuries.

- Store the iron unplugged with the cord wrapped around it.
- Iron on a well balanced board.
- Never leave the iron unattended when in use. Put it on a firm surface.
- Be sure all electrical appliances are well vented and properly earthed.
- Keep cleaning supplies and tools locked up high out of the reach of children.
- Never leave clothes to soak in pails or basins if you have young children.
- Empty all buckets, fluid containers, and sinks immediately after finishing a task. Don't leave buckets unattended.
- Don't re-use large straight-sided, flat-bottomed chemical containers as cleaning buckets.

Dangerously high levels of lead are sometimes found in children. Without early treatment, accumulated lead can cause damage to the brain and nervous system, resulting in behaviour problems, headaches, hearing problems, learning problems, and impaired growth. This is especially true for babies and even unborn children, whose nervous systems are just developing. Young children tend to accumulate high levels of lead because they may put objects that have lead dust or chips into their mouths, and because their growing bodies absorb more lead. A simple blood test can determine levels; even children who appear healthy may have high levels of lead.

Common sources of lead include the following:

- Paint in homes built before 1978.
- Soil around homes, which may be contaminated with flaking paint as well as with the lead that was formerly added to petrol.
- Drinking water from plumbing with lead pipes or solder.
- Antique or foreign-made furniture, toys, crystal, and pottery.
- Industries, such as lead smelters, that release lead into the air.

If you suspect your home may be contaminated, notify your landlord (if you rent) and contact a safety inspector. Do not remove lead paint yourself; it is often more dangerous to remove than to live with. Have a professional do the work, and relocate your family, especially small children and pregnant women, during the process. A few safety precautions you can take immediately include:

- Cleaning up paint chips.
- Washing children's hands before eating and napping.
- Keeping floors, window sills, toys, dummies, stuffed animals, and all surfaces clean.
- Rinsing sponges, mops, and dusters thoroughly after cleaning.
- Removing shoes before entering to avoid tracking in lead from soil.
- Scientific research shows that a healthy diet can help protect children from lead poisoning.

OUTSIDE THE HOME

Outside the home, your child's environment is harder to control. Young children must be constantly supervised to ensure their safety.

Young skin is especially prone to burning, so always put sun block with a sun protection factor (SPF) of 30 or higher on your baby and insist your children wear sun protection. There are non-irritating sun blocks made especially for children. Dress youngsters in comfortable, lightweight clothing that covers the body, including hats that shade the face and ears. Sunglasses with ultraviolet protection are a good idea.

- Be sure your child is away from an automatic garage door before you open or close it. (There are new garage doors that automatically stop if a child or pet is in the way.)
- Keep all chemicals – paints, thinners, pesticides, fertilizer – and all tools up high in a locked cupboard or locker.
- If you have an old refrigerator or freezer, remove the door so children can't get trapped inside.
- Never allow your child to play in the garage or driveway.

As soon as your child is old enough to play outdoors, the garden should be baby-proofed as carefully as the inside of your home.

- Never let a small child play outside alone. Even a baby napping outdoors needs watching.
- Be on the look-out for things a child might put in her mouth: stones, twigs, animal droppings, or mushrooms.
- Keep children away from outdoor barbecues at all times, but especially when in use. If possible, cover propane tanks or lock them up.
- Check your garden for poisonous plants. Remove mushrooms, stinging nettles, and other hazardous plants as soon as they appear. Teach your child never to eat things he finds in the garden unless you tell him it's safe. Common poisonous plants found in the garden include buttercups, daffodil bulbs, ivy, holly, mistletoe, tomato leaves, potato vines, laburnum, rhododendrons, and rhubarb leaves. Brightly coloured berries are especially attractive to young children, but many are poisonous. Be on the look-out.
- Avoid using pesticides or herbicides especially in areas where children play. If you or your neighbours use these products, make sure children are indoors when they are applied, and do not allow children to play on the lawn for at least 48 hours after treatment.

- Don't mow the lawn when young children are around. Never let a child ride with you on a tractor mower. Do not let children less than 12 years old use lawn mowers.
- Put lawn and garden equipment, such as hosepipes, rakes, and shovels, away when not in use.

- Keep the sandbox covered when it's not in use, especially if there are cats in the neighbourhood.
- Change the sand frequently and try to prevent toddlers from putting it in their mouths.
- Be sure that swing sets, jungle gyms, and seesaws are well anchored. They should be set on either soil or rubber padding, not concrete.
- Check that swings are light but strong. The seat should be made of plastic or rubber. The set should be fenced in to keep small children from running close to the swings.
- Don't allow young children to play on trampolines, trapeze bars, or swinging rings, except in special children's gymnastics classes when an instructor is present. Do not buy a home trampoline.
- Slides should be smooth with no protruding seams. They should not be made of metal, and the sides should be raised 10cm (4in). The platform should be protected with sides or guard rails. Be sure the landing surface is soft.
- Children less than 3 years old should not play on seesaws. Older children should use seesaws with others of approximately the same age and size.

Car crashes are the leading cause of death and injury in children between the ages of 1 and 14 years. Most of these deaths and injuries would be preventable with proper safety precautions. A parent's lap is the most dangerous place for a child or infant to be during a crash. From the moment you take your baby home from hospital, use a car seat that meets safety standards, and make sure that it's right for your child's age and size.

- When installing a car seat, follow the manufacturer's instructions carefully. Once you've finished installing a car seat, rock it back and forth to be sure it is secure. Check that the seat is firmly anchored with the car's seat belt before each trip.
- The safest place for all children is the rear seat, especially if you have airbags. Older children should sit in the rear seat with seat belts fastened.
- Never use rear-facing infant seats facing forward or in the front seat of a car equipped with airbags.

- Always insist your child use the harness when sitting in the seat.
- Once your child is in the harness, adjust the straps so that they fit snugly. Be sure they lie flat and are not twisted.
- Check metal parts and vinyl upholstery in the summertime to make sure they are not too hot for your child.
- Once your child has outgrown a car booster seat (at about 23kg [3 stone 8lb]), be sure your car's seat belts fit your child properly. The shoulder strap should go across the shoulder, not the neck, and the lap belt should fit low across the hips, not the abdomen. If they do not, the child still needs a booster.
- Always wear your seat belt; setting a good example is the best way to make sure your child always wears his. Refuse to start the car until everyone is buckled up. If anyone unbuckles, stop as soon as it is safely possible.
- Never, ever leave your infant or child alone in the car. A moment is all it takes for a child to lock himself in, shift gears, release emergency brakes, burn himself on a cigarette lighter, or become overheated. Also, a child alone in a car is a prime target for abduction.

Because the pram itself is used for only a short period of time, prams that convert to pushchairs are now widely available and a better investment.

- Always properly strap your baby into the pushchair, using both the seat belt and the harness. Rolled blankets and towels can be used as bumpers to keep the baby from slumping.
- Be sure that prams and pushchairs have brakes, preferably on both wheels, with the release mechanism located where your child cannot reach.
- Stop using a pram once your child can sit on her own. Babies can lean out and fall while the pram is moving.
- Do not hang bags on the handles of the pram/pushchair.
- If you buy a double pushchair, be sure the foot rest goes all the way across. Separate rests can trap little feet.

Drowning kills many children each year, and near-drowning episodes cause many more children to be hospitalized, many of whom are permanently brain damaged. Extra safety precautions around water are necessary because drowning happens quickly and silently. Boating and swimming are great ways for a family to have fun together, but everyone should know how to swim and follow basic safety rules.

- Children should wear safety-approved life jackets on boats at all times, even when sleeping.

- Never leave your child alone in a swimming area, and never take your eyes off your child while he is swimming.
- Don't allow running, rough play, or riding bikes near the pool. Do not allow glass or breakable dishware in the pool area.
- Do not take a baby in a pool until he is able to control his head, and never fully submerge a baby in water.
- Don't allow children in a hot tub.
- Don't rely on swimming lessons to save your children from drowning. They may forget what to do in a moment of panic.

- Fence in your home pool completely on all four sides and keep the gate locked at all times, even in the winter.
- Install a phone near a home pool so you won't have to go into the house to answer the phone and can call for help if necessary. Alternatively, use a mobile or cellular phone.
- Keep a safety ring with a rope and a pole beside the pool at all times.
- Empty or securely cover paddling pools when not in use.
- Learn CPR. (See First Aid, p. 204.) Research shows that pool-side CPR can save lives – even if you don't do it perfectly.
- Use only battery-operated radios and other appliances by the pool; electrical appliances are never safe near water.

Preventing injury from animals

When bringing a new baby into a home with a pet, do not leave the infant alone with the animal for the first month or two. Observe your pet carefully – feelings of fear or jealousy should give way as he gets used to this new relationship. If you have a child and are getting a pet, wait until the child is mature enough to treat the pet humanely (about age 5 or 6).

- Teach your children that animals are not toys. Most bites come from teasing or too-rough play.
- Make it a firm rule never to disturb an animal when it is eating or sleeping.
- Don't leave small children alone with a pet. They may not recognize when the animal is getting upset or excited.
- Have all pets immunized against communicable diseases.
- Follow laws about keeping dogs on leashes and keep your pet under control at all times.
- Teach your child not to approach an animal other than his own pet. Even if the owner gives permission, the animal may not want a stranger petting it.
- Instruct your child not to run or make threatening gestures if he is approached by a strange or barking dog.
- Teach children to observe wildlife from a safe distance. If you see a wild animal that is injured or acting sick, strangely, or overly friendly, do not approach it. Instead, call your local RSPCA or vet.

Naturally inquisitive and adventurous, children make great travelling companions. Planning, however, is essential. Make sure you know in advance how you'll get from place to place and where you will stay. Try to plan age-appropriate outings: a backpacking holiday, for example, is probably not the best choice for a 3-year-old. If your child is an infant, try to plan the day's activities around her schedule. It is not wise to go sightseeing at her normal nap time. Adolescents and teenagers may enjoy having a friend along on the trip.

- Baby-proof your accommodations – whether at a friend's or relative's house, hotel room, or camp site – as soon as you arrive.
- Check that your hotel caters for children. Some have reliable baby-sitting services, allow children to stay in parents' room free, or have special baby proof rooms complete with cots and changing tables.
- In a hotel room, make sure the mini-bar is securely locked and keep the key out of children's reach.
- Try out any new equipment, such as baby carriers, at home.
- Before travelling outside the country, check with your doctor or practice nurse that your child's immunizations are up to date and whether supplemental immunizations are needed.
- Bring a small first aid kit that includes: a children's pain killer/fever reducer, the medication you normally give your child for colds and coughs, motion sickness medicine, a children's electrolyte solution (for dehydration), sun block and bandages.
- Before allowing your child to swim in the ocean, check water temperature and pollution levels. Make sure the water is free of jellyfish and other marine hazards.
- Encourage your youngsters to wear beach shoes to avoid scratches from rocks, coral, and shells.

- Infants and small children are more likely to suffer ear pain when flying than adults and older children. Schedule a feed during landing. Some doctors may recommend a children's antihistamine and decongestant an hour before take-off and a nasal spray before landing if your child is prone to earache. If your child has a cold, check with your doctor.
- Have young children carry identification with their names and address. Include your name, the airline and flight schedule, and your travel itinerary so you can be located if necessary.
- Children under age 5 should not fly alone, and most airlines do not permit it. If a child under 10 is flying alone, notify the airline.

Cycling is a great way for children to get outdoor exercise, increase coordination, and develop self-confidence and independence. However, cycling can be dangerous. Children under the age of 14 are often involved in injuries. Many of these injuries could be avoided with proper safety measures.

- Parents who enjoy cycling often consider purchasing a baby carrier that attaches to the back of the bicycle. But even the best cyclists can lose control on uneven pavement or be hit by a car. If you do decide to cycle with a young child, be sure the seat is securely attached over the rear wheel, and has a high back, shoulder harness, and lap belt, as well as spoke guards to prevent hands and feet from getting caught in the wheels. An infant bike helmet should always be worn.
- Never let your child ride on the handlebars.
- Wait to buy your child a tricycle until he has the necessary coordination to ride one and the maturity to follow your rules about when and where to ride (usually about age 3).
- Don't buy your child a bicycle until he is physically able to ride one. For most children this is about age 6 (with training wheels). He must also understand the 'rules of the road.'
- Insist that everyone in your family wear a properly fitting cycle helmet.
- Never let your child listen to headphones while biking; they're distracting and block out traffic sounds. Set a good example by not using them yourself.
- Make sure your child's bike is in good repair.
- Teach your child the rules of the road.
- Obey traffic signals and regulations.
- Ride with, not against, traffic.
- Stay to the far left or in a bicycle lane.
- When cycling in groups, ride single file.

Fire injury prevention

Although we all think burns can't happen to us, they can and they do. That is why every family member must be prepared in case of a fire.

- Install at least one smoke detector on every floor. Test smoke detectors regularly.
- Teach your children what to do in case of a fire: where the nearest exits are; to stop, drop, and roll if clothes catch on fire. Practise at least two escape plans several times a year.
- Keep fire extinguishers in the kitchen, all stairwells, and work rooms. Check that they are not expired.
- Put 'child inside' stickers on bedroom windows to alert firefighters to youngsters' whereabouts in case of an emergency.
- Keep fire ladders in upper-storey bedrooms.
- Annually check electrical wiring for fraying, heating systems for safe pressure and venting, and fuses and circuit breakers for the right amperage.
- Keep portable heaters away from curtains and furniture. Only use them for short periods of time.
- Do not allow smoking in the house.
- Always extinguish candles and open fires before going to bed.
- Have your chimney cleaned each year.
- Keep matches and lighters out of the reach of small children.

FINDING CHILDCARE

Because today's family often includes a single parent or two working parents, finding reliable childcare is a necessity. It's also a process that often leaves parents emotionally exhausted. It is helpful to talk to friends and relatives to see what childcare facilities they recommend or if they can recommend reliable baby-sitters. The following may help ensure your child's safety and your peace of mind. The most important tip, however, is to follow your instincts.

Sitters can provide your child with one-on-one attention and the security of home. Because they usually come to your home and have semi-flexible hours, they may be more convenient than a childcare facility.

- Request references and the names and phone numbers of former employers. Call former employers and ask specific questions: How many children did the sitter watch at a time? Did the children like her? Did she ever have to face an emergency situation? Was she on time?
- Ask the sitter specific questions. What would she do if your infant had a fever? What does she like and dislike about baby-sitting?
- Tell her clearly what your views are on discipline. Explain your policies on smoking and drinking around your child, and state at the beginning of her employment whether visitors are allowed at the house.

- Spend time with the sitter and your child and watch how they interact.
- Show the sitter where all fire exits, first aid kits, torch, and emergency phone numbers are located.
- Show her where all baby supplies are kept. Go over the proper way to feed, pick up, change, and comfort your baby. Also tell her what your child's normal schedule is and about any special preferences your child may have, such as listening to a story before napping.
- Occasionally make unannounced visits, especially if your child does not yet speak.
- Treat your sitter as a professional; draw up a contract that includes a job description, hours, salary, and overtime pay, if any.

Childcare centres can be beneficial for toddlers and pre-schoolers because they allow children to interact with others. They are also more affordable than private sitters. Some children, however, get overstimulated in childcare settings.

- Be sure the centre is registered. Ask whether a background check is done on all employees. Inquire at social service agencies to see if any reports or complaints have been filed.
- Inspect the centre. Is it clean? Is it free of hazards? Are there enough toys and books for children? Is there an area with handwashing facilities for changing nappies? Where are nappies disposed of?
- Watch how an employee changes nappies. Does she wear gloves? Does she wash her own and the child's hands? Does she sanitize the changing area when she is through? How does she deal with nappy rash?
- Ask to talk to all staff members who will be in contact with your child. Look at the employee-to-child ratio. Ideally, there should be one adult for every four children ages 2 to 3 and one adult for every eight children ages 3 to 6.
- Insist that naps be taken if the child is there all day.
- If there are outdoor facilities, inspect them. (See Playgrounds and outdoor play equipment, p. 230.)
- Spend time at the centre to see if the children look happy and how they are treated. Be wary of centres that do not allow parents to drop in.
- Make sure that staff members never release children to anyone but the parents unless very specific arrangements are made in person.

The age at which youngsters are emotionally, mentally, and physically old enough to be left alone varies from child to child. Most children and young teenagers feel more comfortable if a friend or sibling stays home with them, rather than being left totally alone.

- Make sure your child knows never to tell anyone he is alone. He should tell anyone who calls that his parent is busy and cannot come to the phone.
- Make sure your children know never to answer the door when they are home alone. Make sure they know how to reach you, the police, and a close neighbour.
- Install a burglar alarm and a panic button in your home.
- Practise what to do in various emergency situations, such as a fire, someone trying to enter the house, and minor scrapes.
- Make short trial runs before leaving your child alone for long periods of time or on a regular basis.
- Call your child regularly and any time you expect to be late getting home.
- Make sure your child understands that being home alone is not punishment but is helping the family.
- Leave an extra key with a trusted neighbour.
- Be sure the house is inviting to your child; leave a few lights on, a note, and a snack.
- A pet can make your child feel more comfortable and be good company.

Protecting children from abduction

A missing child is every parent's nightmare. It is important that your child be wary not only of strangers but also of anyone acting oddly or making unusual requests, because, in most cases, an abductor is someone the child knows.

- Have your child memorize his full name, address, phone number, and parents' names as soon as possible. He should also know how to call 999 and a relative or neighbour, and when it is appropriate to call. As soon as he is able, have him memorize his parents' work places and work phone numbers.
- Keep an up-to-date photo of your child.
- Don't buy clothing with your child's name on it; a kidnapper may use the name to get the child's trust.
- Teach your child never to leave the house or garden without a parent's permission. Having teenagers let you know where they are at all times, including going from one friend's house to another's, will also spare you needless worry.
- Make sure your children know never to hitchhike.
- If your child is outdoors without adult supervision – walking to school, playing – make sure he has a partner.
- Children should avoid any adult they do not know who asks for help, makes friendly advances, or claims to know them or their family.
- Get to know your child's friends and their parents. Do not let your child sleep over at someone's house until you know all the facts: Who is going to be there? Will there be adult supervision? What hazards are in the home, such as a pool or a hot tub?

CHAPTER 6 GUIDE TO FOOD SAFETY

PREVENTING FOOD-BORNE ILLNESS

Although food in the United Kingdom is some of the most abundant and safest on earth, food-related illnesses still happen and reported cases are only the tip of the iceberg. Gastroenteritis is still remarkably common, and babies and small children are among the most vulnerable to advserse effects from food-related illness or food poisoning. Gastroenteritis simply means that the lining of the digestive tract becomes irritated and inflamed, and this leads to diarrhoea, vomiting, or both.

Most gastroenteritis infections are caused by viruses, particularly a virus known as the Rotavirus. However, they are sometimes caused by bacteria, such as pathogenic E coli or salmonella, or by other organisms. The most common types of food-borne illnesses are caused by careless food handling in homes, fast-food restaurants, and other food-service establishments. Germs can enter the food chain by way of water, animal foodstuffs, and even through the air. Cooking should normally destroy any germs; problems arise when cleanliness is poor, or cooking is incomplete. Be particularly careful about hygiene in the kitchen, and in the lavatory. Always wash your hands thoroughly before preparing food and after going to the toilet.

Recent cases of epidemic food poisoning in the UK have almost always followed poor hygience techniques, with the same knife being used to cut both fresh and cooked meats, for instance – a perfect way of transferring bacteria and organisms from the raw meat to the cooked.

While healthy adults can usually shake off the effects of food poisoning in a few days, children may suffer more severe effects. Youngsters can quickly become dehydrated with the loss of fluid in diarrhoea and vomiting. Elderly people and those with chronic illnesses are also vulnerable. Bacteria such as E coli can lead to food poisoning with severe kidney complications that have been fatal in several cases.

You can help protect your children from food-borne illness by following some commonsense rules in buying and preparing food:

- Alert the manager at once if you see unsanitary food-handling in your supermarket or a restaurant (e.g., a food worker picking up meat with bare hands; failing to use gloves when handling baked goods; using a phone then handling food without washing hands; touching hair, skin, and face while serving at the delicatessen counter).

- Wash your hands for at least 20 seconds at a time with hot water and soap before you start preparing food, and wash them again as necessary while you're working. Always wash hands after going to the lavatory.
- If you have a break in the skin, use a waterproof bandage or wear rubber gloves.
- If you wear rubber gloves while preparing food, wash the gloves as often as you would wash your hands (but you don't have to take them off and wash your bare hands as well).
- Clean food preparation surfaces with hot, soapy water then wipe with a weak solution of bleach (60ml [2oz] diluted in 3.8 litres [6¾ pt] of water). Plastic chopping boards can go right in the dishwasher, if you have one, for thorough cleaning.
- When you wash dishes by hand, it's safest to let them air dry.
- Boil dishcloths regularly and clean sponges with bleach. These materials can harbour germs unless kept clean.
- Keep your refrigerator at 5°C (41°F) or below.
- Return food to the refrigerator immediately after serving. Refrigerate freshly cooked food straightaway; don't cool it to room temperature first.
- Use leftovers promptly.
- Throw out food that smells 'off' or looks discoloured. Don't taste it to see whether it's bad.
- Buy food in good condition from traceable sources; be especially cautious about buying food from street vendors.
- Check that packaging is intact and tins are not dented or bulging. Don't look for bargains among bins of tins and packets that have lost their labels.
- Don't buy unpasteurized dairy products or fruit juices.
- Avoid fish and shellfish from noncommercial sources.
- Don't use raw windfall fruit (though it can safely be used when cooked for a long time such as in making preserves).
- Trim visible fat off meats before cooking to reduce levels of pollutants while at the same time cutting down on calories and fat content. Traces of pesticides and other environmental pollutants such as industrial wastes, when present, are likely to be found at higher concentrations in animal fats.
- Generally, choose mild cooking methods (boiling, steaming) to keep potentially toxic chemical by-products at the lowest possible levels. Many foods can be baked or parboiled, then finished off with just a minute or two on the grill to add flavour.

Symptoms of food poisoning

Food poisoning causes symptoms like those of 'stomach flu'. If two or more members of the household have similar symptoms after eating the same dishes, food poisoning is the likely culprit:

- Cramps.
- Nausea.
- Vomiting.
- Diarrhoea.
- Fever.

In most cases, the problem clears up after a few hours without eating (3 to 4 hours for an infant, 6 to 8 hours for an older child). If symptoms are still present after that time, call for your doctor's advice.

PREPARING SAFE FOODS FOR BABIES AND YOUNG CHILDREN

Many people find commercial baby foods convenient and economical. They offer a wide range of flavours and the jars are available in useful serving sizes. Others prefer to save money by preparing baby food at home. For a practical compromise, you may prepare your own baby foods for everyday – and rely on commercial foods for emergencies or when travelling. When buying commercial baby foods, read the labels to make sure the foods don't contain unnecessary additives.

You don't need special equipment to make strained fruits, vegetables, and meats for your baby. Steaming is a good method of cooking because it preserves more vitamins than boiling. But whichever method you choose, follow these guidelines:

- Bananas may be served raw if thoroughly strained; all other fruits and vegetables should be cooked until tender.
- In some regions, beetroot, turnips, carrots, and spring greens may contain high levels of nitrates from the soil. The levels may increase during storage. These chemicals can cause a type of anaemia (low blood count) in babies. Baby food manufacturers test produce to make sure it doesn't contain unacceptable nitrate levels. But since you can't do this at home, it's safer to use only commercial preparations of these foods while your child is eating baby foods.
- Don't give raw honey to a baby under 1 year of age. It may contain spores that can cause serious illness in infants. Honey in processed foods, however, is safe.

- Use the least amount of water for cooking to preserve nutrients. Seasonings are not necessary.
- Cook fruits and vegetables until tender then rub them through a fine mesh sieve. Add a little of the cooking liquid or a few drops of formula to moisten the mixture.
- When you make a large batch, freeze individual servings for future use.
- Refrigerate leftovers promptly and discard partly eaten portions.
- Never refrigerate partly consumed bottles of formula, milk, or juice. Germs transferred from your baby's saliva can rapidly spoil leftovers.
- You can use a microwave oven to cook fruits and vegetables for your baby, but be extremely careful if you reheat foods. Microwaved purées heat unevenly, with pockets of extreme heat and cold throughout the mixture. Allow the food to stand at least 5 minutes and stir it well. Don't feed it to your baby unless you've tested it against your own lips first, using a separate spoon from your baby's.
- Don't heat bottles in the microwave; a bottle warms quickly, evenly, and economically when placed for a few minutes in a jug of hot water.
- Don't use the microwave to prepare meats for puréeing; it gives them an unpleasant texture that may make your baby gag.
- If your family includes pets, keep their food and water dishes out of your young child's reach. Crawling babies and active toddlers make a beeline for pet food. An occasional sampling won't harm your child, but it is not hygienic and pet food is not considered fit for human consumption.

SPECIAL PRECAUTIONS WITH ANIMAL PRODUCTS

Meats and dairy products are more susceptible to contamination from germs than vegetables, fruits, and grains. The meat of healthy animals is clean, but it can provide ideal growing conditions for germs picked up during slaughter, processing, and handling. Meats sold with the skin on, such as poultry, are especially prone to spoilage because germs can stay on the skin even after thorough washing.

- At the supermarket, bag meats separately from fresh produce.
- Refrigerate or freeze raw meat as soon as you bring it home.
- Follow the safe-handling labels on prepacked raw meat and poultry.
- Remove giblets before you refrigerate or freeze poultry.

- Defrost frozen foods in the refrigerator. Don't leave frozen food to thaw on a countertop.
- Use separate cutting boards for raw meats and raw produce.
- When you use a cutting board to prepare raw meat, fish, or poultry, wash it with soap and hot water and rinse it with a mild bleach solution before using it again for any food.
- Knives and other utensils that have come in contact with raw meat should be washed and disinfected before being used again.
- Cook meat to the recommended temperature and use a meat thermometer if you find it difficult to judge whether or not meat is done.
- Beef and lamb can be eaten rare to medium, provided the internal temperature has reached 60°C (140°F), which will kill most food-borne bacteria.
- Don't serve hamburgers rare. Minced meat is handled much more frequently than other meats during preparation and is therefore more likely to be contaminated. Hamburgers should be cooked until brownish-pink to brown in the centre.
- Pork should be thoroughly cooked with no pink colour, to prevent the spread of trichinosis parasites.
- Poultry is properly cooked when the thigh joints move easily and the juices run clear.
- If you stuff poultry, cook it immediately. Better yet, bake the stuffing in a separate dish.

ADDITIVES: MISUNDERSTOOD INGREDIENTS

Food additives are among the most misunderstood food ingredients and worries about additives are generally unfounded. Used properly, as in the majority of cases, additives improve flavour and help preserve food. In fact, many of the food additives that have worrying-sounding E numbers are actually foods or nutrients. Among the most widely used additives are salt, which helps preserve food and make it palatable; sugar and golden syrup, which improve flavour, help retain moisture, and retard spoilage; and ascorbic acid (vitamin C, a preservative), alpha-tocopherol (vitamin E), and BHT and BHA (butylated hydroxytoluene, butylated hydroxyanisole), substances with anti-oxidizing properties, which keep fats from turning rancid.

It's also true, however, that some manufacturers use certain additives needlessly, usually to make food look more appealing. Leaders in this group are synthetic food dyes, which are used purely for cosmetic purposes. In certain special cases, food dyes have been linked to adverse health effects. E102, also called tartrazine, causes allergic reactions in those who are sensitive to it and has been linked to severe asthma attacks in some people with this disease. Additionally, many people who have adverse reactions to aspirin and other salicylate compounds suffer symptoms after consuming tartrazine. Some synthetic food dyes are no longer permitted and now all food labels must clearly state whether any dyes are present, so that consumers may avoid them.

Manufacturers are required to list additives on food labels in order of the amounts present. Following are the characteristics of commonly used additives:

- BHA and BHT, preservatives long used in dry cereal, instant potatoes, active dry yeast, drink and dessert mixes, and food packaging, have been linked to cancer when fed in huge doses to laboratory animals. There's no evidence, however, that the small amounts in our diet carry any risk.
- Enriching additives put back essential nutrients that are present when food is harvested but are lost in processing. White flour and rice, for example, are enriched with B vitamins that are destroyed in milling.
- Fortifying additives are substances that, although not naturally present in a food, are added on scientists' recommendations to make sure people consume enough for health. Vitamin D added to milk, vitamin A added to margarine, and iodine in salt are fortifying additives that help prevent illness.
- Irradiation, a method of preserving food, is classed as a food additive. Some people associate food irradiation with fears of nuclear fallout and radiation sickness. The process of irradiation does not make food radioactive or change the food in any way, however, and some experts believe that irradiation may be a safer method of preservation than many other food additives. Others are unconvinced and irradiation remains a very controversial topic.
- Nitrites are chemicals traditionally used to preserve bacon and other pork products. They help prevent the growth of the bacteria that cause botulism. In the digestive tract, some nitrites are changed into nitrosamines, chemicals that can cause cancer. To keep the risk of cancer low, manufacturers may only use permitted levels of nitrites. When vitamin C and vitamin E are present, lower levels of nitrosamine are produced from nitrites. It may be a good idea to serve

plenty of citrus juice when you offer bacon or sausage for breakfast.

- Monosodium glutamate (MSG) is a flavourless chemical that is used as a flavour enhancer in processed foods as well as in restaurants that serve Asian foods. After eating food containing MSG, some people have experienced unpleasant symptoms including headache, flushing, dizziness, tingling, numbness, nausea and vomiting, headache, and a feeling of pressure in the head and chest. So well known is this reaction that people call it the 'Chinese restaurant syndrome'. No direct link between the additive and the symptoms has been demonstrated, however and some people doubt that Chinese restaurant syndrome actually exists. It may be that certain people are unusually sensitive to MSG, so for them, the wisest choice is ordering foods prepared without MSG. In any case, flavour enhancers are not necessary for food that is carefully prepared and seasoned. There's no need to add MSG to foods cooked at home.
- Sugar substitutes currently allowed are saccharin (300 times sweeter than sugar), aspartame (180 times sweeter than sugar), and acesulfame potassium (acesulfame-K, 200 times sweeter than sugar). Saccharin, which also occurs naturally in grapes, has been in use for many years and has never been linked to serious health risks. A temporary ban was imposed in the United States when researchers claimed that saccharin could cause bladder cancer when given in huge doses to laboratory animals. No such link has been found in humans and the ban is no longer in force. Aspartame, tested more exhaustively than any other food additive, is considered safe for adults and children except those who have the rare inborn disorder phenylketonuria (PKU). Studies have failed to show any adverse effect of aspartame on children's health, behaviour, or learning ability. Acesulfame-K can be used in cooking and baking and is considered safe for all.
- Sulphites are used to slow discoloration, overripening, and spoilage in fruits and vegetables. They are added to fruit juices, soft drinks, dried fruits and vegetables, processed potatoes, and wines. Following frequent reports of severe allergic reactions (especially in people with asthma), the American Food and Drug Administration stopped the use of sulphites on fresh foods in restaurants and salad bars. These chemicals are still permitted in wines and packaged foods, but must be listed on labels if they are present at a level higher than 10 parts per million. Read labels carefully and ask restaurant staff about sulphite content before ordering questionable foods if your child has asthma, eczema, or allergies, or is sensitive to sulphites.

PESTICIDES AND ORGANIC PRODUCE

Pesticides are chemicals used to protect plants from insects, weeds, and fungi. Pesticides have been used in one form or another since the dawn of agriculture, but the availability of inexpensive synthetic pesticides now makes it possible to produce fruits and vegetables on an unprecedented scale. The downside of this is that pesticides linger as trace residues in foods. Many consumers worry that long-term exposure to these chemicals may have adverse effects on health, including birth defects, fertility problems, nerve disorders, weakened immunity, and cancer. In fact, problems in these areas have been seen in studies that examined the effects of high doses of pesticides over long periods. What these results mean for human health isn't fully known, however, since the doses studied were far greater than the levels a human being would normally consume over a lifetime.

Some consumers try to avoid pesticide exposure by buying only organic produce, which has been grown with manure and compost instead of synthetic pesticides and fertilizers. Unlike most produce, foods labelled organic reach the market without the aid of hormones, antibiotics, synthetic dyes, and preservatives. But there are a few risks and other factors to keep in mind when buying organic foods:

- Organically grown produce may pick up pesticide residues from the soil, wind, or groundwater.
- While organic foods may lack certain additives and contaminants, they may not be any more nutritious than nonorganic foods.
- Growers and retailers usually ask premium prices for organic foods, sometimes twice the price of conventional goods, but organic produce tends to spoil faster because it is not treated to inhibit insects and bacterial growth.
- Some organic fertilizers are not sterilized and may carry harmful bacteria.

PURE WATER

Water is needed for every process that takes place in our bodies. Without water, we can't digest our food, absorb nutrients, grow, repair our tissues, regulate our temperature, or get rid of wastes. In short, without water we can't live for longer than a few days.

The water we drink varies in taste and chemical content according to the rock and soil through which it passes. While many people prefer sodium-rich 'soft' water – so called because it lathers well and doesn't leave a grey film – 'hard' water that is lower in sodium is somewhat healthier. Some water-softening systems use potassium chloride. This is preferred by consumers who are following a sodium-restricted diet.

Local water companies maintain purification facilities that ensure our water supply stays free of the germs that once caused deadly epidemics such as cholera, typhoid fever, and dysentery. Occasionally, however, disease-causing organisms still manage to get into water supplies. Because water companies regularly test water for contaminants, they can alert residents when there might be a problem. Pay attention to such alerts; you may be instructed to boil water before drinking it or use commercial bottled water until the problem is cleared up.

Another new threat is a tide of man-made chemicals including detergents, pesticide and fertilizer run-off, industrial effluents, nuclear waste, and many other pollutants. These contaminants may be harmful on long-term exposure. The real danger is that once they enter the water supply, it's hard to get rid of them.

- If you have any doubt about your water supply, contact your water company for advice..

Although lead water pipes are no longer allowed in construction, lead solder can still present a risk even in fairly new homes. To protect your family from lead in your drinking water:

- In the morning, or when you haven't run the water for a while, flush out lead residues by leaving the tap on until the water is as cold as it can get. Do this for every tap used for drinking or cooking.
- Don't use hot tap water for cooking or for mixing drinks for your baby. Hot water dissolves more lead from solder than cold water.
- If you must use a water softener, use it only for your hot water supply. Soft water leaches lead out of solder much more than hard water.

Index

Note: Entries and page numbers in bold type refer to sections that cover a symptom in detail.